The Untold Story Of

ANNIE McKAY

And The

Boston Public School Nurses 1905-1988

*The Formation of the Massachusetts
School Nurse Organization*

Dorothy M. Keeney

Copyright © 2020 – Dorothy Keeney – All rights reserved.

No part of this book may be reproduced, distributed, or by any means, including photocopying, recording, or other electronic or mechanical methods without written permission of the author and publisher.

Important Author Note regarding historical significance:

I am choosing to refer to race in the vernacular of the times as it was related to me by the subject and does not in any way intend to promote racist language.

Published by Derrydamph Publishing House

Book cover design by Lizaa through 99designs
Book interior design by Allan through 99designs

ISBN: 9798640511970

Dedicated to my mother,

May Anne Hall.

I missed her on my journey.

Table of Contents

Introduction 1
Acknowledgements 5

SECTION I – BEGINNINGS

Chapter 1 – The Development of Boston School Nursing 9
Chapter 2 – Annie McKay's Adventuresome Life 25
Chapter 3 – The Way We Were 37
Chapter 4 – Annie McKay at Work with the Instructive
District Nursing Association. 47
Chapter 5 – Annie McKay Becomes Boston's First School Nurse 59

SECTION II – PROFESSIONALIZATION

Chapter 6 – Fresh Start, New Rules, and New Laws 89
Chapter 7 – Boston Public School Nurses: The Early Years. 101
Chapter 8 – School Nurse State Law 1921 123
Chapter 9 – The Beginnings of the
Boston Public School Nurses Club. 133
Chapter 10 – The Boston Public School Nurses
Endure the Depression. 165
Chapter 11 – The Boston Public School Nurses Club Presses On 181
Chapter 12 – Post-World War II School Nursing 217
Chapter 13 – School Nursing During the Polio Epidemics 245
Chapter 14 – Threatened Policy Changes and Voices from the Past 261
Chapter 15 – School Health Restructures in the 1970s 303
Chapter 16 – Boston Public School Nurses in the 1980s. 329

SECTION III – LOOKING FORWARD

Chapter 17 – The First Twenty Years of MSNO 1970 – 1990 375

Chapter 18 – A Midnight Séance 403

EPILOGUE 413

About the Author. 415

Index 417

Introduction

When New York City celebrated the 100th Anniversary of their school nurse program in 2002, the first in the nation, the Massachusetts School Nurse Organization (MSNO) speculated about the introduction of school nursing in Massachusetts. Who was the first school nurse in Massachusetts and when and where did it start? Since I worked as a school nurse in Boston, MSNO asked me to look into this, because in all likelihood, it started in Boston. Of course, it did. After much research, I discovered the stirring details of the introduction of school nursing in Boston in 1905, and the first school nurse, Annie McKay. That ignited my passion to discover more of their story, and ultimately writing this book. As a first-time writer, it has been a huge undertaking requiring me to learn the tools of the craft.

This book attempts to tell the complex story of the early school nurses, prior to becoming the professionals that we know today. "Nursing history is key to understanding the past, defining the present, and influencing the future of nursing," explains Brigid Luskin, RN, PhD, AAHN (American Association for the History of Nursing) President in the May/June 2011 issue of *Nursing Spectrum*. "History gives nurses an identity. Studying nursing history helps us to look at the influence of race, class, gender, and religion on the profession, so we can understand all the influences on what we are today," added Barbara Mann Wall, RN, PhD, FAAN, of the Barbara Bates Center for the Study of the History of Nursing at the University of Pennsylvania School of Nursing in this same issue of *Nursing Spectrum*.

Many issues transformed nurses from the stereotypical doctor's handmaiden, struggling to obtain a respected professional status, to the school nurse who is now the clinical health expert in the school, the health care provider for students and staff while in school, and an advocate for disease prevention and health maintenance, health professional of today. When taking an in depth look at the beginning stages of the school nurse movement in Boston, from the first notes of the Instructive District Nursing Association (IDNA), and from the earliest minutes of the meetings of the Boston Public School Nurses, many of these issues can be recognized. Examples are respect and recognition as an equal professional, pay equity, and a five-day work week.

As a school nurse historian, I will take the reader on this empowering, engaging and emotional journey through the past, to further enlighten the reader

Introduction

about the challenges and struggles over adversity that led to the transformation of Massachusetts school nursing in the 20th century. By the end of the journey, I promise, there will be no more strangers to school nursing.

Book's Format

Regarding the format, this book's 18 chapters are divided into three sections. The first section, *Beginnings*, Chapters 1-5 includes Boston's early school nurse movement. Chapter 1 takes in the history of the first school nurse in Boston, Chapter 2 reveals Annie McKay's personal story, and Chapter 3 covers the early education of nurses. As we go forward, Chapter 4 follows Annie McKay at work at IDNA (Instructive District Nursing Association), and Chapter 5 discusses the early beginnings of school nursing in Boston, with Annie McKay and IDNA.

Section 2, *Professionalization*, Chapters 6-16, incorporates the new nurses hired by the Boston School Committee in 1907. Chapters 6 and 7 look at their management in the early years. The State School Nurse Law is explained in Chapter 8. Starting in Chapter 9, the story is told through the eyes of the emerging Boston Public School Nurses Club, involving their trials during the flu epidemics and the roaring 20s. Chapter 10 explores the nurses through the Depression, Chapter 11 examines the possible transfer of school health services, school nurses dealing with contagious diseases, and their work during WWII. I investigate changing times for women and gender inequity in Chapter 12, as well as school nursing national trends during the 50s, 60s, and 70s. Chapter 13 probes school nursing during Boston's polio epidemics. Chapter 14 explores Boston's problems during the 1960s including new challenges over the consolidation of school health services, the funding and salaries of school nurses, the Racial Imbalance Act, and interviews with school nurses Ann Donovan, Shirley Ericson Garagna, and JK.

Chapter 15 researches the 1970s amid the teachers' strike, nurse caseloads, the postponement of the 1973 school nurse exam, HB 1194, and the school doctor inquiry. Chapter 16, covering the 1980s, is the last chapter recording the Boston school nurses experiences. There were no *Boston School Nurses Club Minutes* available to me after that time. This chapter enquired about the lack of a nurse supervisor, hiring nurse practitioners, Dr. Lamb's problematic report about school nurses, Medicaid reimbursement, and interviews with school nurses K. Marie Clarke, and Carol Almeida Fortes.

Section 3, *Looking Forward*, covers Chapters 17 and 18. Not to be excluded, Chapter 17 looks at the founding and first 20 years of the Massachusetts School Nurse Organization. The book ends in Chapter 18 with A Midnight Séance. After spending so many years researching this book, I imagined this to transpire. It includes a special guest.

This book discusses the evolving role of school nursing in Boston, told through the eyes of IDNA (Instructive District Nursing Association), and the Boston School Nurses Club. *The Boston Public Schools Manual*, *The Boston School Committee Minutes* and *The Superintendent's Notes* are additional resources. Further, I used many nursing journal and newspaper articles from the various times covered for additional support. Timelines in various chapters stress key events that affect school nursing.

Acknowledgements

In closing, I want to thank the research of archivist, Annie Orchanian-Cheff of the Toronto University Health Network, without which my report would not have been able to move forward. The archivist discovered Ms. McKay's original application to the school of nursing from 1891 and is a true friend and supporter of school nurses. My research for this project required me to correspond with many interesting people, and I am indebted to their many kindnesses and professionalism. To name but a few: Ms. McKay's family in Beaverton, Ontario, Canada, including Roberta Mitchell and Dave MacKay; the archivist and librarian in Beaverton; the Visiting Nurse Association of Boston where I discovered the assignment of the first school nurse, Annie McKay; the Red Cross volunteer nurse historian in Washington, D.C. who found Annie McKay's enlistment; nursing archivist Diane Gallagher at Boston University's Howard Gotlieb Archival Research Center which houses the papers of the Instructive District Nursing Association; Boston Public Schools; Quincy School in Boston; libraries at Massachusetts Eye & Ear Hospital, Tufts Medical Center, and Beth Israel Medical Center of Boston; the Boston Public Health Department; Thomas J. Geraghty, Geraghty Assoc. Inc.; Marta Crilly at The Boston City Archives; Dawn Huston, Director Dunbar Library, Grantham, NH; the many research librarians at the Copley branch of the Boston Public Library, including Jenna Collins for her writing assistance.

In addition, I express thanks to Director Anne Smart at the South End branch, and research librarians at the Massachusetts Law Library, State House. Last, I want to thank Kim Gifford's writing group for all of their support and feedback. A final tremendous thank you to my husband, Jim, for his editing, support, and patience during this writing process.

Declaration of Conflicting Interests
The author declared no potential conflicts of interest with respect to the research, authorship, and /or publication of this book.

Funding
The author received no financial support for the research, authorship, and or publication of this book.

SECTION I

BEGINNINGS

Chapter 1

The Development of Boston School Nursing

The Need for School Nurses

It's 1905. Annie McKay strides confidently down Franks Court, a narrow, dirty alley in Boston's South End when she sees a ball pitched towards her. She kicks it back towards the group of shabbily dressed children who sheepishly smile as they recognize their school nurse. Nurse McKay will visit a family that has six absentee students in this neighborhood. A small boy at a neighboring tenement directs her to the family's building. See figure below.

The tenement's small, semi-dark entrance hall harbors a heavy, damp, musty odor that smacks McKay in the face. A closed glass skylight spills some light from the top floor down, easing the darkness. Dressed in her heavy uniform coat, protecting her from Boston's bone-chilling winter, and armed with her nurse's bag, nurse McKay trudges up the steep, dilapidated staircase. Halfway up the stairs, she stops for a minute to catch her breath. The air reeks of urine and beer on her trek to the fifth floor, full of sounds of the many families living in the building, babies crying, doors slamming, and parents yelling at kids, or each other, in unknown, multiple languages.

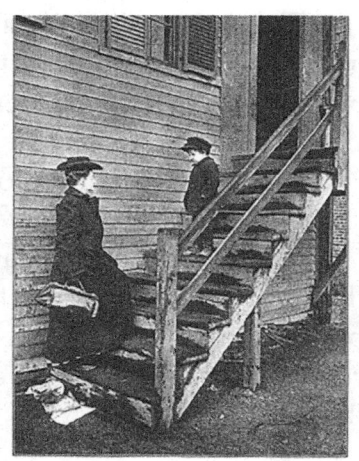

Image courtesy of Boston University Howard Gotlieb Archival Research Center.

Thirty-eight-year-old Annie McKay, a former Canadian schoolteacher, and nurse, additionally trained in New York City, is the first school nurse in Boston. The Instructive District Nurses Association (IDNA), a precursor to today's Visiting Nurse Association, assigns her as their most experienced nurse to a pilot program, privately funded, in partnership with the Boston School Committee. The program intends to assist school physicians in reducing a 13 percent school absentee rate, during an era in the early 1900s marked by widespread infectious disease and poor sanitation.

Imagine, one afternoon as the area's school nurse, McKay visits the home of an absentee Syrian student who has scabies. The strategy with this visit is to teach the mother and the children how to treat scabies, also known as, "the itch," and prevent another outbreak in the family. Scabies is a skin infection resulting from infestation with the itch mite. It occurs worldwide, is predisposed by overcrowding and poor hygiene, and can be endemic.

At the top of the stairs, she catches her breath again and then knocks on the door. Mrs. Abadi, a slight woman with charcoal grey hair, and pallid skin, with six of her nine children, answers the door. There is some giggling going on, and the smaller children push to be in front. Nine children and their parents are cramped into this two-room apartment. The six children that are gathered in the front room with their mother have acquired scabies.

The children's lesions are mostly resolving. Nonetheless, one little boy, dressed in a suit of underwear with long sleeves and legs is still scratching a crusted lesion on his wrist. McKay reviews the treatment with his mother.

"That is a splendid outfit that you are wearing," McKay says to the boy.

"I hope he had a cleansing bath using soap and a wire brush before applying the sulfur ointment that I left earlier with you. The ointment has to be applied to his body twice a day for three days. The outfit that he is wearing is excellent, and he can wear thin cotton gloves at night. His clothes soon will become permeated with the ointment."

She comments, "On the evening after his last treatment, he should take another scrub bath using soap and a stiff nail brush. After that, he can put on clean clothing. Do you have any questions?"

Mrs. Abadi doesn't seem to understand. Her eyes stare at the floor. One of the girls quickly translates McKay's instructions for her mother. Mrs. Abadi's eyes light up. The corner of her mouth quirks up. She replies in a language that McKay doesn't understand, but her daughter translates, "I have put it on for two days and nights and have one more day."

"Good, Mrs. Abadi. You are doing a fine job. A cold cloth might help with the itching, but please boil the cloth afterward." See figure below showing areas where scabies is usually found (Malasanow, Barkauskas, Moss, & Stoltenberg-Allen;193).

McKay reviews the importance of decontaminating the bedding and the clothing. She advises Mrs. Abadi of the need for "prolonged boiling" of the family's underwear, clothing, and bedding to kill the mites and the eggs. Mrs. Abadi shows McKay her washing tub and clothesline that hang outside her window. Secretly, the nurse wonders how this slight woman could scrub all that wash. Perhaps the older girls help her.

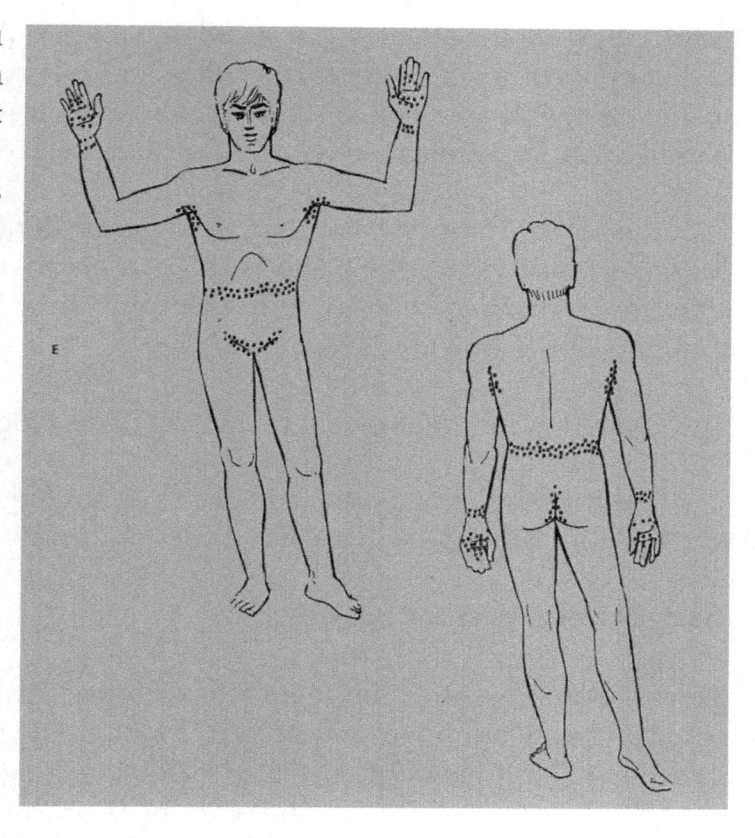

Simultaneously, McKay further explains the importance of simple hand washing and sanitary techniques to both the children and their mother, with the assistance of Mrs. Abadi's daughter again doing the translating. No doubt the nurse knows that this will not be as simple as it sounds since all the families on the floor share one bathroom at the end of the outside hallway.

Privately, Annie McKay compares this family to her own, as she was one of ten children growing up in rural Canada. Yet, she thinks, they had clean, fresh air and so much space to safely run around. Now, McKay sees people crammed in everywhere. Snapping quickly back to the present, she advises Mrs. Abadi that the children can return to school the following Monday. The mother takes in a deep breath, and replies, with a sigh of relief, that she will be glad, for it distressed her to have all of them around aimlessly at home.

Standing at the top of the stairs outside of the apartment, Annie McKay can feel her heart still pounding after her conversation with Mrs. Abadi. She looks at the fob watch on her uniform, a gift from her late father, and tells herself to move along. Holding on to the wobbly banister, Annie McKay again negotiates the stairs to the street, reminding herself to use the fumigation room at the district office this evening.

The school children have continued their ball playing in the alley during nurse McKay's home visit. As she leaves the house, she immediately thinks again of the smell of freshly mowed hay, birds chirping, and open fields. In the alley, those thoughts flee as quickly as they came.

"Are they coming to school tomorrow, Miss McKay?" The boys want to know.

"Be gone with you now lads," she says, smiling. "You are good boys. Go home and eat your dinner. I will see all of you tomorrow, eh."

Treatment for Scabies and Fumigation

Still used today, 5% sulfur ointment was the only treatment available at that time for scabies.[1] Fumigation was required if the nurse suspected that she was exposed to infection. This treatment consisted of disinfecting themselves and their clothes, changing into fresh garments and washing their hair with soap, water, and corrosive sublimate as an antiseptic. Does that sound like fun? McKay had a long night ahead of her. In Chapter 4, learn more about the various features of the fumigation room.

History of School Health Services

School Health Services in the United States followed the development of public health and school nursing in England and Europe. In fact, the U.S. was late to the game.

---

[1] Finnerud, C. W. (1929, February). Common Diseases of Children. I. *The Elementary School Journal, 29,* 461-462. Retrieved on March 20, 2019. https://www.jstor.org/stable/995412

Other countries, such as France, as early as 1837, mandated health supervision of students. Brussels, in 1874, became the first city to obtain the services of doctors for schools and establish a regular system of health inspections. In 1892, London appointed Amy Hughes, the first school nurse in Europe.[2]

In the United States, it was Boston that led the way in 1894 to improve the health care for school children by implementing the medical inspection of students in schools using physicians. Boston's Board of Health developed this pioneering system. About 80 physicians, then called medical inspectors, were employed and charged with visiting schools in their district, once daily. They checked on students referred by their teachers and suggested medical or surgical treatment when necessary. The inspectors screened students to identify and exclude from school those with serious communicable diseases such as scarlet fever, diphtheria, pertussis, chicken pox, and mumps. Later on, the list expanded to include parasitic diseases. If found ill, the inspector excluded the student from school to protect the other school children.

The system's major shortcoming soon became apparent: it hinged on referrals from teachers. Some teachers cared more about their students' health than others. A second drawback of the program resulted in students excluded from school without providing enough follow-up care to ensure that they would return to school promptly after receiving treatment.[3] The Boston School Committee then grew increasingly concerned by a high rate of absenteeism among students being excluded from school due to medical reasons. Simultaneously, in the early 1900s, school enrollments across America were expanding under President Teddy Roosevelt. His party's progressive, reform labor movement brought more children into the classrooms who had previously labored in mills and factories.

The Development of Boston School Nursing

School nursing as a profession in America dates back more than 100 years. In 2005, Boston school nurses and the Massachusetts School Nurse Organization both celebrated

---

[2] Wold, S. (1981). *School Nursing, A Framework for Practice*. North Branch, MN: Sunrise River Press, Pages 5-6.

[3] Herlihy, E.M. (Ed). (1932*). Fifty years of Boston - A Memorial Volume. Issued in Commemoration of the Tercentenary of 1930.* Pages 468-9.

a century of school nursing in Boston. They gathered to honor a key figure in Massachusetts nursing history, namely Annie McKay, Boston's pioneering first school nurse, initially introduced earlier in this chapter. One hundred years ago, she accepted the Instructive District Nursing Association's (IDNA) challenge to become the first school nurse in Boston, thus making Massachusetts history. Nurse McKay was appointed on December 6, 1905, to a pilot project placing a nurse in three Boston schools, namely the Quincy, Andrews, and Way Street Schools.

Her legacy in Boston's public schools lay in making a free education accessible to more children and especially for scores of immigrant children to pursue an essential aspect of the American Dream. Her pioneering work also helped to establish a system of health assessment, intervention, and follow-up for all school children that is still enjoyed today.

Across America, in the early 1900s, cities struggled to find ways to further improve the health and medical care of students. New York City established a school nursing program in 1902 when nurse Lillian Wald, Director of the Henry Street Settlements, placed a nurse in a public school to improve the health of students. Three years later, in 1905, the Boston School Committee, deeply troubled by the 13 percent rate of absenteeism in their schools, developed a partnership with IDNA. They agreed to assign Annie McKay in a privately funded program to supplement the work of physicians in those previously named schools in the South End area of Boston.

Many issues affected early school nurses before they became members of the profession that is known today. From the first notes of IDNA and the earliest minutes of the meetings of the Boston School Nurses, a few key issues emerge. These include respect and recognition of nurses as a professional equal to other medical and education professionals, defining their practice, a workweek limited to five days and pay equity. These early nurses faced challenges and struggles with obstacles put before them. It became the fabric of their being.

These problems transformed nurses from being the stereotypical doctor's handmaiden, struggling to obtain a respected professional status, to the school nurse who is now the clinical health expert in the school, the healthcare provider for students and staff while in school, an advocate for disease prevention and health maintenance, and promoter of academic success for students. All of this is essential to the understanding of school nursing's past. As nurses grasp these influences, they can better understand why and what they are today, and how to forge an informed present and a dynamic future.

Come along with me on this journey. Allow me to introduce myself. I am a retired Boston school nurse after having worked 20 years as a school nurse serving a high school, a middle school, and multiple elementary schools. Sixteen of those years were at the Thomas Edison Middle School, Brighton, Boston, MA. Let's go together. The train is leaving the station. Hop on board.

Boston's History

It is important to understand some of the factors that affected the health of McKay's students, including child labor, and their environment. The mortality statistics at the time reveal a grim story and underscore the seriousness of the problems.

The Boston Health Department in 1907 released the following infectious disease report:

Mortality Numbers

Children 5 years and over to 36-year-old adults
Deaths as the result of infectious diseases:

- Diphtheria and Croup (144)
- Scarlet Fever (49)
- Typhoid fever (64)
- Cerebrospinal meningitis (169)
- Whooping Cough (43)
- Measles (29)
- Smallpox (0)
- Cholera (130)
- Septicemia (blood poisoning) (87)
- Erysipelas (Streptococcus bacteria skin infection) (45)
- Intermittent Fever (2)
- Dysentery (20)

In its annual report for 1907, the Board of Health listed the total number of deaths as 11,686 in a population of 609,757. The death rate per year was 19.16 per

1,000 inhabitants. At the same time, this rate was 26 percent higher than in the previous year but 34 percent lower than the average of the last ten years.[4]

Consumption (tuberculosis) was listed separately. Pulmonary tuberculosis recorded 18.40 deaths per 10,000 population in 1907.[5] These statistics demonstrate the main problems associated with contagious diseases that prevailed in Annie McKay's day.

By comparison, a report of Health for Boston 2012-2013 revealed the following:

Boston-Leading Causes of Death 2012-2013

- cerebrovascular disease - 34.6 per 100,000 residents,
- cancer -181.6 per 100,000 residents
- diseases of the heart -749 per 100,000 residents
- infant deaths per 1,000 live births -5.9 per 100,000 residents
- homicide per 100,000 residents - 9.4 per 100,000 residents
- substance abuse deaths per 100,000 residents -181.6.

These numbers give an entirely different picture of the population's health than what was occurring in 1907. Vaccines developed since then have decreased the number of new cases of infectious diseases and consequently, the number of mortalities. For instance, in 2012, nationwide, the Centers for Disease Control reported 41,000 new cases of whooping cough, including 18 deaths. Most of these deaths were in children under one year of age. Compare that to the 43 deaths in Boston alone in 1907.

The Inner City

Boston by the early 1900s had grown and developed from an agrarian area where cows grazed on the Boston Common to a crowded city filled with fast-rising tenements, the beginnings of slums, and unprecedented social conditions and disease.[6] In

---

4   Boston Health Department. *Annual Report, 1907.* (1908) Pages 1, 3-5. Boston Municipal Printing Office.

5   *Thirty-Sixth Annual Report of the Health Department of the City of Boston 1907.* Retrieved from https://babel.hathitrust.org/cgi/pt?id=mdp.39015069390162;view=1up;seq=65, 43.

6   Bromberg, C. (Ed.). *Revolutionary Care Then and Now. A History of Tufts New England Medical Center, Founded in 1796.* Page 15.

the last part of the 19th century, due to the economic downturn in 1873, wealthy homeowners fled to the suburbs of Roxbury and Dorchester. The South End of Boston, for example, changed from an area of elegant, brick, bow-front townhouses into a district of lodging and tenement houses. This change coincided with a time of massive immigration to the United States, caused by large-scale financial crises, food shortages, and political unrest abroad. Though these immigrants coming to the U.S. came as legal immigrants, the situation is somewhat analogous to the tide of illegal immigrants from Central America streaming over our southern borders in the early 21st century.

One of the problems inherent in this Boston area was dampness, since much of the land had been filled in dating back to the 1600s. Boston's burgeoning population outgrew the original peninsula, forcing the city to develop more land. Starting in 1858, a train from Needham arrived about every 45 minutes, day and night, for 30 years with a load of gravel to fill the odorous tidal marsh known as the Back Bay. It created 459 acres of new land including all of the Back Bay, plus some of the South End, filled to an average depth of 20 feet.[7] In the political climate of today, environmentalists might be very distressed with a similar vast landfill project.

More specifically, the area around Tyler Street which was the site of McKay's first three schools was not as formally "laid out" as were the elegant South End areas surrounding Blackstone Square and Union Park. The original construction of buildings began to be altered both in front and in the back, and additional stories were added as well. This kind of development resulted in vast overcrowding, and slums arose.

Families lived in the dark and even wet basements for low rent. Bathrooms had an insufficient flushing supply and served upwards of fifteen to thirty people. There were no bathing facilities. In some tenements, a shaft furnished the only light and air for rooms, including bathrooms. Ventilators at the top of the stairway shafts and rooftop windows were generally kept closed. There was no area even to wash clothes. All of these circumstances led to unsanitary conditions. In response to this environment, the city opened in 1898 free, public

---

7   Campbell, R., Vanderwarker, P. (1992). *Cityscapes of Boston-An American City Through Time.* Boston, MA: Houghton Mifflin Co. Page 78.

bathhouses for bathing, which became very popular.[8] See an example of housing in the image below.

If the parents in a tenement-dwelling family were sick and unable to go to work, they, in turn, were unable to pay their rent and buy food for the family. Parents did not intentionally keep their children out of school, but they needed their children to earn additional income to feed their family. In Boston, children worked as peddlers, delivery boys, scavengers, and toiled at processing factory goods in the home called homework. They helped out the family as best they could.

Scavenging was a common form of collecting wood, either for the family or for sale. A report from the Massachusetts Child Labor Committee said that "small boys and even girls, permeated to the skin with dirt, their ragged clothes torn by nails, piled up great loads, heavy enough for two union laborers to carry, and dragged or struggled under them for a mile or two." Dr. Joel E. Goldthwait reported in a paper cited by the Committee mentioned above that those children had been "permanently injured by the constant strain of carrying loads continuously for long distances."

Child scavengers also played and picked over dumps of ashes, garbage, and other refuse with their fingers. Their short backs were bent so low that their heads almost touched the trash, and at the same time, they inhaled the dump's vile odor. The Massachusetts Child Labor Committee reported that 2,128 children from one Boston

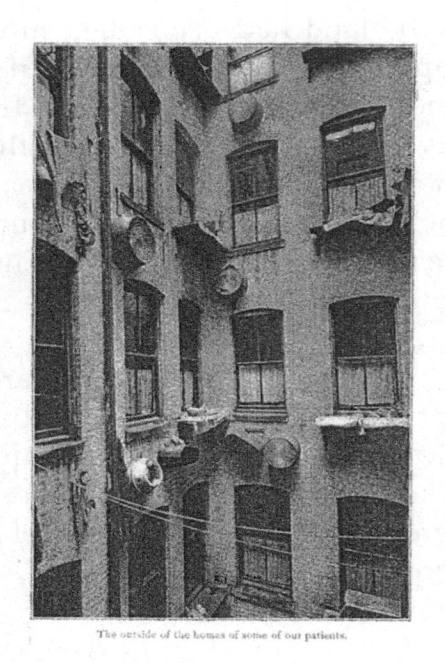

---

8   Woods, R.A. (1898) *The City Wilderness A Settlement Study* (1970 Garrett Press ed.). New York, N Y: Garrett Press. Pages 62-66.

school district regularly engaged in this practice.[9] See the image below showing children at the dump.9

"Homework" described the practice of bringing factory goods intended for sale to the home to be further processed. This involved the mother, who was in charge, and the children. It consisted of long hours, low wages, unsanitary conditions, and child labor. The critical point was that it exploited women and children. Despite the union's protest against this practice, asserting that it depressed wages paid in factories, and undermined their efforts to improve wages and relieve unsanitary factory conditions, this custom persisted well into the 1920s.

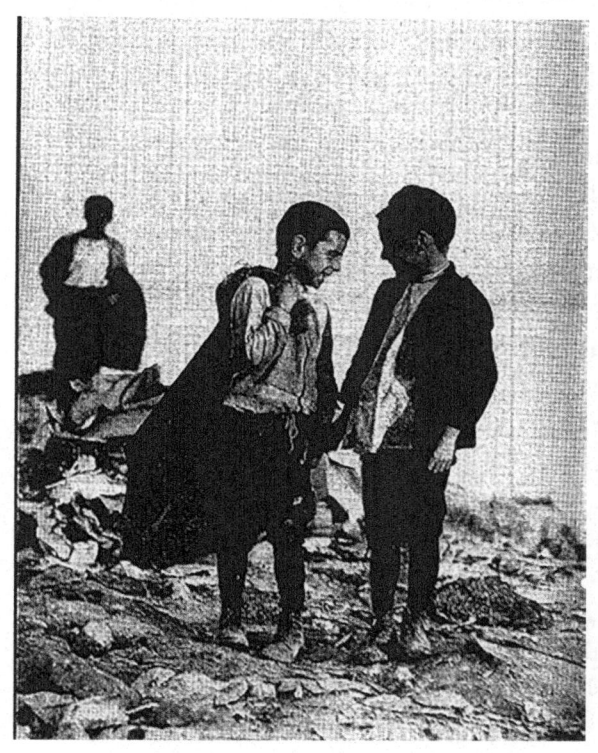

To some parents, the era's child labor laws seemed unreasonable, especially to those immigrants accustomed to family work in the fields. Here, Massachusetts law required children to attend school between eight and fourteen years of age. On the other hand, when children were absent from school, they were denied the opportunity to learn the skills needed to participate in modern American society. At the time, two out of ten U.S. adults could not read or write. Only six percent of all Americans had graduated from high school. Undoubtedly, all of these issues contributed to the poor health, poor nutrition, and socio-environmental problems afflicting McKay's students and families. In Chapter 9, child labor will be discussed in more depth.

Social Reformers of the Times

The question arises, who were these social reformers that we have referred to, and

---

[9] Macieski, R. (2015). *Picturing class: Lewis W. Hine photographs child labor in New England.* Boston, MA: University of Massachusetts Press. Page 224.

what prompted them to demand change? Newspaper archives from this era tell of a Mothers' and Fathers' Club organized in November 1901 for a threefold purpose of studying the problems of parenthood, to put into everyday practice the results of these studies, and to lend a hand to others. Within a short amount of time, they became active in the movement to introduce nurses to the schools.[10]

Over the next few years, the meetings of the Mothers' and Fathers' Club had programs on literature for children, connection with the schools, summer outings and work for needy children, and child labor laws. They maintained that if the new immigrants were taught and acquired high moral values, they would become better citizens.[11] Also, the Mothers' and Fathers' Club held rummage sales to earn money for the annual Christmas parties and two weeks of summer vacations they gave to the underprivileged children from the settlement and charitable institutions.

At this critical point, an influential person traveled from New York to speak to the Club on November 28, 1904. It was no less than Lina Rogers, the first school nurse, appointed in New York City in 1902. She accepted a promotion there in 1904 to become supervising school nurse. At this meeting, Rogers related how the city looked after the health of its children using school nurses. In New York, during the first month after Rogers's appointment, she administered 80 treatments, made 137 home visits, and returned 15 children to school, some of whom had been out for a full term. The New York City Board of Health was so pleased with these results that they appointed 12 more nurses the following month.

Dr. Durgan, Chairman of the Board of Health in Boston, expressed his support on this occasion and at other events for utilizing skilled nurses to care for the schools' needy children. With the introduction of nurses, he believed much of the contagious disease spreading then through the schools could be averted.[12]

---

10   Great National Park. (1902, February 21) *Boston Daily Globe* (1872-1922), 7 Retrieved Dec. 9, 2007, from ProQuest Historical Newspapers *Boston Globe* (1872-1924) database. (Document ID: 689385582). P. 7.

11   Ibid.

12   School Nursing: Miss Lina L. Rogers of New York Explains the Work to Mothers and Fathers Club. (1904, November 29). *Boston Daily Globe* (1872-1922) 8. Retrieved April 2, 2008, from ProQuest Historical Newspapers Boston Globe (1872-1922) database. (Document ID: 707635822).

Lina Rogers revisited Boston to speak on the benefits of school nurses at the Massachusetts State Conference of Charities on November 8, 1905. At this time, she relayed the costs involved in the employment of school nurses in New York City. In 1903, the New York City Board of Health appropriated $30,000 for the work, providing 27 nurses at a salary of $900 a year, who took charge of 131 schools with an attendance of 200,000.

George H. Martin, then Secretary of the Massachusetts Board of Education, said the results justified the expense. A large number of children failed school vision and hearing tests, which severely hampered them from receiving their education. Martin asserted that it was possible to remedy these conditions when they were brought to the attention of the parents and a physician. He followed by saying that while school committees and health boards were generally favorable to a system of thorough medical inspection, they did not have the finances to support it: "An awakening of public sentiment is needed, and it may be necessary to enact some compulsory legislation, as has been done in some other states."[13]

Yet another organization envisioned the placement of nurses in the Boston schools and helped provide the framework for their future. The Hawthorne Club, named after the noted writer Nathaniel Hawthorne, developed an after-school and summer program for school-age children in 1902. *Children's House, A History of the Hawthorne Club* revealed that besides story reading, the Club gave classes in proper hygiene, homemaking, basketry, woodworking, cooking, job training, and tutoring, just to name a few. As was common among settlement houses at that time, the Club had homes in Natick, and later Winthrop to take the underprivileged children for a summer vacation away from the hot city. The prevention of tuberculosis particularly interested them, and they were instrumental in the establishment of the Boston Association for the Relief and Control of Tuberculosis in 1903. At various times, they presented programs and set up health exhibitions at the Quincy, Andrews, and Way Street Schools, which would later become Annie McKay's assignment.

Their 100-year-old wooden cottage was located on 3 Garland Street, a short walk from the Way Street School. *Children's House* described the Way Street School

---

13   Nurses in Schools. Dr. Samuel H Durgin Makes Appeal for Them. (1905, November 9) *Boston Daily Globe* (1872-1922), 10. Retrieved December 9, 2007 from ProQuest Historical Newspapers Boston Globe (1872-1924) database (Document ID; 694156112)

"as a small, unsightly school at the edge of the railroad tracks.[14]" Because of the poor condition and location of the school, the Boston School Committee granted permission for "Play Sessions in the Hawthorne Club." At that time, a schoolteacher, one in the lead and one in the rear, would march the children (74 from one classroom) from the school to the Hawthorne Club playground for a play hour once a week. The Hawthorne Club observed that this playtime resulted in healthier looking children. They concluded it was their efforts in working with the Instructive District Nursing Association (IDNA) that brought a nurse to the Way Street School. For several years a trained nurse came to the Club to give hygiene classes. Whether this nurse was from IDNA is lost to historical speculation.[15] However, the groundwork was being laid for the introduction of school nurses.

The Influence of Societal Organizations

By the end of 1905, Boston, still upset with the 13 percent rate of absenteeism, followed the lead of two other American cities, first, New York in 1902, and Los Angeles in 1904, and looked to nurses to supplement the work of physicians. IDNA, one of two organizations, though apparently unknown to each other, had for some time felt the need for and importance of nurses' services in the public schools. Both organizations separately petitioned the Boston School Committee for permission that each might place at its own expense a trained nurse in a school district. The Mothers' and Fathers' Club of Boston then reached an agreement with IDNA to the extent that the Club would pay IDNA each year the necessary money for the maintenance of a nurse. This nurse was to be known as the Mothers' and Fathers' Club Nurse, but she would be under the supervision of IDNA. Subsequently, IDNA invited the president of the Club, Mrs. Mary Pamela Rice, to become a manager of IDNA.[16]

In her annual report for the year, February 1906, IDNA Superintendent Nurse, Martha Stark, reported that one of the managers donated $700 as an experiment to

---

14 Robinson, L.V. (1937). *Children's House - A History of the Hawthorne Club*. Boston, MA: Marshall Jones Co. Page 80.

15 Robinson, L.V. (1937). *Children's House - A History of the Hawthorne Club*. Boston, MA: Marshall Jones Co. Page 80.

16 *Instructive District Nursing Association Board of Managers Report, November 1905*, Box 8, Folder II, Boston Visiting Nurse Archives, Howard Gotlieb Archival Research Center, Boston University.

pay for a nurse in public schools for one year. Another section of the report stated that Walter C. Baylies contributed $700 to pay for a nurse's salary for one year's work in the public schools.[17] Several years later, in 1912, another newspaper article reported that a member of the Hawthorne Club as mentioned earlier assured the salary of Massachusetts first school nurse.[18] Whether this person is one and the same is difficult to surmise at this time, but it is safe to say that contributions and endowments supported all of IDNA's school nurses.

In response, specifically, the Boston School Committee on November 14, 1905, announced a new "experiment" in the following manner:

"Permission is hereby granted the Instructive District Nursing Association, and the Mothers' and Fathers' Club of Boston, respectively, to place a trained nurse in the Quincy and Wells Districts for the purpose of supplementing the medical inspection of the schools by the Board of Health by personal effort among pupils and parents in matters of sanitation and hygiene. Said nurses to be under the supervision and direction of this Board, their employment to be without expense to the city, and to be terminated at the pleasure of the Board.[19]"

Accordingly, the Instructive District Nursing Association, with the consent of the Boston School Committee, placed in their words "one of our most experienced nurses" on December 6, 1905, in the South End area of Boston.[20] Thus enters Annie McKay. In Chapter 2, we will look at Annie's early years before her pioneer nursing journey begins.

---

17 *Twentieth Annual Report of the Instructive District Nursing Assn. for the Year Ending Jan. 31, 1906*. P. 7.

18 Work of the School Nurse: Usefulness Proved in the Public Schools (1912, July 7) *Boston Daily Globe* (1872-1922), 53. Retrieved December 9, 2007, from ProQuest Historical Newspapers Boston Globe (1872-1924) database. (Document ID: 729249992).

19 Apollenio, T.D. (1905, November 28). *City of Boston In School Committee.*

20 *Instructive District Nursing Association Board of Managers Report, November 1905*, Box 8, Folder II, Boston Visiting Nurse Archives, Howard Gotlieb Archival Research Center, Boston University.

Chapter 2

Annie McKay's Adventuresome Life

Dave MacKay (note the different spelling) a cousin of Annie McKay, said she desperately wanted to "get out of the bush." As will be seen, she accomplished that and much more. He made these remarks in 2010, when he and his daughter visited Boston. They came to view the plaque placed by the Massachusetts School Nurse Organization in 2009, on the historic Washington Street building to commemorate where Annie lived in the early 1900s.

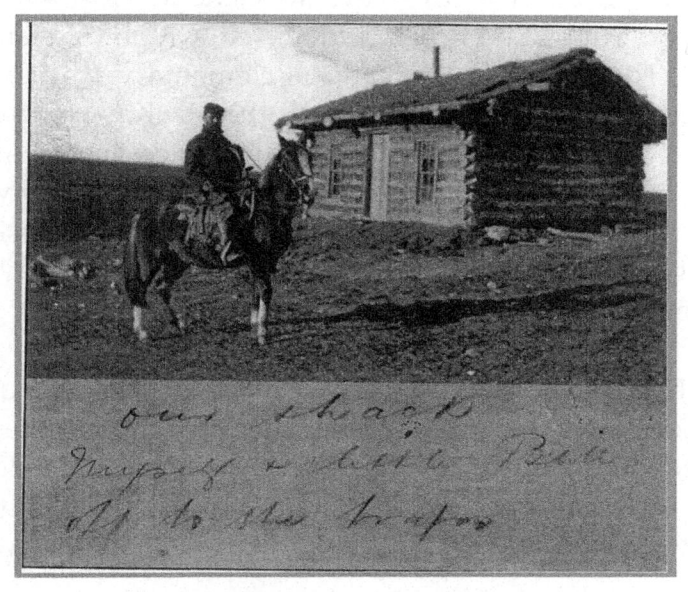

The House Where Annie McKay Was Born
Photo courtesy of Dave MacKay

A look into Annie McKay's life provides insight into her early childhood, growing up in a rural area, her zeal for travel, her sense for adventure, her passion for education in her nursing career, and her later years. My inquiries have revealed that Annie McKay was born on July 29, 1867, in a humble log house in rural Beaverton, Ontario, Canada, the sixth of ten children of Angus MacKay and Rebecca Fraser. Beaverton, on Lake Simco, is located 65 miles (104.6 km) north of Toronto, which itself is on the much larger Lake Ontario. On the south bank of Lake Ontario is the U.S. See the figure on the previous page -The House where Annie McKay was born.

Correspondence with Annie McKay's remaining family and the Beaverton Thorah Eldon Historical Society disclosed that her grandfather had emigrated with his small children from Scotland to Canada in 1830. They boarded a small ship and endured the rough, cold waters of the Atlantic and traveled into the interior of Canada to start a new life. The 1881 Canadian Census found the family with ten children living together on the farm. At that time, the Census listed Annie as 13-year-old Ann (1881 Census). To this day, the family uses the spelling of "MacKay" in contrast to Annie's early choice spelling of "McKay" as seen on her nursing school application. Over the years, however, she reverted back to using "MacKay" as her family name.

Annie's 1891 application to the Toronto General Hospital Training School for Nurses asked questions about her primary education. She answered that she attended SS No. 3, Thorah, probably the local elementary school, and the Toronto Collegiate Institute. The family memoir recalls the MacKay children walking three miles each way to school, regardless of the harsh Ontario winters. As was the custom of that era in rural areas, if students did well in their studies, they were encouraged to attend secondary school. Frequently, these schools were not within commuting distance, requiring the students to board. Therefore, Annie McKay left home in her teens to further her education.

As noted in her application, Annie McKay attended the Toronto Collegiate Institute, now known as the Jarvis Collegiate Institute, located in downtown Toronto. "Founded in 1807 during the frontier days of Upper Canada, it is the oldest secondary school in Toronto with over 200 years of tradition."[21] It is interesting to note, that the first school nurse in the U.S., Lina Rogers, likewise a Canadian, also

---

21 *Jarvis Collegiate, Toronto, Canada.* Retrieved from http://schools.tdsb.ca/jarvisci/.

attended Toronto's Jarvis Collegiate Institute. In all likelihood, they were not in the same class, as Lina was three years younger than Annie, but if they knew of each other, what a coincidence that would be.[22]

It was commonplace at that time for the older children in large families on small farms to leave their homes to make their livelihood elsewhere, and that is what Annie and several of her siblings did. Both her parents passed away in 1899. Interestingly, Annie trained as a schoolteacher and taught school before she decided to enter nursing. The Canadian census of 1891 lists an Annie McKay, age 24 living in Toronto, working as a teacher, which falls in line with what we know of her. Undoubtedly, her experience with children contributed to her later success as a school nurse.

Records from the Toronto General Hospital School of Nursing show that Annie McKay was one of the 53 who were accepted out of 647 applications to the class. On her application in 1891, she stated she is 5'3," has a fair complexion, and has brown eyes. She graduated in 1894 at age 27 (See her Nursing School Application on the next page).

"On ordinary evenings" relates the family memoir, "there were enough people in the MacKay family to organize card games." A coal-oil lamp provided light, making it possible to have lively conversations, read newspapers, and write letters. The family memoir tells a story of older brother Ronald bringing his younger sisters Tena and Jenny to a dance and party in 1892, but there's no mention of Annie. Would she have been out tripping the light fantastic (dancing) if she were home? We will never know.

Do Canadian's have an accent? Western and Central Canada apparently speak the same way as what is known as General American English. Ontarians speak with the more rounded British pronunciation. They seem to add "eh" to the end of their sentences and shift the pronunciation of some vowels. For that reason, in the movie Argo, they taught Americans to pronounce "Toronto" with the second t sounding like a d. Therefore, Annie McKay would have spoken a little differently from the Boston accent.[23]

---

22 Pollitt, P. (1994). Lina Rogers Struthers: The first school nurse. *Journal of School Nursing*, 10(1), Page 34.

23 Canadian Accent Influences. Retrieved from http://tvtropes.org/pmwiki/pmwiki.php/Main/Canadian Accent Influences

Young women, coming from rural farm areas as Annie McKay, were considered the most exceptional candidates for nursing, commented Betsy Beattie in her book about Canadian women living in Boston. Beattie described a rural farm girl as a, "physically strong, hard-working girl who nevertheless was deferential and responsive to the efforts of her supervisors to mold her into an obedient, self-sacrificing, and refined young woman." She continued that their parents brought them up with a sense of responsibility to family needs, accustomed to hard work, and "untouched by the temptations or comforts of the big city.[24]"

Annie's Nursing School Application

---

24 Beattie, M. (2000). *Obligation and Opportunity: Single Maritime Women in Boston 1870-1930.* Canada: McGil-Queens University Press.

Annie McKay became a part of history when we find her again in an entry in *The Victorian Order of Nurses for Canada, 50th Anniversary 1897-1947*. They recorded her as one of the original nurses admitted to Canada's first visiting nurses on April 6, 1899, to Vernon, British Columbia, western, rural, Canada.[25] We shouldn't be surprised as she developed into an independent, self-reliant, and adventuresome woman.

After that, Annie McKay found her way to Boston following a time in New York City. A large migration of single Canadian women ventured to Boston in the late nineteenth and early twentieth century in search of employment. The numbers of women leaving were equal to or surpassed that of men. At one point, more people were leaving Canada than immigrating to Canada. The farms no longer needed the daily work of young females, as in churning butter, since there were expanded operations on farms leading to farmers raising more commercial crops. However, the young people that left for the big cities were expected to send home some of their earnings. It was a way for families to preserve their farms and their way of life.[26]

When the Instructive District Nursing Association (IDNA), a precursor to today's Visiting Nurse Association, employed Annie McKay in 1901, she listed her credentials as the following: Graduate of Toronto General Hospital; Graduate of Victorian Order Training School, Toronto; District Nurse for Victorian Order (VON) for two years; Graduate of Woman's Hospital in New York; and Graduate of Massachusetts Charitable Eye and Ear Infirmary, Boston.[27] She, therefore, had accumulated extensive postgraduate courses in community health and general medicine. Later on, in Boston, she would meet up again with her former superintendent from VON, Charlotte Macleod.

On a manifest from a Buffalo checkpoint on the U.S.-Canadian border in 1927, Annie declared that she came to the U.S. in 1902. Given the many times that she

---

25 Gibbon, J.M. (1947). *The Victorian Order of Nurses for Canada, 50th Anniversary 1897-1947*. Montreal, Canada: Southam Press. Government of Canada. (2014, April). Page 39.

26 Beattie, M. (2000). *Obligation and Opportunity: Single Maritime Women in Boston 1870-1930*. Canada: McGil-Queens University Press.

27 *Twenty-First Annual Report of the Instructive District Nursing Association for the Year Ending January 31, 1907*, Box 10, Boston.

traveled back and forth, perhaps she lost track because she must have first arrived in the U.S. around 1900.

Living in Boston

A Boston City *Directory* in 1902 provides insight into McKay's whereabouts at that time, as she was listed as "MacKay, Annie, nurse, rms. 31 Dartmouth." Historic Dartmouth Street still exists in the South End area of Boston, looking much as it did back then, with bow front brick houses lining both sides of the street. However, from about 1890 on, the stately residences had changed from being single-family homes to rooming houses. Later, Boston demolished 31 Dartmouth Street around the 1980s to make a place for a pocket park that remains today.

A lodging house, then, consisted of several private rooms on a single floor with a bathroom to share. Generally, they were quite sparse, with a window, bed, bureau, mirror, and maybe a sink if you were lucky. IDNA's Superintendent's notes tell us that several nurses who worked there lived at 31 Dartmouth Street; moreover, the building included new technology, a telephone. Since Annie was still new to the city, she must have enjoyed the companionship of her fellow nurses. To obtain an idea of how much she paid for rent, *The City Wilderness* contained some estimates for a room as going from $1.00 per week to $5.00 per week, depending on size and accommodations.[28]

By 1905, however, we found that McKay had moved about four blocks west from her former address, to 1521 Washington Street, a handsome stone-fronted apartment building, again in the South End that still stands today.[29] Even nowadays, it is considered a distinguished building with its first floor finished off for stores. At this address, Annie had her own apartment, larger, of course, than her previous room. To quote *The City Wilderness* again, an apartment would rent from $4 to $25 for the best, per week.[30] Given that Annie's salary at IDNA was $600 a year, we can

---

28 Woods, R. (1898). *The City Wilderness, A Settlement Study.* Boston: Houghton, Mifflin and Company. Page 102.

29 *Boston Directory*, (1906). p. 1190. Boston, MA.

30 *Twenty-First Annual Report of the Instructive District Nursing Association for the Year Ending January 31, 1907*, Box 10, Boston.

deduct that she must have been paying on the lower end rather than, the higher.[31]

The Boston Directory classified Annie McKay as a nurse, living there as "do," meaning that was her work and home. A reference librarian at the Boston Public Library said this meant that she also probably cared for an individual in the apartment building. This was not surprising, for she was an unmarried woman, living on her own, and most likely needed extra money, perhaps to remit to her family in Canada.

The building, 1521 Washington Street, has survived the era of elevated trains built on Washington Street in 1901 and removed in 1987. It has also withstood the threat of the wrecker's ball and urban redevelopment that bedeviled the South End until the end of the 1970s. Would you believe a ride on the elevated trains cost five cents back then?

We don't know what Annie McKay did in her spare time, but there is a family-owned restaurant/bar on Berkeley Street, JJ Foley's that has been at that spot since 1909. The owner reports that it would have been proper for a group of ladies during that era to sit at a table for a night out. If it was the correct thing to do, she probably did.

One might also imagine that Annie McKay may have sat down in her apartment, with the noisy, elevated Orange-line train screeching by her windows, and composed a letter to her family that perhaps went something like this:

Dear Family,

How is everyone? I am living in a lovely apartment in a safe area of Boston. My days are fulfilling, working for the Instructive District Nursing Association (IDNA) and giving nursing care to poor, sick families in their homes.

Now, IDNA is starting a new experimental program with the City of Boston where they are sending a nurse into the schools intending to reduce absenteeism. They have chosen me as the nurse to start the program. Perhaps they selected me because I was a schoolteacher in Toronto and did nurse training in New York

---

31 Instructive District Nursing Association. (1901) *15th Annual Report for the Year Ending 1-31-1901*. Retrieved from ocp.hul.harvard.edu/dl/www.004487784. Pages 6-7.

City. My supervisor said I was their most experienced nurse for the job. I am really pleased with my new assignment. As always, I will give it my best effort.

Regarding the children, when I visit the homes, sometimes they are playing out on the streets when they should be in school. So, it is no surprise that Boston schools have a high absentee rate.

I am really becoming fond of this city. It has a cosmopolitan flair, so much running about, not at all like Beaverton. In comparison, I like it more than New York City, as it is smaller, but still has many things to do. There is a church that I enjoy, First Presbyterian Church just a stone's throw from my apartment. It reminds me somewhat of the Old Stone Church back in Thorah. We walked up to the Boston Public Library to see their new murals of Sir Galahad standing alongside his golden tree by one of America's famed artists, John Singer Sargent. I have never seen anything like that. It was so empowering and engaging!

Since I am going to a lecture this evening, I must sign off. I miss you all and will come home for my vacation in August. Please write a few lines to me.

Cheery bye,
Annie[32]

Do we feel the urge to write back? I submit that I do. I would say to Annie McKay,

"All is well back in Beaverton. Even though much of what people learn about history is told through the paintings of famous people, or those who held lofty, leadership positions, history is filled with examples of significant yet largely unknown individuals who made unheralded achievements, and you may become one of them."

Following her period of school nursing, Annie McKay remained in Boston and worked with tuberculosis patients in area hospitals and other health agencies. However, by 1909 and 1910, the *Boston Street Directory* finds that Annie McKay had returned to rooms at 31 Dartmouth Street.[33] Instead, the Boston Street Directory

---

32 *The South End Almanac* (1924) Directory of churches, 12,13. Boston. South End Improvement Society.

33 *Boston Directory*, (1909, 1910). p. 1163. Boston, MA.

does not list her for 1911-1912, or in 1914. What happened here to make her return to one room? In answering that question, we must construe her circumstances. It could have been the noise and soot from the elevated train, a deteriorating neighborhood, the expense of the apartment, and the need for more companionship. Perhaps she was not receiving the fee from the apartment neighbor for whom she had been caring. Then again, she may have returned to visit Beaverton during these times.

Comparison annual salaries at that time were a city clerk's compensation at $1,512.50, and domestic live-in help received $432.81 separate from the food, uniforms, and lodging which was included.[34] As mentioned earlier, Annie's salary at IDNA was $600 a year. What choice would you have made if you were in Annie's situation?

During World War I, the family revealed that Annie McKay served as a nurse with the American Expeditionary Forces overseas. The U.S. Armed Forces were unable to corroborate that information. However, the American Red Cross has records of an Annie MacKay joining the Paris Committee (American Red Cross Nursing Service) in 1918, in Paris, which they considered unusual. Generally, applicants joined in the States. Jean Waldman, the volunteer nurse historian for the American Red Cross in Washington, D.C. checked their records, and commented that this is only the second time that she found a nurse joining that way.

Annie McKay received American Red Cross Nursing Badge number 16989. The attractive red and blue uniform of the Red Cross drew many young women to its cause as much as for patriotism. On her application, she entered French as her second language. The family verified that she was indeed fluent in French. Being a nurse and knowing French

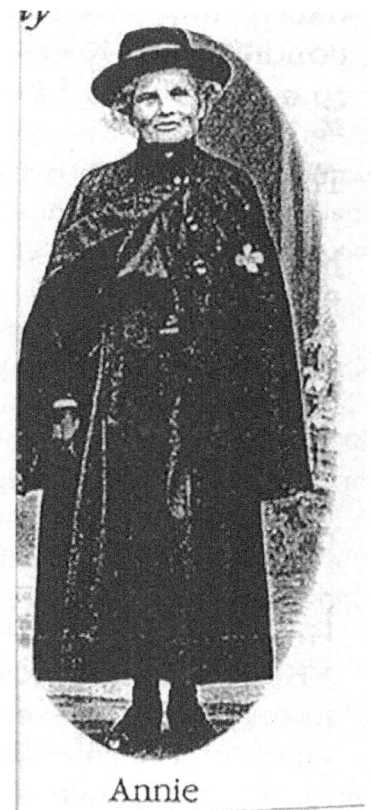

Annie

Annie McKay in her Red Cross uniform

---

34   Public Documents of Massachusetts. (1907). *Bureau of Statistics of Labor*. Vol. II pgs. xxvi, 107-111. Retrieved from http://books.google.com/books?Id=K_kWAAAAYAA&pg=PA660&dq=fireman+Salaries+in+Boston=1906+Source.

would have made her very valuable in the war effort. It was also noted that she was a non-naturalized citizen. The First World War must have been yet another journey and experience for her (See the image above, Anne McKay in her Red Cross Uniform. Photo courtesy of Roberta Mitchell).

Like so many other people, she apparently yearned to be part of a world historical moment. During World War I, the American Red Cross recruited 20 million people, working through their chapters, with their calls to patriotism and service to give aid to military personnel. Their 18,000 nurses provided the majority of medical care during this war. They witnessed enormous destruction in both France and Belgium. It was a war that killed, maimed, and injured servicemen on an industrial scale.[35] Unfortunately, we know little of what encompassed Annie McKay's service in World War I. A family member, who knew more of her experience, died a year before this inquiry.

Efforts to locate a passport for her have proved fruitless. After making inquiries into Canadian passport policy, the reason is understood. The modern type of Canadian passport was only first issued in 1921. Previously, Canada followed the British model, as the country was part of the United Kingdom. British passports, first disseminated in 1862, were called a Letter of Request. This was then updated in 1915, to become a ten-section single sheet. Probably, they grandfathered older passports for several years. Sadly, the Canadian government kept no records of their first passports, and any that were kept have been lost.[36]

However, with the help of the American Canadian Genealogical Society in Manchester, NH, a passport application has been found for an A. E. McKay in 1898 within Great Britain's collections in the category for travel and migration, with no age given. Whether or not this is authentic is left to speculation.

Family Memoir

A member of Annie McKay's remaining family, Jean MacKay, was ambitious enough

---

[35] *Rallying a Nation: American Red Cross advertising during World War I.* (2014, June 13) Retrieved from http://www.aef.com/on_campus/classroom/case_histories/3002.

[36] *History of Passports.* Retrieved from http://www.cic.gc.ca/english/games/teachers-corner/history-passports.asp.

to write a family memoir and included a chapter about the three sisters in the family. Frequently, during the 1920s, Annie visited her family in Canada and seemed to be on hand when any medical emergency arose. This is how she told her story.

"I had scarlet fever when I was six, and she was there to nurse me through it. I made a complete recovery but, ungrateful little bugger that I was, I was furious with her (Annie) because, in her zeal to get rid of all articles which might harbor germs, she burned my favorite book, 'The Wizard of Oz.' She was also on hand and worked unstintingly when my mother was sick before she died in 1930. Annie was a very dedicated woman. After my mother's death, Annie stayed on to keep house for my father. She was a good nurse, but the same couldn't be said for her housekeeping! She was a well-meaning soul, and she did a lot for me, like providing me with enough money to go to art school.[37]"

Another family member, Roberta Mitchell, shared an account of her family recollections:

"In 1919, her brother Jack and his wife Lillian were taken ill with flu and pneumonia. Their three children, Lillian (7), Jean (6) and Jack (2) were taken ill with scarlet fever. Aunt Annie traveled to Alberta to nurse the family, but only the parents and one daughter Jean recovered." (This is the family member, Jean MacKay, who wrote the preceding memoir).

After retirement, Annie McKay returned to Canada to spend her golden years. When her brother Jack died in 1937, Annie went to live with her sisters Tena and Jennie and brother Angus in Shanty Bay, near Beaverton. In 1944, at the age of 77, she passed away in her native Beaverton. She was laid to rest in the Old Stone Church cemetery, and from there, she would undertake her final journey.[38] Annie's nursing education served her well in her life, allowing her to be an independent woman, nurture family relationships, travel extensively in North America and Europe, and indeed to experience more of the world beyond Beaverton. In Chapter 3, we will explore the early education of nurses.

---

37   MacKay, J. *Family History*.
38   Obituary. (1944, September 28) *Beaverton Express*.

Chapter 3

The Way We Were

> "No man, not even a doctor, ever gives any other definition of what a nurse should be than this- 'devoted and obedient.' This definition would do just as well for a porter. It might even do for a horse. It would not do for a policeman."
>
> - **Florence Nightingale**[39]

The Early Education of Nurses

My inquiry into the education of Annie McKay, led the archivist Annie Orchanian-Cheff of the Toronto University Health Network, to discover Annie McKay's original application in 1891 to their School of Nursing. Orchanian-Cheff has turned into a true friend and supporter of school nurses. She sent a report from The Toronto General Hospital Training School for Nurses from 1894, which not only gives us an idea of Annie McKay's education but also focuses on the early education of nurses. The documents illuminate how these young women were influenced to become more like the Victorian woman; in short, a vision of a nurse who is an angelic, demure, subservient, and dependent woman. Since that era, nurses have worked diligently to change that model to become the strong, competent, resourceful health professional of today.

---

[39] Nightingale, F. (1860). *Science quotes by Florence Nightingale*. Retrieved from http://todayinsci.com/N/-Nightingale_Florence/NightingaleFlorence-Quotations.htm *Notes on Nursing: What it is, and What it is Not* (1860). 200.

The report opens with the history of the school that began in 1881. Though the Toronto Hospital Training School for Nurses, in conjunction with the Toronto General Hospital had goals of educating and training nurses, it states that their main goal was the care and nursing of the sick in the various wards of the hospital. To quote from these reports: "Our work and methods of instruction during 1894 have not differed materially from that of other years. It consists in the usual class teaching, in elementary anatomy, physiology, and hygiene, by the Superintendent and her Assistant, together with a very complete course of lectures, extending from October until July." In other words, the hospital needed an inexpensive source of workers.

The report continues: "For these lectures, the Training School is indebted to many of the most prominent members of the medical profession in our City, who, notwithstanding their arduous labors, and numerous engagements, have always most cheerfully given their valuable services as lecturers and examiners." The report introduces a series of educational talks given by the hospital physicians on the following subjects: two on dermatology, two on the eye and ear, two on gynecology, four on obstetrics; four on contagious diseases; one on hygiene; eight on surgery and surgical appliances; one on the nose and throat; and also, on medical nursing.

A discussion of the 647 applications that were received during 1894 followed. Of those applications, only 53 were admitted to the training school, though on further inspection, just 22 were found to be suitable to become pupil-nurses, what today we would refer to as student nurses. In that group, another four dropped out. There were another four graduate nurses in the school.[40]

After completing their school year and examinations, the students received their certificates of qualification to be a trained nurse. The graduates accepted a variety of positions, totaling about 202, all acceptable to the school. For example, their nurses received employment with private families, as lady superintendents, or head nurses of hospitals, or as foreign missionaries.

Another passage records a situation in which one of their graduates displayed

---

40   Suively, M. (1894). *Report of the Toronto General Hospital Training School for Nurses for the Year ending October 31st, 1894*. Pages 1-2.

selfless heroism. She had received a call to help a family where the entire household, numbering five in all, was suffering from the dreaded disease smallpox. Without any help whatsoever, this nurse cared for the family through sickness and death, ignoring her own personal needs. "To her praise be it said - she was faithful to her trust.[41]"

This raises the question of whether nurses would do this kind of service today. As reported in the August 13, 2014, *The Boston Globe*, American nurses were donning protective garb known as a Tyvek suit, followed by rubber boots, an apron, a gown and another pair of gloves. The outfit was complete when a hood with a clear plastic front was added to the head, plus an air-filtering device was attached to the waist. They would be working directly with those infected and dying from the Ebola virus in Africa. At that time there was no proven cure or vaccine to combat the disease, so they were definitely taking dangerous chances regarding their own safety. As a consequence of caring for patients during this Ebola crisis, despite wearing the protective gear, both nurses and physicians came down with the disease.[42]

Another example is the highly contagious coronavirus, circumventing the globe in March 2020, hitting 182 countries. President Trump says he sees nurses selflessly running into hospitals, donning their protective gear, eager to start their shift. They are risking their own health during the uncertainties and fears of this time. The epilogue to COVID-19 is yet unknown.

A later report of the Toronto Hospital Training School for Nurses in 1905 illustrates the growth and appeal of nursing as a profession. An astounding 666 applicants applied for admission to the training school, of which 39 were ultimately accepted and admitted on probation. They then trimmed them down to 25, followed by one who left the program. Each year, there was an increase in the number of postgraduate nurses, or staff nurses on duty in the private and semiprivate wards. For instance, there were 22 such nurses on duty at one time during 1904. Of course, the report said they were paid for this work.[43]

However, the report continues, several times, five of their post-graduate nurses

---

41   Ibid. Page 3.

42   Freyer, F. (2014, August 13). A 2-pronged ebola mission. *The Boston Globe*, pp. A1, A5.

43   Suively, M. (1905). *Report of the Toronto General Hospital Training School for Nurses for the Year ending September 30th, 1905*. 1.

volunteered to work without pay on the public wards.

"We welcome this evidence of the truly professional spirit in our nurses and trust that every effort may be made to foster its growth. Not so much for the benefit which the Hospital may derive as for the nurse herself, who must ever strive to cultivate such qualities as compassion, charity, and self-sacrifice which have been the outstanding virtues which have marked the true nurse in all ages, making her calling a noble and beneficent, rather than a commercial one.[44]"

Generally, people who are compassionate about their work are willing to go the extra mile. This is still true today demonstrated by the doctors, nurses, delivery people, and checkout staff to name a few who are working tirelessly for our health and wellbeing during this coronavirus era.

Duties of the 1887 Floor Nurse

Annie McKay might have encountered some, if not all, of these regulations in her training at Toronto's School of Nursing; how she liked them will never be known:

Duties of the Floor Nurse – 1887
"In addition to caring for your 50 patients, each nurse will follow these regulations:

- Daily sweep and mop the floors of your ward; dust the patients' furniture and windowsills.
- Maintain an even temperature in your ward by bringing in a scuttle of coal for the day's business.
- Light is important to observe the patient's condition; therefore, each day fill kerosene lamps, clean chimneys, and trim wicks.
- Wash windows once a week.
- The nurse's notes are important in aiding the physician's work. Make your pens carefully. You may whittle nibs to your individual taste. (Making a writing instrument)
- Each nurse on day duty will report every day at 7 a.m. and leave at 8 p.m., except on the Sabbath on which day you will be off from noon to 2 p.m.

---

44   Ibid.

- Graduate nurses in good standing with the director of nurses will be given an evening off each week if you go regularly to church.
- Each nurse should lay aside from each payday a goodly sum of her earnings for her benefits during her declining years, so that she will not become a burden. For example, if you earn $30 a month, you should set aside $15.
- Any nurse who smokes, uses liquor in any form, gets her hair done at a beauty shop, or frequents dance halls will give the director, of nurses, good reason to suspect her worth, intentions, and integrity.

The nurse who performs her labors, serves her patients and doctors faithfully and without fault for a period of five years will be given an increase by the hospital administration of 5 cents a day, providing there are no hospital debts that are outstanding.[45"]

1890 Nurses: Woman of the Hour

In 1902, Annie McKay listed as one of her credentials a postgraduate course at the Massachusetts Charitable Eye and Ear Infirmary, now called the Massachusetts Eye and Ear Infirmary. Many thanks are extended to Mary E. Leach, Director of Public Affairs, who was kind enough to research their archives, and forward a copy of *"Massachusetts Eye and Ear Infirmary, Studies on Its History, Nursing Education, 1895-1925."* This report follows the development of nursing education and hospital staffing in Boston around the period when Annie McKay attended the course, approximately 1900-1902.

There is no record of Annie McKay, however, having taken a course at this institution. For that matter, no records have survived of any nurse who took postgraduate study there. On the other hand, the hospital recorded every physician's name who took a course there. This further demonstrates the low regard that women were held in, and the prevailing dominance of men over women and doctors over nurses at that time. During this era, women had minimal property, inheritance, or marriage rights, and could not vote.

It must be noted that as early as 1873, Linda Richards became America's

---

[45] Holder, L. (2014) Nursing through the generations. Nursing Excellence e-Edition, Issue 8. Retrieved from www.childrencentral.orgPRESSROOM/PUBLICATIONS/NURSINGEXCELLENCE8Pages/NursingThroughGenerations.Aspx

first officially trained nurse when she graduated from the one-year training program for nurses at the New England Hospital for Women and Children.[46] *The 19th Annual Report* in 1893 of the Boston Training School for Nurses, attached to Massachusetts General Hospital described what the student nurse was taught to do. She received instruction on: "the dressing of burns, sores and wounds, the preparation and application of fomentations, poultices, cups, leeches and of minor dressings; (a topical substance as a poultice treatment for pain that uses a warm moist application) the giving of baths; and the principles of massage, with practical exercise." In addition, how to take care of the patient's room, including making beds, and proper airing of the room; how to care for an invalid, and convalescent patient; the construction, and application of bandages, and splints; how to treat emergencies, and the use of stimulants; and lastly, the preparation and serving of food. All of these lessons were then combined into the nurse being able to monitor the patient closely, keeping track of their diet, medications, intake, and output of fluids, and general body functions.[47]

By 1890, the medical profession generally welcomed the professionally trained nurse sometimes called "woman of the hour." However, not all physicians held that opinion, as noted in these remarks taken from a reading of the time:

"The doctor's responsibility as to the nursing service is like that of a captain to his ship...nurses were often conceited and too unconscious of the due subordination owed to the medical profession, of which they are a sort of useful parasite... with the right sort of notions of their duties, they will eventually prove a blessing to the sick of all classes of the community... nursing is the natural vehicle for women in medicine.[48]"

In 1889, a group of aural surgeons (an otologist, an MD focusing on conditions of the ear) requested the hiring of a professionally trained nurse for the Massachusetts Eye and Ear Infirmary. Many local area hospitals at the time adhered to the practice of hiring untrained personnel. Superintendent, Dr. George Stedman, MD, then

---

46 Judd, D., Sitzman, K., & Davis, G.M. (2010). *A history of American nursing trends and eras.* Sudbury, MA: Jones and Bartlett. Page 41.

47 How nurses are trained. *Boston Daily Globe (1872-1922)*; Feb 22, 1893; ProQuest Historical Newspapers Boston Globe (1872-1924) Page 10.

48 Snyder, C. (1984). "Massachusetts Eye and Ear Infirmary, studies on its history, nursing education, 1895-1925, Boston, MA. Page 1.

responded that to employ a trained nurse would cost $12-$14 per week compared to their current practice of paying an untrained nurse $4 per week. He maintained it would be more economical to hire a professionally trained nurse only in the instances when one would be needed for exceptional surgical cases, which was not often.

The hospital hired a new medical superintendent, Dr. Farrar Cobb, MD, in 1895. He embarked on a plan to make long-overdue changes in management and patient care. He found the hospital in horrible shape. In his mind, there were not enough nurses to care for the patients efficiently. One of the head nurses could neither read nor write, and the wards and beds were filthy and unsanitary. His changes included hiring a Superintendent of Nurses to develop the nursing education program, plus a plan to train nurse's aides. Perhaps what they really needed was a safe staffing amendment. That amendment was passed in Massachusetts in 2004, which would require acute care hospitals to establish and maintain safe, flexible, minimum RN-to-patient ratios.[49] However, in the climate that prevailed in 1895, Dr. Cobb's plans were dramatic steps forward.

The Post-Graduate nursing education program consisted of a four-month course. They required the students to wear a uniform of the school, for which they were charged, work three weeks on night duty, and paid them $15 per month. The program flourished and by 1914 doctors and the new social services department offered as many as 114 classes and lectures. Dr. Cobb increased the length of the program to five months and set the salary at $72 for that period.

Additionally, Dr. Cobb presented to nurses' aides a probationary period of three months. If they did well, he offered them nine more months work, and then encouraged them to apply to a nurses training school. They offered a salary of $15 per month and reached a peak wage of $20 per month, plus room and board. By 1915, the hospital excluded nurse's aides from direct nursing care of patients, other than bathing.[50]

By 1915, a new Superintendent of Nurses, Mary Coonahan, arrived on the scene,

---

[49] *Massachusetts Nurses Association* (2004) Legislation and Politics. Safe staffing. Retrieved from: http://www.massnurses.org/legislation-and-politics/safe-staffing/p/openitem748.

[50] Snyder, C. (1984). "Massachusetts Eye and Ear Infirmary, studies on its history, nursing education, 1895-1925, Boston, MA. Page 2.

who had a forward vision for nursing. She insisted that not only should nurses care for the patients, but they should also teach the patients and the public what can be done to maintain hearing and vision. After graduating from this program, the former nursing students from both here and abroad carried this contemporary knowledge with them to their new positions. This was an example of good preventive care. Another innovative idea was to allow student nurses from Massachusetts General Hospital Training School for Nurses to intern at the Infirmary for 60 days to study eye and ear nursing. Coonahan hoped that similar arrangements would be made with other area hospitals. The program proved successful.

Unfortunately, in 1917, international affairs took center stage, as the intervention of World War I severely affected both the nursing and medical staff. The government called many to active duty, leaving a small team that could not maintain the extensive program of lectures and bedside demonstrations. After the war, many more professions opened up to women, which were also less physically demanding than nursing. With the telephone and typewriter becoming standard office technology for the time, businesses became a more attractive place to work as compared to making beds and emptying bedpans. Can you blame them? This created a scenario where fewer women were entering the nursing field. In response, Superintendent Coonahan envisioned a nursing education program where the "students (were) to be relieved from the laborious hospital housework, so destructive to the energy and purpose of the woman who wanted training in the care of the sick." As a result, this plan would leave her students more free time to study.

The program at the Massachusetts Charitable Eye and Ear Infirmary continued to grow, including the appointment of a full-time instructor of nursing theory, Abby Helen Denison. By writing a book entitled "A Textbook of Eye, Ear, Nose and Throat Nursing," Denison accomplished another first. She became the first woman, and moreover a nurse, to author a book on this subject.

This nursing education program stood in sharp contrast to many hospital schools of the day where students frequently received no education, little equipment, and where they considered the young nursing student not a student, but "only as a worker." On the average, a student nurse toiled 52 hours a week, and night schedules could be, as long as, 84 hours a week.

Florence Nightingale, the Crimean War's beloved "Lady with the Lamp" as she was called, became a legend in her own time, long recognized as the founder of modern nursing. She intended nurses training schools to be autonomous, but this did not happen as administrations placed them under the control of hospitals. "Nursing students replaced the ward maids who had preceded them, and the salary of the maid became the educational stipend of the student. Once grafted onto the domestic sphere of the hospitals, nursing education became subordinate to the needs of the hospitals.[51]" Male and medical domination of the fledgling nurses trying to establish themselves as a profession was well underway. Nurses were "trained" as opposed to "educated." As Miss Murphy, one of my instructors always said, "Dogs are trained, you are educated."

In sharp contrast by 1870, the move to improve medical education of physicians coincided with the growth of American universities, seeking to make them equal to those in Europe. The universities encouraged research and the development of scientific knowledge. By 1893, John Hopkins University required all incoming medical students to have a college degree. Medical schools, built hospitals as a place where medical students would learn how to care for patients, and the two were run as a cooperative entity.[52]

Now the obstacles that molded and shaped early 20th-century nursing can be recognized. These same challenges would follow nurses throughout this era. Every journey is made up of one step at a time, and in the nurses' quest to progress from a domestic person to a professional, at times, they were only "marking time." In the interim, Annie McKay climbed aboard the wheel of fortune to make her mark on school nursing.

---

51 Donna, M.E., Hawkins, J., Van Ryzin, U., Frienman, A., & Higgins, L. (1995). Nursing in Massachusetts during the roaring twenties. *Historical Journal of Massachusetts* 23(2), 135. Retrieved from http://www.westfield.ma.edu/mhj/pdfs/Doona%20combined.pdf. Page 135.

52 Starr, P. (1982) *The social transformation of American medicine*. New York, NY: Basic Books. Pages 113-116.

Chapter 4

Annie McKay at Work with the Instructive District Nursing Association

A newspaper in 1907 wrote these comments about some of the people living in Boston's tenements:

"They cooked, ate, and slept in the same room, four to a room. Not a man, woman, or a child in the entire block could boast the exclusive use of a bed, and some considered themselves lucky to be one of five huddled up on a mattress at night instead of stretching out on the floor. Cleanliness is an unknown quantity; no money is available for bread, yet liquor seems abundant.[53]"

The Beginnings of the Instructive District Nursing Association

The Instructive District Nursing Association (IDNA) began in 1884 when Abbie Howes, a member of a prominent Boston philanthropic family and a supporter of the Women's Education Association traveled to England to study their system of district nursing for the poor. Two years later, with the support of doctors from the Boston Dispensary, Howes launched IDNA in Boston, Massachusetts. The name, The Instructive District Nursing Association, contained the words instructive, and district nurse. They wanted to convey that the district nurse or what we now call

---

53   What District Nurses Do. (December 12, 1907) *Boston Evening Transcript*: 10. Retrieve from https://attachments.cityofboston.gov/?f=26431&fid=8638f87e

visiting nurse would be a teaching nurse and demonstrate to the entire family how to care for their own using cleanliness and hygienic principles. It was the first organization in this country to offer home health care for the poor who otherwise could not afford it.

After a few years with their number of home visits increasing, IDNA rented a room at 2 Park Square to develop a more efficient organization. The influence of Florence Nightingale played its part in the development of IDNA through their communication with the Metropolitan Nursing Association of London (MNA), England. It was Florence Nightingale who said, "that a district nurse… must be of a yet higher class and of a yet fuller training than a hospital nurse." She considered community health nursing a higher calling. A newspaper of the era quotes Florence Nightingale as saying, "the district nurse is a health missionary.[54]" In a letter to the fledgling Victorian Order of Nurses (VON) in Canada in 1898, Florence Nightingale stressed that a district nurse did not have the doctor close at hand to refer to as a hospital nurse, nor did she have the use of hospital equipment for assistance. Consequently, this nursing specialty required a nurse with a more independent character, high morals, and special education in district nursing supplementing their hospital training[55]

The Metropolitan Nursing Association of London (MNA) recommended to Howes that only "ladies" care for the sick poor as opposed to people of a lower class because they embodied cleanliness, respect, and served as an example of improvement for the patient. Florence Craven commented that the district nurse must have a love of the poor and a real desire to lessen their misery in an 1889 British article, proofread by Florence Nightingale.[56]

Abbie Howes received these suggestions from Emily Mansel of the MNA. Mansel's comments were carried in "District Nurses and Their Work," Nursing Record, 1888:

---

54   Instructive District Nursing Association (IDNA), Reports, IDNA Collection, Box 10, Folder 3. Box3, Folder 3.

55   Gibbon, J.M. (1947). *The Victorian Order of Nurses for Canada, 50th Anniversary 1897-1947*. Montreal, Canada: Southam Press. Pages 35-36.

56   Howse, C. (2009). The reflection of England's light. In P. D'Antonio (Ed.), *Nursing History Review*, Official Publication of the American Association for the History of Nursing (pp. 47-69). New York, NY: Springer Publishing Company. Page 54.

"Many come to the work with grand and high-flown ideas. For a time, they seem to enter into it, but when they find that the work is of an exceedingly practical character, the novelty wears away, and interest fails. These do not make good district nurses. What we want are good women, with earnestness and steadfastness of purpose. Women who are prepared to throw their whole heart into the work.[57]"

The Boston Dispensary, located on the corner of Ash and Bennet Street, an area where Tufts Medical Center now stands, consisted of a group of physicians dedicated to the care and treatment of the poor. The Dispensary embarked upon a new, more efficient system of providing health care through outpatient or ambulatory clinics. After dividing the city into ten districts, the Boston Dispensary assigned a physician to each region to provide medical and surgical care. Concerning medical and surgical issues, IDNA's nurses followed the physician's orders assigned to the district. Consequently, these orders permitted them to give follow up care to the patients.[58] A visit from the nurse had to be requested through the IDNA office or through the Boston Dispensary.

Regardless, there were several differences between Boston IDNA and their English counterparts. The English system required a six-month training period for a trained nurse, working under the direct supervision of their district superintendents. By contrast, the Boston system had no training period save for a probationary period of two to three months of service. Another prerequisite of both systems required that new recruits must be graduates of a training school for nurses. Preference, however, was given to graduates of a Boston training school who received positive recommendations following personal interviews. Notice the immense difference in preparation for visiting nurses between the Victorian Order of Nurses (VON) in Canada, which was modeled on the British system, and the new IDNA nurses. Remember, as mentioned in Chapter 2, that Annie McKay was a graduate of the VON in Canada.

The nurses worked eight hours a day, Monday through Saturday, with a starting time of 8:30 AM. Their compensation was $40 for the first two-months' probation, followed by $45 per month for the next nine months, and finally $60 per month after that. The organization furnished the nurses with their uniforms, except for

---

57   Ibid. 53-54

58   Bromberg, C. (Ed.) *Revolutionary care then and now A history of Tufts-New England Medical Center founded in 1796.* Page 12.

the collars and aprons which they supplied themselves. Additional compensation included $5 per month for carfares, and $2 per month for the charwoman, who would clean up an apartment when needed and wash the patient's clothes. They received one month's paid vacation as well.[59]

Another issue at IDNA involved layperson managers. Managers generally were affluent, philanthropic persons who would have donated a minimum of $100 to IDNA, thus entitling them to that position. IDNA nurses reported directly to their managers. As a result, they had no direct nursing supervisor. The nurses gave required oral and written reports of their work at the office each week to the managers. They kept these reports on file.

Obvious problems developed in this arrangement, because a nurse should not be supervised by a layperson who lacked knowledge of nursing practice. A layperson could manage the nurse on non-nursing duties, for example, whether she arrived at work on time.

According to her contract, the Superintendent of Nurses in 1900 also reported to the Board of Managers, that consisted mostly of lay people. Though she was responsible for the work of her nurses and could even suspend a nurse, she could only recommend their dismissal to the Board of Managers. Management required the Superintendent to wear a uniform. The new Superintendent who came in June 1901, was Martha H. Stark, a former East Boston visiting nurse, who reportedly, had an unsympathetic personality.[60] She would remain in that post for ten and a half years.

The Arrival of Annie McKay

Into this motley assembly, Annie McKay arrived in October 1901.[61] At this point,

[59] *Twenty-first Annual Report of the Instructive District Nursing Association for the Year Ending January 31, 1907*. p. 14.

[60] Howse, C. (2009). The reflection of England's light. In P. D'Antonio (Ed.), *Nursing History Review, Official Publication of the American Association for the History of Nursing* (pp. 47-69). New York, NY: Springer Publishing Company. Page 67.

[61] *Committee on Supervision of Nurses* 10/27/1897--May 1905. IDNA Collection, Box 8. Instructive District Nursing Association of Boston Collection, Howard Gotlieb Archival Research Center. Boston University (hereafter IDNA Collection) Divers Good Causes, *Boston Transcript*, August 11, 1906. IDNA Collection, Box 3, Folder 3.

Annie McKay was a seasoned visiting nurse, accustomed to being independent, working, and thinking on her own. Consider how she must have felt about lay managers accompanying her and physicians on visits as they sometimes did. Did they have specialized education and life experiences that contributed to the goal of the visit? Did they understand the objectives of what she was doing and why? I rather doubt it. We do know that physicians so disliked the practice of layperson managers tagging along, that it was eventually discontinued.

A commentary from a monthly meeting of IDNA's Committee on Nurses, dated November 1901, stated that Ms. McKay was doing well during her probationary period. The staff records in December 1, 1901, listed Annie McKay as working in the Central area of Boston. They referred to Annie McKay as the "Victorian Order Nurse," since she had worked for Canada's Victorian Order of Nurses, and said she was doing outstanding work. Besides giving nursing care, nurses were encouraged to keep record books, report cases of contagious diseases, and cases of handicapped children.[62] See the image below - a 1902 picture of the Instructive District Nursing Association.

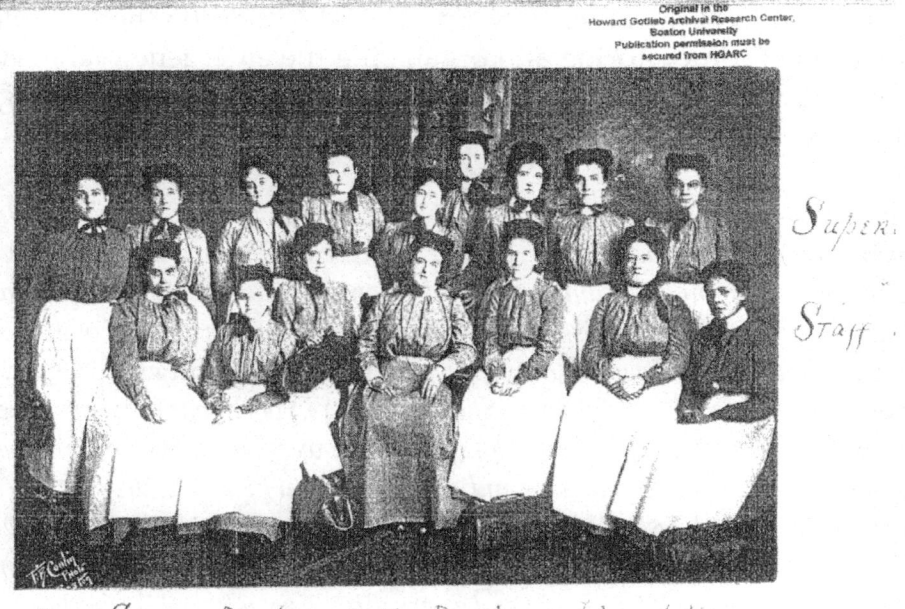

62 Ibid.

At the same time, however, mention was made that the theoretical nurses' training was more significant in the United States than in Canada. What did they mean by that? Not enough academics or practical experience? Nonetheless, the doctors said about McKay, "there was none better," and that patients were devoted to her.[63] Despite these remarks, as we shall see, IDNA would reach out to another Canadian nurse to run a new program.

Over the next few years, the Superintendent's report chronicles a very busy Annie McKay, seeing a variety of patients, including children and adults with tuberculosis, pneumonia, gastro-intestinal problems, and postpartum visits. She visited the many children who were predisposed to tuberculosis at the Hawthorne Club, an after-school Settlement House program. "She spends a great deal of time with each of her patients, resulting in the necessity of putting in long hours to cover her work assignment. In the same way, the doctors meet her on time to go out on their initial visits together."

New technology swept into the rooming house where Annie McKay resided, namely, a telephone, at her 31 Dartmouth Street address. Annie probably enjoyed the companionship of the other IDNA nurses who boarded there. Apparently, she was responsible for monitoring and organizing the emergency calls after 5:30 PM. One of Superintendent Stark's reports described a case that a visiting nurse was sent out to cover, perhaps Annie McKay.[64]

January 17, 1905. Miss Marion Bate, 114 Huntington Ave. Phthisis (pulmonary tuberculosis), acute attack of grip. I called this case at 7:30 in the evening and found the young woman in a dreadfully dirty condition. She had been ill three days and was vomiting a dark green vomitas. She was under opiates, and on account of the vomiting, no nourishment could be given her. She is said to be a singer at Park St Church and is reported as having a beautiful voice. She was living in one room in an apartment kept by Mrs. Johnson. This was no place for her as there were other roomers, and the young woman must have the best nursing and care. So, for that night and the next day specials were put in. Then I beseeched of the doctor to send her to the hospital, so after many vainless attempts, we got her in the City Hospital last night Wednesday, January 18 at 11:20 at night. She is 27 years old and a very attractive nature. Her mother was with

---

63 *Superintendent's Monthly Reports to Miss Cordner, 1901.* November 16, 1901. IDNA Collection, Box 9.

64 *Superintendent's Report from March 16, 1905.* IDNA Collection, Box 10, Folder 3.

her for a little while, but she was one of the very helpless women who are very much in the way. The report from the City Hospital tonight is that the young woman is most uncomfortable and very ill. As the doctor's diagnosis was phthisis, I notified the Board of Health this AM, and they fumigated the room in the lodging house so that nobody else could be infected. I think there is a question in the diagnosis as to what she really had now although tubercular.

At that time, tuberculosis was also called consumption, because it seemed to consume people from within, with a bloody cough, fever, pallor, and a long relentless wasting away. Other names for it included phthisis, the Greek name for consumption meaning decay, waste away. Originally thought to be an inherited disease, Germany's Koch found that it was caused by a bacterium and was infectious. This discovery won him the Nobel Prize in Medicine in 1905. Still, no one had found a cure for tuberculosis. Boston reported the death rate was 21.75 per ten thousand people, though a steady decrease from earlier years.[65] As noted, tuberculosis was widespread among those living in overcrowded housing conditions.

Additionally, physicians prescribed opiates indiscriminately to treat a variety of disorders, but mostly to relieve pain and induce sleep. The corner drug store sold marijuana, heroin, and morphine over the counter. It was not until the Harrison Narcotics Tax Act of 1914 that the Federal Government regulated the distribution of these drugs, by requiring a prescription from a licensed medical doctor. In addition, it required the medication label to disclose the exact contents in the bottle of "alcohol, opium, cocaine, morphine, chloroform, marijuana, acetanilide, chloral hydrate or eucaine.[66]" Today, though many people disagree, several states are now allowing marijuana to be used legally for medicinal and recreational purposes. Our state laws regarding drugs often reflect the changing social standards of behavior.

Nursing Workforce Issues

During Annie McKay's time, the nurse washed the patient, provided them with clean clothes, monitored vital signs, such as temperature, breathing, and heart rate, and

---

65 *Boston Health Department Reports 1909.* City Document No. 18. p. 44.

66 Keeling, A.W. (2007). *Nursing and the Privilege of Prescription. 1893-2000,* 9-13. Columbus, Ohio: The Ohio State University Press. Retrieved from https://Ohiostatepress.org/Books/Book%20PDFs/Keeling%20Nursing.pdf.

kept watch on their diet and other body functions. Additionally, she probably applied cold compresses, or hot medicated cloths called poultices, when needed, demonstrated to the family how to boil dishes contaminated with tuberculosis germs, communicated with the doctor, and without a doubt, tidied up the room, bringing renewed order to the house. As a result of these interventions, the patient regained more of their health and self-respect and would feel better about themselves.[67]

Miss Stark noted that despite Annie having a cold, she nevertheless, was able to work. However, Stark expressed concerns about several of the staff. One nurse, she thought, was not entirely self-reliant enough to use good judgment when needed. Superintendent Stark considered using her as a substitute a few times and then placing her elsewhere. Other nurses, she believed, were not strong enough for this kind of work, despite supporting statements from their doctors that they were. Yet another nurse, she said, was overweight, having a difficult time managing the stairs, getting out of breath. Was this the reason that the doctor would not make home visits with her? One more nurse appeared not robust enough for patient home visits. Similarly, a further nurse looked tired from worrying about a sick relative. Still, there was a nurse who thought district nursing was not that appealing to her, but, regardless, she wanted to continue. What appealed to her were the "interesting deliveries" at home with the mother. See the image below - IDNA nurses boarding the Floating Hospital for Children (Prinz).

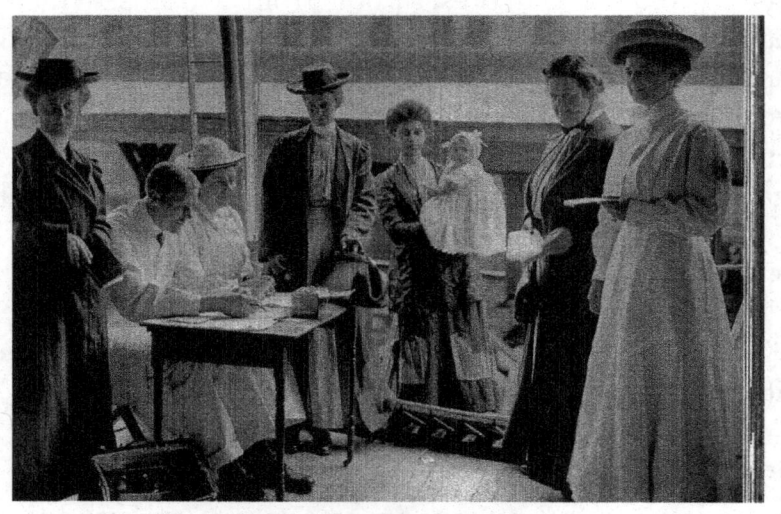

The Floating Hospital for Children

[67] *Meeting Address, November 11. 1911* IDNA Collection, Box 2, Folder 6.

So, it continued on with doctors not meeting regularly with the nurses or not meeting every day or wanting to make visits in the afternoon at 4 PM, as opposed to the morning, which did not give the nurse time to provide nursing care. Simultaneously, nurses found waiting 15 minutes for a doctor very time consuming.[68] These entries indicate that there were problems amiss in the management of IDNA.

Regardless, IDNA continued to grow and needed to have larger quarters. They purchased a house in 1906 at 561 Massachusetts Avenue, in the area known as Chester Square, already run down, having lost its luster, between Tremont Street and Shawmut Avenue. An article in the *Boston Evening Transcript* described their new headquarters; "in front (of the house) is what was magnificent Chester Square with its park, fountain and a score of towering elm trees.[69]" It was located about seven short blocks west from McKay's apartment on 1521 Washington Street. The large, brick townhouse, still stands today, but has subsequently been divided into condominiums and sadly, the elm trees have all died from disease. See the image below - IDNA.

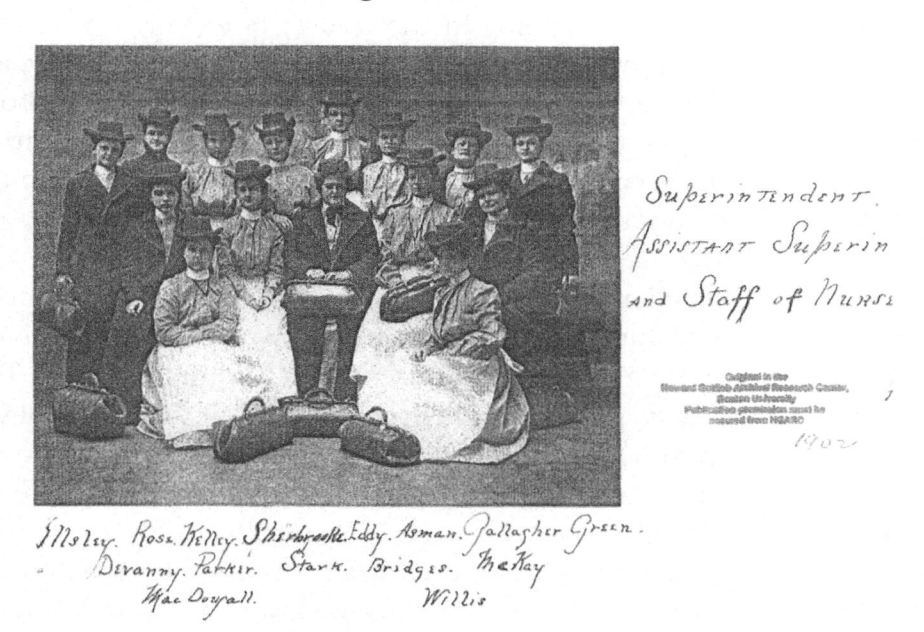

From here, IDNA launched the first school for the study of district nursing. They employed Charlotte Maclead, a Canadian nurse who had studied with Florence

---

68 *Superintendent's Report from 8/22/1905-9/22/1905*. IDNA Collection, Box 10, Folder 3.

69 Hurd, C. *Boston Evening Transcript* September 22, 1906. The Nurses House.

Nightingale to run the school. Interestingly, she was the first superintendent of the VON in Canada, so Annie McKay would have known her when she was in their training program and as a district nurse.[70]

Having acquired the Massachusetts Avenue facility, everything for IDNA was now located under one roof. A physician or the general public could telephone any time of the day or night, 24 hours a day, weekends and holidays, and receive immediate service. Their programs of free nursing care, or whatever the patient's family could afford, and instruction on hygiene had proved to be very useful to the community in improving the sanitary conditions of the city. Their new home consisted of four floors of large rooms and a basement. The first floor, known as the parlor, contained the director's room, the sitting room, and the dining room. The second floor included the offices and the superintendents' room. The third and fourth floors remained as bedrooms and storage areas.

One of the most exciting rooms in the house, however, was the fumigation room, located in the front of the basement, while the kitchen, laundry, and furnace rooms comprised the back of the basement. This room, measuring about 10 by 20 feet contained shelves, chairs, table, and a large formaldehyde lamp. If a nurse suspected that she might have been exposed to infection, she had to fumigate herself here before she could roam throughout the rest of the house.

Fumigation consisted of disinfecting themselves and their clothes, changing into fresh garments, and washing their hair with soap, water, and corrosive sublimate as an antiseptic. Each of the ten district houses had a fumigation room. *The American Journal of Clinical Medicine* gave some instructions on fumigation. They suggested boiling garments exposed to infection for one hour. The nurse followed this by taking a bichloride bath. Knowing how to use a formaldehyde lamp required skill and comprehension. After it was lit, you had to work quickly to escape the room because the vapors irritated the eyes. It required leaving the room closed for six to eight hours, with all vents closed, sealing the windows and doors, then opening the doors and windows to air the place for 12 hours before occupying it.[71]

---

70   Penney, S. (1996). *A Century of Caring - The History of the Victorian Order of Nurses for Canada*. Ontario, Canada. VON. Page 27.

71   *The American Journal of Clinical Medicine. Vol.23* (1916). p.542. Retrieved from http://books.google.com/books?id=RdgAAAAAYAAJ Page 542.

They used a formaldehyde solution as a disinfectant since it was lethal to most bacteria and fungi, including their spores. Formaldehyde is carcinogenic, so it is used now in different forms. Can you imagine all of the nurses running around boiling their clothes and taking a bath with corrosive sublimate? It must have achieved wonders for their hair and skin. This same article referred to earlier in the *Boston Evening Transcript* goes on to say that sunshine was the best disinfecting agent. Thank goodness, we have improved disinfecting agents today. A bit of comic poetry[72] made the rounds and was printed in the *Maritime Medical News* in 1897:

> We have boiled the hydrant water
> We have sterilized the milk
> We have strained the prowling microbe
> Through the finest kind of silk
> We have bought and we have borrowed
> Every patent health device,
> And at last the doctor tells us
> That we've got to boil the ice.

INSTRUCTIVE DISTRICT NURSING ASSOCIATION

BOSTON

This Association furnishes trained nurses for daily visiting of the sick poor in their homes.

Services given free when patient unable to pay. Small charge made when patient can pay.

No physician need be without a nurse. These nurses respond to the call of any physician who makes application for them. Night nurses furnished for emergencies.

Any one desiring a nurse may apply at the **House of the Association, 561 Massachusetts Avenue.** Telephone 539 Tremont.

IDNA Notice - Image courtesy of Boston University Howard Gotlieb Archival Research Center.[73]

---

72 Penney, S. (1996). *A Century of Caring - The History of the Victorian Order of Nurses for Canada.* Ontario, Canada. VON. Page 32.

73 *Superintendent's Report from March 16, 1905.* IDNA Collection, Box 10, Folder 3.

The visiting nurses made at least 68,761 recorded home visits to needy families in Boston in 1905.[74] This is another story of one of those visits.

> *April 13, 1905, Teacher from the Washington School, Miss Murphy, Norman St, West End, Mary Marcissni 49 Hale Street. This child's mother is ill with cancer, and the child is being kept at home to take care of the mother, and the teacher applied to us to know-if we would look into the matter. The Massachusetts law that a child cannot be kept at home under 14 years of age to work in the family was being ignored so we sent the District doctor and nurse there and then reported it to the Associated Charities and the Provident Association and they allowed so much to be given to the family to put someone in to do the work, or the child would be taken from them. The father is a fruit vendor, and the brother works in a cracker factory, and when they both work, they earn about $15, but just now they are not working on steady time.*[75]

Think how difficult it must have been for the family, a mother fighting a devastating disease, and a father desperately looking for work. In their distress, they left their young daughter in charge of the household instead of sending her to school. They needed IDNA's intervention that offered them guidance and social services.

The stage is set, and all the characters are in place. The curtain rises on the next act when Annie McKay takes the leading role as Boston's pioneering first school nurse.

---

74 *Twentieth Annual Report of the Instructive District Nursing Association for the Year Ending January 31, 1906.* p. 16.

75 *IDNA Collection, Box10, Folder 3. Superintendent's Report from March 16, 1905.*

Chapter 5

Annie McKay Becomes Boston's First School Nurse

The Nation

The year 1905 turned into another significant year in the history of the United States. Flamboyant Theodore Roosevelt occupied the White House and won the Nobel Peace Prize for his involvement in the mediation of the Russo-Japanese War. The Treaty of Portsmouth was signed in Kittery, Maine, ending this war and promoting the ideals of peace. A new progressive spirit was attacking immigration, technology, social equity, and the economic status quo. Keen inventors like Alexander Graham Bell, Henry Ford, and Thomas Edison almost completely altered our nation by forever rearranging the way society operated. The telephone, automobile, electric light, and the moving picture made the old way of life impossible. Technologic winds of change swept the nation. Social change was inevitable.

Here are some United States statistics from 1905: the average life expectancy was 47 years; only 14 percent of homes had a bathtub; only 8 percent of homes had a telephone; 2 out of 10 adults couldn't read or write; there were only 8,000 cars in the U.S., and barely 144 miles (232 km) of paved roads; and sugar cost 4 cents a pound.[76] Hardly believable!

---

76 *Chautauqua History Comes Alive*, New Hampshire Humanities Council 1905.

Boston Launches School Nursing

Boston was a fertile field for reform work. As an outgrowth of this new movement, the Boston School Committee developed its pilot program for school nursing. This was accomplished by a collaborative agreement with the Instructive District Nursing Association (IDNA), precursor to the current Visiting Nurse Association. For this new assignment as first school nurse, IDNA chose their most experienced nurse, Annie McKay.[77]

Boston selected the South End, one of its poorest districts, as the first site of the pilot program. The overcrowded tenements filled with unsanitary conditions blighted this area, which contributed to the poor health, poor nutrition, and socio-economic problems that affected the families living there. If Annie McKay didn't improve the 13 percent absenteeism rate in her district, the program would be eliminated. The Boston School Committee, aware of the financial commitment of school nursing, wanted to see some positive outcomes before taking any further steps. As has been pointed out earlier, they were not paying for this pilot program, since it was being paid for by private organizations. What benefits would Annie McKay bring to the school children and their families? The next few months would be revealing.

Boston's pioneering experience of placing nurses in schools got under way on a cold 24° F (4.44 C), clear to partly cloudy day, not quite the beginning of winter.[78] On the morning of Wednesday, December 6, 1905, Annie McKay set out from her Washington Street apartment to go to the Quincy School, to meet Superintendent Stark. Together, they would make their introductions to the principal and staff and discuss plans for what McKay would do, their shared goals of increased school attendance and healthier students.

McKay's mind must have been reeling with plans. In her anticipation, she might have dashed off a letter to her family the night before, telling them again of her daunting new position, and that she hoped to live up to the great faith that IDNA

---

[77] *Twentieth Annual Report of the Instructive District Nursing Association for the Year Ending January 31, 1906.* pgs.7,15,16.

[78] Weather. (1905, December 6) *The Boston Daily Globe* (1872-1922), p. 1. Retrieved January 26, 2015 from ProQuest Historical Newspapers Boston Globe (1872-1924) database.

had placed in her. Perhaps she took a quick stroll in Blackstone Square Park, across the street from her apartment house, reviewing again the next day's activities and her expectations. Whether she had any second thoughts or any seeds of doubt about launching this new program and her role in making history we will never know. No records have survived of any journals that she kept, if she had one at all. We do know that she was passionate about her work as will be seen as her story unfolds. Did she make any promises? I speculate that she privately thought, "I think I can turn this around." Will we ever be able to ask her?

Superintendent Stark's notes open on December 6, 1905 with Miss Stark accompanying Miss McKay on her first day at the Quincy School. They spoke with Headmaster Alfred Bunker, and in Stark's own words, "introducing a wedge" as a great deal of tact had to be used. It seems that she didn't want to progress too fast as Mr. Bunker might get confused as, "he is rather old." Everything is relative. They agreed on the terms for how McKay would see children who were identified as being ill or at risk of developing illness. At this school, they would be sent to McKay, whereas at the Way Street School, which had only three rooms, she would go into the classroom and inspect the children. McKay would then take the children to the area assigned to the nurse for further inspection, evaluation, and treatment as necessary. For children with defective hearing, or vision problems, she would make a home visit. The role is developing for a "school nurse."

Annie McKay's Schools

Annie McKay's schools were located in the South End area of Boston. The original Quincy School opened in 1847 and is still standing today on 90 Tyler Street. The location is in an area now known more commonly as Chinatown. A plaque on the building discloses its history as a school. It was named after Josiah Quincy, the second Mayor of Boston. The renowned educator Horace Mann conceived the design of the curriculum and structure of the building. Since the area schools were crowded, the new school was formulated for boys.

At the time, it was the first school in the country, and thought to be very progressive as well, giving each teacher their own classroom, where students were separated by grade, and each had their own desk. The building contained 14 rooms and a hall, adding up to 12,413 square feet. The old public school closed in 1976 and the building became the home of the Chinese Consolidated Benevolent Cultural Center. At the present time, it is a thriving community center, home to many local

Chinese organizations. A new replacement school opened in 1976, displaying bright yellow and red children's characters at its roofline, is located on nearby Washington Street in Chinatown, one block from Tufts Medical Center.

The Andrews School was located on Genesee Street between Harrison Avenue and Albany Street, and the Way Street School was situated on Way Street, three blocks away, also between Harrison Avenue and Albany Street. Built in 1896, the Andrews School contained nine rooms, covering a site of 19,761 square feet. It was named after William T. Andrews, a member of the Primary School Committee. In comparison, the Way Street School, erected in 1850 contained only three rooms, covering a site of 2,508 square feet. It was closed around 1928.[79]

As mentioned in Chapter 1, locals described the Way Street School as, "a small unsightly school on the edge of the railroad tracks.[80]" This area of the South End was known as the "New York Streets," named after cities in New York State. The three schools that Annie McKay visited were in a seven-block radius of each other. Though streetcars were available, she probably walked briskly between her schools, as she was accustomed to walking the fields in Beaverton. When urban renewal became fashionable in 1957, Boston closed the Andrews School and demolished buildings in the entire area. [81]

Gloria Ganno, a lifetime Bostonian, then a resident of the "New York Streets" still remembers attending the Andrews School, a grade one through grade three school. She recalls how disruptive it was for her family to be dislocated and her neighborhood destroyed when the New York Streets were demolished. A sprawling building housing the *Boston Herald* newspaper complex filled the area of the cleared land. But as change is inevitable, the newspaper within the last few years has been printed elsewhere at a lower cost, therefore making that building irrelevant. Recently demolished, that building has become a new apartment complex calling itself "Inkblock" with 24-hour concierge, a high-end grocery store, and restaurants.

[79] *Documents of the School Committee of the City of Boston – 1901*. (1901). Boston, MA: Boston Municipal Printing Office. Page 28.

[80] Robinson, L.V. (1937). *Children's House – A History of the Hawthorne Club*. Boston, MA: Marshall Jones Co. Page 80.

[81] Seasholes, N.S. (2003). *Gaining Ground - A History of Landmaking in Boston*. Massachusetts: MIT Press. Page 252.

Constructed on its footprint, the area is going through yet another transformation. Has the South End gone full circle? Will all the working-class families return to the area? What does the reader think?

The Quincy School

Up until a few years ago, the Quincy school remained as it had been for over a hundred years. A large, weathered, straight back wooden bench still sat outside the main office, a veritable antique at this point, where probably disobedient schoolboys and their parents waited for a talk with the principal. At one side of the school, there was a boy's staircase and when the school became coed, a girl's staircase on the other side. We can still imagine hearing the patter of little feet running up the stairs, and the sounds of excited children, jostling and giggling, laden with boot bags and book bags, so thrilled to be in school.

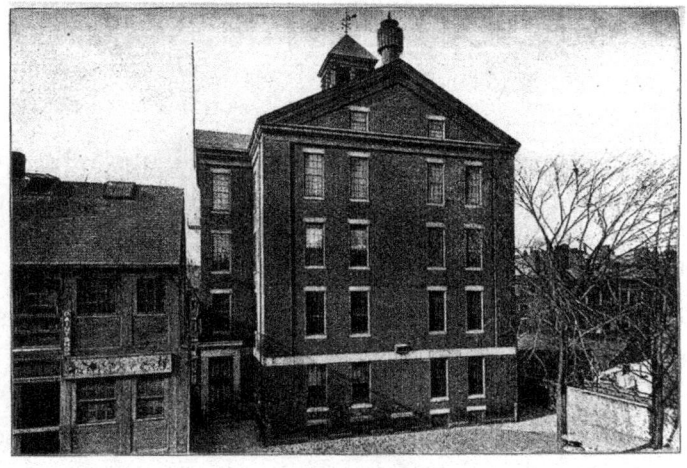

QUINCY SCHOOL.

Quincy School
Photo courtesy of Boston Public Library Photo Collection

Massachusetts law required children of this era to attend school between eight and fourteen years of age, but this was difficult to enforce. Student attendance at the Quincy School for June 30th, 1905 was at 87 percent. The enrollment included

607 students.[82] The ethnic makeup of the Quincy School was Jews, 19 percent, Irish, 31 percent, other foreigners, 18 percent; and Native Americans, 32 percent (presumably white and African Americans, but not American Indians).

Smallpox vaccination was a requirement and strictly enforced. In 1855 Massachusetts passed *The Act to Secure General Vaccination* (Chapter 414, Section 2) that read, "The school committee of the several towns and cities, shall not allow any child to be admitted to, or connected with the public school, who has not been duly vaccinated." The General Court followed with another law in 1894 stating that students that were not "duly vaccinated" would be excluded (Acts, 1894. Chapter 498, Section 9). "Duly vaccinated" was not defined until a later date.

The schools played an important role in the assimilation of this generation into America. Teachers at the time felt that there should be a closer relationship between school and home, but that was hardly possible for the individual teacher because each had 50 students. By contrast, the enrollment at the new Quincy School was 808 students, with attendance at 98 percent.

Work of the School Nurse

The school nurses worked closely with the school physicians who were appointed by the Department of Health. The school physician, called medical inspector, worked in an area in the school assigned to them where they could see referred children. A physician visited the school generally every day and advised but did not prescribe medicine. In cases of suspicious contagious and infectious disease, the school physician recommended the exclusion of children from school and outlined the conditions for readmission to school. It became the responsibility of the school nurse to see that the student and their families carried out the school physician's recommendations.

Parents were consulted before the child received any treatments. If a child had their own doctor, that physician was consulted for whatever was needed. Communication became easier as phones became more available and were used in hospitals. If the child did not have their own physician, they were taken to the various local hospitals or dispensaries for treatment of their condition. Frequently,

---

82   *School Document No. 8. Primary Schools -Concluded.* Semi-annual Returns June 30, 1905, p. 18.

these conditions amounted to faulty vision and hearing, or having their tonsils and adenoids removed, or a general referral. The school nurse also dealt with nose, throat, pulmonary, skin cases, pediculosis, plus medical and surgical issues. If, at all possible, these visits to the clinics were done on Saturdays.[83]

Instructions and Treatments Used by the School Nurse

Regardless of the circumstances, nurses made home visits to impress upon the parents the importance of medical care. Frequently, the nurse just taught the family simple techniques of self-help, hygiene, and how to protect themselves and others from disease.

During this time period, the few medicines that doctors used to treat illnesses were available to the public in drugs stores. As it happened, there was very little difference between home remedies and what a physician prescribed, since basically both only offered symptomatic relief. Skilled nursing care frequently used the same medicines such as cough medicines, analgesics for pain, and antipyretics for fever. That also included standard medical treatment. In comparison, a pharmacist in a drug store could compound and distribute a drug, but not advise customers on how to use them.[84]

Health providers considered these treatments standard for that time. Doctor's would have prescribed them, and Annie McKay would have used them in school and demonstrated to families how to use them. When a child was excluded from school because of parasites, nits, ticks, or pediculosis, now what we would call head lice, they would receive a note from the headmaster saying at the medical inspectors request, that he or she remain at home until the disease is cured. See the image below - Treatment for Head Lice – Rx for Petroleum.

---

83   *Daily Notes from Superintendent Stark*, Instructive District Nursing Association: November 20, 1905 -January 1, 1908. Instructive District Nursing Association (IDNA).

84   Keeling, A.W. (2007). *Nursing and the Privilege of Prescription. 1893-2000,* 9-13. Columbus, Ohio: The Ohio State University Press. Retrieved from https://Ohiostatepress.org/Books/Book%20 PDFs/Keeling%20Nursing.pdf

Rx for Petroleum to Treat Head Lice

Boston's Board of Health had a standard method of treating head lice, using crude petroleum that could be obtained easily at the drug store. Various kinds of crude petroleum have been used down through the ages for the control of ticks. Step one: wet the hair with crude petroleum; keep it on for three hours. Step two: wash the whole head with warm water and soap, repeat the process for three successive days. Step three: comb through the hair with a fine-tooth comb soaked in vinegar to remove the nits. The family repeated this procedure until there were no more nits. Some reported that using hot vinegar was more effective at removing the nits. If it would make it easier, school nurses advised the family to cut the student's hair short and treat the other children in the family as well, as they were most likely affected. When they completed these steps, they could return to school. That was clearly a lot of work.

The New York City Department of Health had instructions on how to treat common ailments for their school nurses also. Here were some examples:

Favus – Ringworm of Scalp: Mild cases were to be scrubbed with tincture of green soap, epilate the area, meaning remove the hair, then cover the area with flexible collodion, a syrupy liquid that dries to a transparent film. It was used as a topical protectant, applied to the skin to close small wounds. For more severe cases, they were to brush the area with tincture of iodine before adding the flexible collodion.[85]

Impetigo - Bacterial skin infection, lesion evolves into a honey-colored crust. Remove crusts with tincture of green soap; apply white precipitate ointment. (Because of its mercury content, this ointment is no longer produced).

Conjunctivitis –Irrigate eyes with a solution of boric acid. This treatment was done in school and several times at home.[86]

Annie McKay's Address at Annual Meeting, 1906

The Annual Report *of the Instructive District Nursing Association* in 1905 documented the nurses' work in the public schools as one of their achievements. The nurses collected data on the work they did, the same as they do today, but of course, now they use computers. Their salary was $40 per month for the first month probation, $45 for the next two months, $50 for the next 9 months, and $60 per month thereafter. IDNA supplied them with uniforms and $5 per month for car fares. These wages were somewhat comparable to what was offered to hospital nurses as discussed in Chapter 3. As was the fashion of the times, their uniform included a long, dark colored coat and brimmed hat, making them recognizable on the street as a visiting nurse. A white apron covered their long dress of blue and white pin striped, cotton muslin with puffed elbow sleeves.

IDNA's Annual Meeting, on February 28th, 1906, was open to the public, and according to an article in *The Boston Transcript*, many people came to hear of all the good work going on in the community. The nurses served tea after the meeting.[87]

---

85   Farlex. *The Free Dictionary*. Retrieved from http://medical.com/flexible+collodion

86   Rogers, L.L. A Year's Work for the Children in New York Schools. *The American Journal of Nursing*. Vol. 4, No. 3 (Dec. 1903), pp. 181-184. Retrieved from http://www.jstor.org/stable/3401724

87   Great Power for Good. (1906, February 28). *Boston Transcript*, Instructive District Nursing Association of Boston Collection, Howard Gotlieb Archival Research Center, Boston University, IDNA Collection, Box 4.

Annie McKay was their featured speaker. McKay's observations and comments give us an intimate view of tenement life in America at that time. She remarked, "these two and a half months of the work have convinced me that the public schools do more to elevate the moral tone and improve the manner of living in the poor districts than all other agencies combined." She commented further, "they need someone who can visit the homes to try to induce the parents to help them in their plans for the children's welfare. That there is a field for a school nurse in the poorer districts is, I think, beyond a doubt."

McKay held the opinion that the inroads made by the school nurse through home visits improved the family's standard of living and contributed to a better educated community to join the new industrialized America. While she acknowledged the good work of several agencies in the schools and with families, she believed the school nurse working with the schoolteacher had a unique opportunity since the school nurse saw the child directly and developed a friendly relationship with the child.

In her talk, McKay focused on children's health and considered that their needs in the poorer wards of Boston were sometimes neglected. Whether this was due to parental "ignorance and superstition" or just postponing their duties, the result affected the children's welfare. Whatever their origins, she said, people in the poorer communities held a variety of superstitions, such as taking frequent baths led to tuberculosis. They had a fear of fresh air and had a general lack of knowledge about what food to feed their children.

McKay must have captivated her audience by sharing stories of the children she worked with. She disclosed the story of a boy examined by the school doctor because of a discharge from his ear. Immediately, the doctor referred the student for further treatment and asked McKay to advise the parents of this need. McKay spoke with the parent's through an interpreter. The mother relayed that three years ago when she was immigrating to this country from Russia, she was not allowed to go aboard the ship at Liverpool because the child had an enlarged head, or "water on the brain" called hydrocephalous. Fearing the end of her immigration, she took him to a doctor in London, where they performed a procedure on his ear to drain the water out of his brain. Since that time, his ear has had a discharge, and she was afraid if the discharge stopped, her son would develop the "big head" again. After much pleading with her, the mother promised McKay that she would seek treatment. The story ends well, with a neighbor's daughter given the responsibility of taking the boy to the dispensary every day for six weeks to find that the ear had finally healed.

She also relayed another situation referred to her. This boy had bald spots on his scalp with no growth of hair. It was probably tinea capitis, commonly known as ringworm, a condition where there is a loss of hair on the scalp. Despite receiving advice from several doctors over a two-year period, the parents never followed the treatment for more than a few days. It took McKay's intervention to return the child to the Boston Dispensary to restart treatment again and subsequently allow him to return to school. She hoped that the combined efforts of herself and the child's teacher would keep the mother and student returning to the Boston Dispensary until the student was cured. He lost two years of valuable education that would be unthinkable today.

McKay continued with another case where the school sent the boy home in October because he had the "itch" known as scabies, a contagious skin infection resulting from infestation with the itch mite. The mother had dutifully taken him for treatment, but when home, did not thoroughly understand how to give the treatment, resulting in no cure. When McKay checked on him, she thoroughly reviewed again how to administer the advised treatment, and the boy returned to school the next week. Another case of scabies was referenced in Chapter 1.

The single issue that absorbed most of her time was children with poor eyesight. She recounted that she visited the homes of all of the children and relayed to their parents that they could not see the board in school, or had difficulty reading, asking the parents to take their children for an eye examination over the Christmas vacation. The parents promised that they would, but sadly only one of the sixty-six parents followed through and brought their child for the examination. Since they were all willing for their children to have the exam, she took all of them to the Dispensary, going in groups of five or six.

Once again, she visited the homes of the children that required glasses, and most of the parents agreed to purchase the glasses. In contrast, the parents were not as agreeable when they discovered that the fitting of glasses required drops to be put in the eyes that caused a momentary blurring of vision. She reported there existed a strong prejudice about putting any medicine in the eyes that led to even a momentary change in vision. As a result, some of the parents remained undecided about their children's glasses.

McKay's account continued with the number of "throat cases" and those children that required an operation to remove infected tonsils and adenoids. Though by this time, seven operations have already been performed, superstition stepped in again to delay parents in making their decisions. Parents in her district had the irrational belief that operations should not be performed in the cold weather, so she said, "we must wait for warm weather before doing much about it."

Two of the main objections to the introduction of school nursing, McKay believed, were the school nurse would irritate the parents and would be acting as a physician. On the contrary, she related, she never experienced any resentment from the parents on her visits. Frequently, McKay received messages from parents asking her to make a home visit to further explain how to execute a treatment, or in the case of pediculosis, head lice, how to treat the whole family, or observe while the nurse treated the student. She asserted that in no way had the nurse assumed the responsibilities of a physician. "The school doctor is always ready either to visit or give advice," she said.

The doctors at the Boston Dispensary, which was close to her schools, readily saw a student from the school as soon as they arrived. She referred kindly to the assistance of the physicians and staff at the Boston Dispensary, who were always eager and willing to treat the school children free of charge. "Whatever work has been done for the school children has been possible only through their assistance." Note how she graciously thanked the physicians for their work.

Annie McKay's Workday

Imagine being shadowed for a day by a journalist from dawn till dusk! Well, Clara Stanwood, a journalist, followed Annie McKay for an article published on April 4, 1906, in *The Boston Transcript*. In a way, Annie McKay must have been flattered. I wonder if she anticipated this would be an outcome of her new assignment. By the time they published the commentary, Annie had been working for four months in the new nursing specialty, school nursing, though the journalist refers to her being on the job for only three months. Therefore, they published the piece a month after the collaboration at the schools occurred.

The account began with nurse Annie McKay working in the teacher's lounge called the "teachers retiring room" with a seven or eight-year old boy named Tommy, who had a bruised finger at the old Way Street School. The journalist,

Clara Stanwood, couldn't help but notice the easy rapport, with smiles exchanged, between the student and the nurse as she dressed the boy's finger and inquired about how he acquired the injury. Along the way she managed to advise him about his behavior in defense of himself.

After examining some other children, McKay and Stanwood left the Way Street School, and went off to the Andrews, one of her other schools. The location of her office here, in the basement, didn't upset the nurse, because McKay said, "We shall have something better by-and-by." Annie though, easily set up her work area with the use of a wooden box that one of the teachers helped her acquire. She arranged her necessary equipment obtained from her nursing bag. The "nursing bag" that she carried contained a removable linen lining, record cards, instruments, disinfectants, bandages, alcohol lamp, absorbent cotton, pins, Vaseline, stimulants, a small amount of crude petroleum for insect bites, note slips, pencil, Board of Health postcards, carriage orders, and car tickets.[88]

Then Annie McKay proceeded to tend to the children waiting for her, removing sticky bandages with the utmost care, and focusing on soaking one finger, so as to prevent the loss of the fingernail, and cause as little pain as possible. Meanwhile, a little ruckus was occurring among those waiting, one boy kicking another in the ear. The nurse responded with, "Here, Dominic you be filling this dish." The boy dutifully filled the basin with the required water and returned to the nurse. The journalist noted that the nurse had previously been a schoolteacher. The nurse treated all the children sent to her at this location and moved on to her next stop.

Annie McKay's office, if it was that, in the large Quincy School on Tyler Street was on the top floor next to the principal's office. Clara Stanwood described its location at the end of the corridor in a sunny area where Annie had easy access to the roof. I can imagine seeing her taking the thin, drawn, malnourished children out to the roof to inhale some deep breaths of clean, fresh air they so desperately needed. But on that day, with her newspaperwoman companion, she ministered to the children waiting for her.

---

88 Great Power for Good. (1906, February 28). *Boston Transcript*, Instructive District Nursing Association of Boston Collection, Howard Gotlieb Archival Research Center, Boston University, IDNA Collection, Box 4.

At this school, water was available from the principal's office, but Annie used the alcohol lamp in her nurse's bag to heat it. Since her area was close to the principal's office in this school, they probably quickly became acquainted. That may have been one of the reasons why, at a later time, the principal, Alfred Bunker, testified on the need and support for school nurses to the legislature.

After tending to children with bruised feet, referring one to the dispensary doctor, another boy arrived breathless after running up the stairs. He requested that the nurse talk to his father about obtaining glasses, since the father was not convinced that he needed them. She agreed to visit the home and speak with his parents.

Another boy with a very sore and throbbing thumb that he caught in the door became the last student of the day. Every day he dutifully came to the nurse to dress his finger, and she did this with great sensitivity and careful judgment. It would not be surprising to hear her singing under her breath a soothing melody, *Flow gently, sweet Afton*, a popular Scottish song by Robert Burns, when she was concentrating on something.

Despite Annie's best maneuvers with this dressing, the boy sobbed out a few times, called out the nurse's name, and then at the end, thanked her very much. Miss Stanwood noted, "Nearly all of them are grateful like that, because they are poor." In other words, the children would not have received this care, or it would have been much delayed, if there was no school nurse.

By now it was two o'clock, and Annie McKay was anxious to leave the Quincy School, as she had made some home visits that morning even before she met the journalist. McKay would be meeting some children at the Boston Dispensary; the majority of whom she would say needed prescription eyeglasses. Working as a school nurse for just three months, she had referred a large number of children for eye exams. Over 70 children had received prescription eyeglasses. This phenomenon had amazed those at the Boston Dispensary, and they had made arrangements to help pay for the cost of the glasses for those who otherwise could not afford them. However, though some parents had paid the wholesale price for the glasses, they had still requested gold frames for their children's glasses instead of the steel ones, and the nurse had to explain to them delicately, they would then have to pay the full price. Another task for this nurse.

However, that was not all that occurred during these visits to the dispensary. Many times, these parents didn't speak fluent English, but could understand some English. Despite this, once they arrived there, they became bewildered and disconcerted. McKay stepped in and helped them unravel their dilemma, whatever it might be. She said, "I sympathize with them. They are not stupid, as they may appear, but merely confused."

The nurse commented on some other issues surrounding dispensary visits. McKay expressed concern that many parents sampled medical advice, received free care, but followed few of their suggestions. She complained that the parents used some medicines, but never enough to affect a cure. "When the child is ordered for dispensary examination, they will take him not alone to the dispensary, but to two or three in different parts of the city. This thing ought to be systematized," said the nurse, "so the patronage of the dispensary shall be limited to certain districts. As it is, many people run about and consult several physicians, and perhaps the child is not treated at all." She said this frequently happened when doctors prescribed an operation to remove enlarged tonsils and adenoids, the recommended treatment of this condition at the time.

At this early point, we can say with hindsight that McKay recognized the problems of patient access to medical care, and how to pay for health care. The nation is still grappling with health care overhaul today. As of this time, the U.S. has a medical plan called Obamacare, named after our 44th president, Barack Obama, with which many are dissatisfied. What is the answer? Some have suggested as a possible solution to use the teamwork and medical home-managed concept approach. Rather than just have your doctor, a collaborative team would work together to meet immediate, but very important, long-term medical issues or preventive strategies tailored to each patient's needs. We are still confronted with these challenging issues requiring complex solutions that hopefully will become more apparent to us in the near future.

Subsequently, after completing her work at the Boston Dispensary, McKay continued her day by following up on some issues that would be best addressed by a home visit. She stressed the importance of reporting on children who had been dismissed from school to see that they were administering the treatment properly. The nurse would advise the mother how to do the necessary treatment and check the medicine if one was prescribed. More often than not, the prescription bottle had been put away and forgotten about. At times, it required giving long explanations to the mother to encourage her to follow the nurse's instructions. These interventions undoubtedly produced a faster cure, returning the child to school earlier than under the program without a school nurse, which pleased both the families and the headmasters.

One of these visits was to a Syrian family of nine children infected with the "itch," presently called scabies. This case is explained in detail in Chapter 1 and the children would be returning to school. Next, McKay visited a Russian family with a baby with sore eyes. The baby's brother in the kindergarten brought this case to McKay's attention at school. Though the mother could not understand English, her daughter from the elementary school acted as interpreter for the nurse's instructions. She investigated yet another child in this building to see how she liked her new glasses prescribed for her strabismus, more commonly known as cross-eyes. McKay found her managing quite well.

And so, her visits extended into the dinner hour when she called upon a home, with the mother just returning from work. The boys were absent from school for several days, unbeknownst to the mother. They were playing hooky. Aha! The mother responded quickly that she would send them to school the very next day, or she would be sending them away where they would have to go to school. Annie McKay almost certainly looked at the boys, who at this point most likely had been hanging their heads sheepishly, and told them, "They would never have a better friend than their mother. They had better go to school while they lived with her than to go away." Was she speaking from her own experience? I believe so.

Image at right - Two nurses making a home visit down a crowded, debris strewn alley

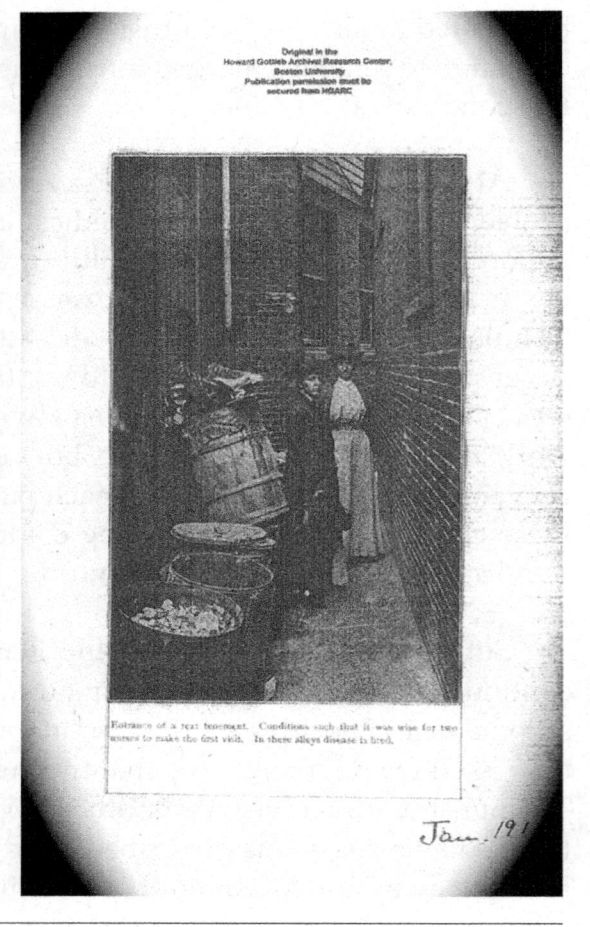

Once again, she was on her way. This time she visited a home where a very pale and thin boy had been absent for several days because of gastrointestinal problems. This perplexed the nurse until the mother happened to say that he drank tea all the time and did not eat any food. I wonder if the mother did likewise. The article does not go into detail about the conversation that must have followed between the mother and the nurse, but I feel for sure that Annie McKay advised her to start feeding the child more nourishing food.

However, after the visit, the nurse exclaimed, "Oh, this matter of food. That is what I have to talk about all the time. It is late hours and improper food more than anything else that makes the children disordered." She went on to talk about children drinking too much coffee, staying up to 11 o'clock, maybe even outside at that hour. She believed she had convinced some children to eat good quality food, not to drink coffee, to go to bed earlier, and to exercise, to be ready to learn in school. There is a certain timelessness of Annie's conversations with children. School nurses across America still converse with students every day about being in school, healthy, safe, and ready to learn.

From there, they ventured off to an obscure tenement to confer with the mother of a girl who desperately wanted to attend a trade school to study the art of being a milliner. Annie McKay would make an appointment with someone that would advocate for the young girl's application.

A final visit to a tailor shop to speak with the father of the boy from the Quincy School, who had asked her to convince his father of the young boy's need for glasses was to no avail since his father had left for dinner. Now she had completed her day, after making six home visits in the evening not counting the ones she made before she arrived at school. This was like a long day's journey into night. The journalist must have been tired also, as I am assuming Annie McKay was, locating the children's homes, trudging up the many flights of stairs in her heavy winter coat, and carrying her nurse's bag. By the time she reached the top floor, she must have been out of breath and perspiring. Regardless of the weather, I can verify as a former public health nurse many years ago, that the stairwells, doubtless, would reek of the unpleasant odors of urine and beer. During these visits, McKay proceeded to nicely cajole the families to follow her directions for the better health of their children and themselves.

At the close of this article, Clara Stanwood, the journalist, asked her readers if this new position was worthwhile. She thought that it definitely was and declared that the question and answer to it, "will soon face the city of Boston.[89]"

After only eight weeks on her job in the Quincy School District, McKay had already seen 215 cases in school, and made 576 home visits. As has been pointed out in the *Boston Transcript* article, though the school day started at 9 AM and finished at 3 PM, McKay made home visits to the families both before and after school, late into winter afternoons already darkening to twilight. Were there concerns about her safety? To compensate for this extensive time involved as a school nurse, IDNA gave McKay Saturday afternoons off!

Soon, IDNA added a local children's philanthropic organization, known as The Hawthorne Club to her assignment to visit, check on the children, and confer with their physician. Records from the Hawthorne Club also refer to a play that was written by a Miss MacKay and later produced by the membership.[90] Nonetheless, the, "experiment" of using McKay proved successful and records of the day show that teachers, parents, children, and medical inspectors praised the new program.

Quincy School's Floggings

The headlines screamed, *Bunker Tells of His "Bad Boys" Defends His Whipping Record in South Cove District*.[91] This article ran in the *Boston Daily Globe* about two and a half months after Annie McKay started at the Quincy School. The write-up referred to the Headmaster, Alfred Bunker, who commented that the, "school is hard to manage requiring him to inflict whippings." There were 456 floggings among 568 boys since September 1, 1905. The school surpassed the record of any Boston Public School for floggings.

The Headmaster whipped the schoolboys for offenses such as truancy, snowballing in the streets, fighting in the streets, stealing from passing wagons, and direct disobedience to a staff member. "We are not only trying to teach arithmetic and geography, but we are trying to build up character to make good citizens," claimed Mr. Bunker. He continued on to say that they deal with the boys' behaviors in school and keep them out of the courts. A frequent complaint he received from

89   Stanwood, C. Nurses in the Schools. *Boston Transcript* (April 4, 1906). IDNA Collection, Box3, Folder 3.

90   *The Hawthorne Club, Boston, Massachusetts, 1910-1912*. (1912). Boston, MA: The Metcalf Press. p.13.

91   Bunker Tells of his Bad Boys (1906, February 20). *The Boston Daily Globe* 1,4. Retrieved from ProQuest Historical Newspapers Boston Globe (1872-1924).

his teaching staff was that he was too soft on the boys when he whipped them. They argued that if he hit the students harder, they would have fewer instances of bad behavior (Bunker Tells of his Bad Boys).

What exactly is a flogging or whipping? The dictionary describes it as, "beating with a whip or strap or rope especially as punishment, with blows commonly directed to the person's back." It apparently was an accepted form of punishment, but just the same, the Boston School Committee was looking into it. Annie McKay never mentioned bruises from flogging in her speech or newspaper interview. Were the bruised students sent to her for first aid? Would she have offered a cold compress? No doubt, she would have advised the student to stop the aggrieved behavior and stay out of trouble. More than likely, she witnessed similar scenes during her own schooling. This account does provide us some insight and a glimpse into the social history of early 20th century school life. It surprised me to find that school flogging is still practiced in 19 states.

The Superintendent's Notes and Other School Nurses Assignments

Let us follow the notes of IDNA Superintendent Stark and track the progression of the school nurse program. Stark commented that McKay had done a great deal of home visiting to prevent the spread of contagious diseases such as measles. McKay met with Dr. Fairbanks of the Hawthorne Club every two weeks to report on the 16 children who attend their after-school program. Both the teachers and the headmaster were very pleased with her work. Superintendent Stark wrote that McKay was not tired, and she does not think she has overworked her. See the image below, Annie McKay at work. (Picture courtesy of Roberta Mitchell)

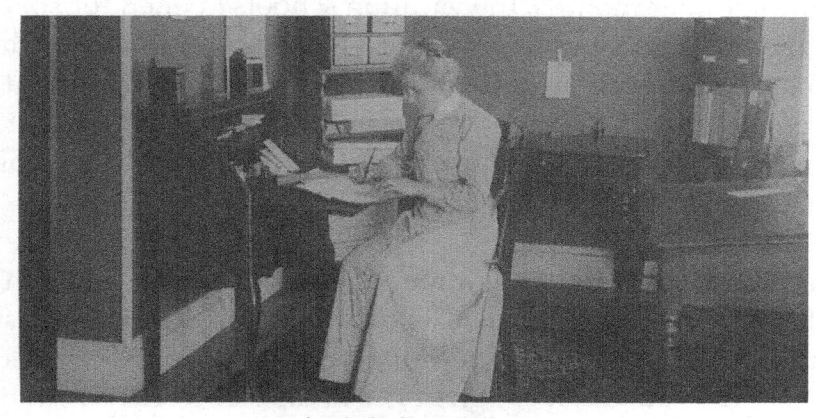

Annie McKay at Work

More than six weeks after Annie McKay pioneered school nursing in Boston, IDNA placed another nurse, Henrietta A. Willis, the Father's and Mother's Club Nurse, in the Wells District, Boston's West End on January 18, 1906. Her assignment included four schools, the Wells, Emerson, Mayhew and Winchell Schools. Stark and an assistant stayed with Willis for three days to orient her and the school staff to the new program. Mrs. Rice, the layperson manager for the Wells District, thought Miss Willis looked tired and might be overworked. However, Miss Willis said she felt terrific. Stark writes that as Miss Willis becomes more familiar with the work, the job won't seem as difficult and she would start to see some positive results.

On the other hand, Stark commented that McKay did not like writing reports and was not as methodical about keeping records as Miss Willis. Both of them preferred to keep records on the students via a card. The April school vacation found them doing follow-up work with the children at the Boston Dispensary and making home visits. If they had any extra time, they reported to the IDNA office.

Stark's reports in 1906 found that the students in McKay's classes were not responding as well to hygiene and cleanliness as those students in Miss Willis's school. "I have been in both their homes and have noticed their clothing," she remarked. That was a curious entry describing the clothing. She must have accompanied both nurses on a home visit. What was suggested to the families? Despite Stark's reports however, Headmaster Bunker and teachers were still pleased with McKay's work. These accounts raise the question of the relationship between McKay and Stark, but this is momentarily put to rest when McKay gets sick with a severe case of the "grippe" during the first week of April 1906.

During the summer months, the vacation schools opened for six weeks. IDNA tested all of the children's eyes, and where there was a school without a school nurse, neighborhood charities stepped in to take the children to various hospitals to have their eyes checked. In cases where the children required retesting, the children were brought to IDNA three times a day for three to four days to place drops in their eyes, requiring a lot of work for IDNA.

As the summer passed in 1906, Annie McKay went on vacation on August 1 for one month. It was not surprising that when she returned, she requested a change in assignment for the reason that she did care for schoolwork any longer, which she was granted. Instead, Stark assigned her to district work in East Boston. In her place in the Quincy school district would be Miss Rose, who had been off duty for an extended period of time because of her brother-in-law's illness. She was told if she did not report she would forfeit her position. Miss Rose would leave district work six weeks later. McKay would temporarily fill in again, to be replaced by Miss McDougall, a substitute nurse. McDougall was waiting for her probation period to be completed and accepted as a regular nurse.

Meanwhile, the Superintendent of Schools sent out a letter to the principals that Miss Stark of IDNA had permission to visit the various schools in the city to supervise and assist the nurses that they employ at their (IDNA's) expense in the schools. They were to cooperate with her to the extent that, in their judgment, it was to the advantage of their school.

Miss Willis became ill in September 1906. Was she perhaps overworked? Stark described the method of communication between the school staff and the nurse to be used in all schools. There would be a box inside the door where the staff could place a note to the nurse with the name of the referred student and classroom. She continued that there would be a place in each building where the nurse could see the child and set up her supplies, usually in the sunny part of the basement. Couldn't she think of a better place than that?

By September 1906, IDNA assigned a third nurse to the school nurse program. Fannie Carter became the nurse for the Bowdoin and Phillips School Districts (West End). Stark spent one week with Carter in her new assignment to introduce her to school nursing. By November, Stark claimed that Carter was too sociable with the school staff, talked too much, and needed close supervision. The principal of one school did not allow Carter to enter the classroom. The nurse only saw students selected by the principal.

By November 1906, Stark notes that they started to use volunteers. These volunteers proved to be a great help to the nurses taking the children to and from the hospital. They were completely subordinate to the nurse. Miss Mary Dexter developed into a very good assistant for Annie McKay. The key aspect was that under this new program, the child was not sent home and did not miss valuable school time (*Daily Notes from Superintendent Stark*). Stark has enforced a new rule that when a nurse leaves one school to go to another school she will leave a note saying where she is going, so she can be easily found.

Now look at the sequence of events so casually described here. This entry relays a change in procedure affecting both physicians and nurses. IDNA's Executive Committee voted that nurses no longer would accompany physicians on their visits and instead it would be left to Superintendent Stark to communicate with the physician and pass the information on to the nurses. Beforehand, however, this was not discussed with either the Boston Dispensary or the nurses, which upset both groups. One of the doctor's concerns was they would be unable to examine women without a nurse present. Nevertheless, their protests were overruled, and the new system was put into effect.[92]

Stark's modus operandi in this incident led to the following state of affairs: within a year seven nurses who had worked for the association for one to six years had resigned, along with the vice president, treasurer, and two of the managers.

Subsequently, in December 1906 Annie McKay delivered a talk regarding her schools' scarlet fever cases at Miss Mason's house, one of the Board of Managers at IDNA. Miss Carter at the Bowdoin School needed some supervision as to where to keep her supplies, as they were found to be in a dirty place. As a result of finding brooms and dustpans where the medical supplies were, Stark had a consult with the janitor.

A new doctor at the Bowdoin School wanted both the nurse and the teacher to write out his records for him, thus saving him time. In addition, he requested the nurse to do whatever treatment he required, disregarding the nurse's limitations. Stark decided to review with Carter her scope of practice, in case she would forget.

The entry for January 1907 says simply for an unexplained reason, Miss McDougall did not relieve Annie McKay who remained as school nurse in the Quincy District until the end of the school year. Stark reported that Annie McKay had large numbers of daily dressings besides home visits, hospital cases, and taking children to Dr. Fairbanks office, who specialized in pediatric tuberculosis.

January 28, 1907, saw the start of another nurse, Miss Bridges, in the Hancock school district, North End. Stark spent four days showing her the ropes. Then on February 3, Stark spent another few days orienting Miss Illsley in the Eliot school

---

[92] Howse, C. (2009). The Reflection of England's Light. In P. D'Antonio (Ed.), *Nursing History Review Official Publication of the American Association for the History of Nursing* (pp. 47-79). New York, NY: Springer Publishing Company. Page 66.

district, North End, where the school doctor held an unfavorable opinion about the addition of school nurses beforehand. For that reason, "our reception was not quite as welcome." However, "after proceeding most carefully," he has appreciated the work accomplished by the school nurse, as have the principals and teachers.

A problem arose at the Eye and Ear Infirmary where the students and volunteer helpers were asked to stay in line instead of being brought to the front of the queue as had been the plan previously. This scenario caused the children to be out of school for a longer time. Stark marched over to check with the hospital superintendent and found that more than one of the volunteers had disputes with prominent doctors there. The doctors themselves decided that the children could wait online. After a talk with the Superintendent, he allowed the prior queue plan to continue. As a result, Stark contended that one school nurse could only handle no more than two volunteers.

By the end of February 1907, IDNA, with Ms. Stark as Superintendent of Nurses, had on its own five nurses working in six of the public-school districts, comprising 19 schools.[93]

By May, IDNA reported that the Father's and Mother's Club was late in paying their bill, where they supported Miss Willis in the Wells district. Plans were being made for nurse coverage for summer schools. The Father's and Mother's Club didn't know if they would keep Miss Willis on during the summer. On the other hand, Miss McKay and Miss Illsley would continue in their districts. The Phillips and Bowdoin Schools' relationship with their nurse came to an end when school closed on June 21, 1907.

Report of the Commission: Health of Children[94]

Despite the pleas of social agencies and various individuals, the Boston School Committee still needed convincing concerning the need for school nurses. Therefore,

---

93 *Boston School Reports* Instructive District Nursing Association of Boston Collection, Howard Gotlieb Archival Research Center, Boston University (hereafter IDNA Collection), Box 1.

94 *Report of the Commission Appointed June 1906, To Report on Matters Relating to the Health of Children Attending the First Three Grades. (1907)*. (School Doc. No. 2-1907). Boston, MA: Municipal Printing Office.

shortly after the appointment of McKay in December 1905 and Willis in January 1906, the Boston School Committee appointed in June 1906 a Commission of five physicians to study the health of the 40,000 children in the first three grades within the Boston Public Schools. They limited their study only to those matters pertaining to children's health. They accomplished this task by visiting 24 of the 386 primary and grammar schools and two special schools, both old and new, in all parts of the city, and interviewing teachers, headmasters and the Board of Health. Their plans did not call for examining the children.

Some of the problems encountered were the lighting, lack of toilets, and overcrowding in the older buildings. Unfortunately, some buildings had no electric lights, still using gas jets without globes, which used up valuable oxygen in the room. The arrangement of windows offered little natural light, causing eyestrain. The Commission commented that because the classrooms were so dark, children were not able to read the large writing on the blackboards from halfway across the room. As has been noted earlier, Annie McKay found helping the children with poor vision demanded much of her time.

In some primary classrooms, the normal class size comprised a colossal 45 students. However, some classrooms had as many as 60 or 70 students in one room. A room full of that many students was very hard for one teacher to manage, even with an assistant. The students would receive very little attention. They suggested, though this was not in their realm of expertise, to separate the slower children into special classes or assign them designated tutors, since they slowed the progress of the class.

The report continued that crowded classrooms could be a potential place for catching the latest cold. Viruses were spread by airborne droplets. In a January 27, 2015 article in the *Wall Street Journal*, Dr. Susan Rehm, reported that a person who was coughing, sneezing or talking could infect others from as far away as six feet (1.83 m), and these viruses can survive on surfaces for two-eight hours. She is Vice Chair of the Infectious Disease Department at Cleveland Clinic. Early 20th century classrooms had neither hand sanitizers nor sinks with running water to wash hands.

When it came to what they referred to as the medical inspection in schools, the Commission explained that doctors were to visit the schools every day, and follow-up on any children who the teachers thought needed to be checked by the doctor. After the doctor examined the child, a report was given to the teacher or the headmaster, who relayed that to the parents. The doctor would not treat the child.

On the other hand, the Commission had some thoughts on this program, saying, "that this is not an inspection by physicians, but by teachers. Yet the medical profession is held responsible.[95]" They commented further that there was a big difference in the teachers' attitudes toward the program. Some were very observant of the children's condition and behaviors, while others were uninterested and unconcerned. To illustrate the differences, one school of 300 children had not called for the doctor's services in one year, and it was hard for them to imagine over that length of time the school did not need a doctor.

The Commission noted that one of the main duties of the medical inspectors was the detection of the contagious diseases of childhood, especially diphtheria, scarlet fever and measles. However, they said, the role of the medical inspector had been developed to include all conditions pertaining to the health of children, and whatever the child's condition was, the school doctor's job ended after the child was examined and the parents notified. No-one knew if the child had been treated, if the advice given had been carried out or ignored. The result was that the child remained out of school for sometimes-trivial ailments for weeks at a time.

Their report, published in January 1907 suggested that a properly qualified nurse, "would not only find the children showing symptoms of physical distress, but would see to it that that they were quickly and properly treated, and returned to school at the earliest possible moment.[96]"

Continuing on, the report, referring to the two nurses in service in the South and West End, stated:

> They have amply demonstrated their value. In these school districts a much larger number of pupils needing medical assistance has been found. Treatment has been carried out efficiently, either through the family physicians or the hospitals... The greatest value of the nurses' service is outside the school building at the homes of the pupils. She explains to the parents the physical defects of the child and advises them as to what had best be done.

---

95   *Report of the Commission Appointed June 1906, To Report on Matters Relating to the Health of Children Attending the First Three Grades. (1907).* (School Document No. 2-1907). Boston, MA: Municipal Printing Office. Page 16.

96   Ibid. Page 18.

If the parents have a family physician, the school nurse would see to it that his orders are carried out. The report concluded with these recommendations:

"That competent trained nurses be appointed to supplement the work of the medical inspectors."

The Boston School Committee accepted the recommendation. IDNA's last school nurse went off duty August 8, 1907. In IDNA's *Annual Report for 1908* they noted the nurses work in the public schools for 1907. They saw 2,375 cases, administered 6,052 treatments, and made 2,822 home visits. Stark reported that she had meetings with the Superintendent of Schools, Dr. Harrayton, on the transfer of school nursing services to the Boston Public Schools (BPS).[97] The Superintendent of Schools remained disappointed that none of the school nurses wanted to take the required exam to work for the BPS, because the school system valued their work. Of the new nurses that the BPS hired, Stark commented they knew nothing about district nursing or making home visits.

After the transfer of school nursing to the BPS, Annie McKay continued to work for IDNA as a nurse with the Relief and Control of Tuberculosis Association in conjunction with Massachusetts General Hospital. McKay went off duty December 21, 1907.[98] Stark reported that McKay was going to take up massage. The question is would McKay have stayed longer if she and Stark had a better working relationship? Bear in mind, McKay liked the independence of community nursing. That answer is left to historical speculation.

Later, in 1911 Stark applied for the position of Director at IDNA but was turned down and then resigned. Apparently, her management style left much to be desired. The Board of Managers said that she had, "no true administrative power"; "a suspicious nature"; "a tremendously quick temper"; "does not get along with other workers well"; and "tampers with the truth."

In later years, IDNA always referred to their introduction of nurses in the public

---

[97] *Twenty-second Annual Rept. of the Instructive Dist. Nursing Assn. for the Year Ending Jan. 31, 1908*. p. 22

[98] *Daily Notes from Superintendent Stark*, Instructive District Nursing Association: November 20, 1905 -January 1, 1908. Instructive District Nursing Association (IDNA).

schools as an example of their pioneer work. In the long term, the transfer of voluntary funded programs such as this to municipal government was the best solution.

As of September 1907, the Boston School Committee began employing their own nurses for their student population of 106,370.[99] They appointed a total of 34 nurses and a nursing supervisor for the elementary day schools.

School nursing became a success because school nurses showed they did make a difference in helping children become healthy and staying in school. Documentation and collection of data, in other words evidence-based practice, just as school nurse Annie McKay did over a century ago to demonstrate to the Boston School Committee the connection between nursing interventions and educational outcomes, is mandatory for Massachusetts school nurses today.

Miss McKay's pioneering work of more than one hundred years ago in improving the health care of students and their families constituted another step up the ladder of the American dream. Her legacy in the public schools was to make our system of universal education more accessible to additional children, and especially for the scores of immigrant children who follow yet today, thus making them productive citizens. With the stroke of her appointment, a system of health assessment, intervention and follow-up for all children within the school system was established. This step also created a new nursing specialty, that of school nurse, which we know, would undergo many challenges during the intervening years.

A blog on the website of the American Association for the History of Nursing commented that much of what people learn about history tends to focus on those who were founders of institutions or held lofty leadership positions. However, the history of nursing is filled with examples of significant, yet largely unknown individuals who have made noteworthy contributions to nursing history. Annie McKay's experiences illustrate this point.

Now another chapter unfolds the school nurses' untold story. We will watch as the Massachusetts legislature takes steps to improve children's health care. IDNA's involvement with school nurses has ended, but endings can be the start of new beginnings. So, stay on board as another journey begins, that of the Boston school nurses.

---

99   *School Document Report Number 12*, June 1908. p 5.

SECTION II
PROFESSIONALIZATION

Chapter 6

Fresh Start, New Rules, and New Laws

Fresh Start, New Rules, and New Laws

Not one of the nurses would take the exam.[100] The year was 1907, but not a single one of the IDNA nurses took the exam to work as a school nurse for the Boston Public Schools. Whatever their reason was, salary, joining another bureaucracy, taking a test, working in damp, dark basements and broom closets, or working with children and families, no one would take the test. Each of us has a set of scales-many sets, in fact, continually weighing the pros and cons of every behavior. How will this help? How will this hurt? They made their decision. Let's review the background of how this situation developed.

State Requires School Physicians - 1906

At a meeting of the State Conference of Charities in 1905, Dr. Samuel Durgin, Chairman of the Boston Board of Health, made a plea for nurses in the Boston schools. Secondly, he mentioned that statewide, medical inspection in the schools existed in only 14 towns and cities outside of Boston. These were Andover, Arlington, Brookline, Cambridge, Chelsea, Fall River, Malden, Marlboro, Melrose, Milton, Newton, Waltham, Wellesley, and Winchester. The board of health in most of these

---

100 *District Superintendents Reports.* May 1907. p. 7. IDNA Collection, Box 9, Instructive District Nursing Association (IDNA) Reports, Instructive District Nursing Association of Boston Collection, Howard Gotlieb Archival Research Center, Boston University (hereafter IDNA Collection).

towns carried out the work which had to do chiefly with contagious diseases. The suburbs of Milton and Marlboro mandated the school committee responsible for medical inspections. In Marlboro, the local woman's club bore the expenses.

Durgin contended that Boston public schools enjoyed physicians visits daily, but medical inspections in Newton only occurred three times a year. In Waltham and Winchester, similar to Boston, the medical inspectors covered not only contagious diseases, but also other physical defects that affected children's ability to do their schoolwork. In comparison, the director of physical training in Andover considered himself capable of performing the whole area of medical inspection.[101] As a result, Massachusetts schools accomplished medical assessment in a variety of ways.

Next, Durgin brought up the problem of expenses saying, "The sentiment school committees and health boards are generally favorable to systematic medical inspection, but they find it difficult to get money for it from city councils. An awakening of public sentiment is needed, and it may be necessary to enact some compulsory legislation, as has been done in some states.[102]"

Therefore, the state made some effort to address the situation, though not wholeheartedly. In 1906, Massachusetts passed a law requiring school physicians called *Acts of 1906, Chapter 502, An Act Relative to the Appointment of School Physicians*. It mandated the school committee in every city and town in the Commonwealth to appoint one or more school physicians to each public school unless the board of health had already accomplished this, or plans were in place for the board of health to perform this.

The physician's duties required that he was to examine all children referred to him, and any child returning to school who had been absent on account of illness or unknown cause who did not have a certificate from the board of health. Also, he would examine any child who showed signs of being in ill health or had a contagious disease unless the child had already been dismissed by the teacher. The school committee would notify the parents or guardians of a child that is ill or has

---

101 Nurses in Schools: Dr. Sam H. Durgin Makes Appeal for Them. Medical Treatment of the Pupils Under Discussion. Plea for Nurses in Schools. Results Justify the Expenses. *Boston Daily Globe (1872-1922)*. November 9, 1905:10. Available From: ProQuest Information and Learning, Ann Arbor, Accessed December 7, 2007, Document ID 694156112.

102 Ibid.

defects. Whenever a child showed symptoms of smallpox, scarlet fever, measles, chickenpox, tuberculosis, diphtheria, influenza, tonsillitis, whooping cough, mumps, scabies or trachoma, the child was to be sent home immediately by a safe means of transportation, and the board of health notified.

Additionally, the law required teachers to test the vision and hearing of every child once a year, notifying the parents of the results and keeping a record of it. The state board of health would be furnishing the equipment needed for the testing. Each individual town would be required to appropriate the money necessary to comply with this act.[103]

The law was a disappointment. Note the absence of any mention of school nurses. The school physicians were going to accomplish all of the conditions so casually described on their own. A prominent social worker of the time, Robert Woods commented that the majority of students left school after elementary school, never going on to high school, despite being capable of accomplishing more. The doctors and school nurses had become another gatekeeper for school attendance.

Soon after, in 1910, the law was amended. *Chapter 257 An Act to Provide for Medical Inspection of Working Children between the Ages of Fourteen and Sixteen.* It added that the school physician must examine children who were applying for an age and schooling certificate, and certify that the child was in good health, and was able to do the work that he wanted to do. It further explained the minor must be able to read and write legible simple sentences in English. If the minor could not read, the minor must attend an evening school until an evening schoolteacher approved his reading ability.[104]

Nurses Law: Chapter 357

Boston would be among the pioneering cities in developing a school nurse program to supplement the work of the school physicians. In order to move forward after the decision of the Boston School Committee to hire their own nurses, the city was

---

103 *Acts and Resolves of Massachusetts 1906. Passed by the General Court of Massachusetts in the Year 1906.* Chapter 502. Massachusetts: Wright & Potter Printing Co. State Printers. Page 680-681.

104 *Acts and Resolves of Massachusetts 1910. Passed by the General Court of Massachusetts in the Year 1910.* Chapter 257. Massachusetts: Wright & Potter Printing Co. State Printers.

required to pass a law known as Chapter 357 of the Acts of 1907, *An Act Relative to the Appointment of Nurses by the School Committee of the City of Boston, May 3, 1907*. The law was divided into three sections. Basically, Section 1 covered the appointment of a female supervising nurse and female district nurses, as many as they thought they would need. Their job was to assist the school physician in the city schools, follow their directions, and give instructions to the students for promoting their health.

The law further stated in Section 2, that the "nurse" should have taken a course or be a graduate from a hospital or similar institution after studying nursing for at least two years. She also must show the school committee evidence that she was a person of good character and was in good health. Finally, she must have passed an examination given under the direction of the school committee "designed to test the applicant's training, knowledge, character, experience, and aptness for the work.[105]"

Before this clause was agreed upon, the Senate exploded into debate, ultimately deciding to alter Section 2 of the original legislation for Boston school nurses. The bill would now read that it was only necessary for an applicant to satisfy the school board that she would make a good nurse. As a result, the section requiring a diploma from a hospital or other such institution was removed. This caused a hullabaloo with the originators of the bill because they claimed that it gave the school board too much leeway and raised the possibility that they might just appoint political favorites instead of competent nurses.

Change brings challenges. The doctors, nurses, and school board members who developed the bill contacted their legislators to have the original clause reinstated. As a final argument, the group mentioned above cited the successes of the New York City school nurse program last year in discovering 150,401 cases of contagious eye diseases and 306,025 cases of contagious skin diseases. They pointed out that their role in arresting these conditions was proof of the value of school nurses as opposed to their expense.[106] Their arguments proved successful in overturning the changes made in Section 2.

---

105 *Acts and Resolves of Massachusetts 1907. Passed by the General Court of Massachusetts in the Year 1907.* Chapter 357. Massachusetts: Wright & Potter Printing Co. State Printers.

106 State House Affairs. Gov Guild to Name Superior Court Judges This Week. *Boston Daily Globe (1872-1922).* April 14, 1917. ProQuest Historical Newspapers Boston Globe (1872-1924) pg.32.

Section 3 of the law addressed the expenses of the nurses. The Boston School Committee (BSC) would appropriate $10,000 for the remainder of the year and each year after that at a rate of two cents per one thousand dollars of the real estate valuation upon which the City Council based its appropriations. The Boston City Council held the purse strings and still does. In the future, they would assign that same rate to pay for the school nurses.

The salary for nurses set a minimum and maximum rate with increases every year until the maximum was reached. The supervising nurse's annual salary was set at $924 to start, with a maximum of $1,116, whereas the salary for the nurse now referred to as "assistant nurses" was $648 with a maximum of $840.[107] Was this similar to Annie McKay's when she worked at IDNA? An article in the *Boston Daily Globe* at the time recounted that the Boston School Committee would set aside $25,000 a year to pay for the school nurses.[108] See the image below - *The legislation appointing nurses to the Boston Public Schools.*

This law was especially meaningful because it laid the groundwork for the school nurse position. In the ensuing years, the exact details might temporarily be forgotten only to be remembered when someone researched it to provide a response when their very existence was challenged.

Superintendents Reports 1907

Written examinations are required at so many

---

107   *Proceedings of the School Committee of the City of Boston* (1907, May 27) p.78. Retrieved from https://archive.org/details/proceedingsofsch1907bost/page/78

108   School Nurses. Number Fixed at 21 by the Committee. *Boston Daily Globe (1872-1922).* May 28, 1907; ProQuest Historical Newspapers Boston Globe (1872-1924) pg. 8.

stages in life, and they can be a chore. So, it was for the first school nurses. At that time, 1907, schoolteachers in the Boston Public Schools were required to take exams in the subjects they would be teaching. Thus, the Boston Public Schools required a series of tests covering health, nutrition, and the welfare of children.

Unfortunately, none of the early exams can be found today, nor do we know precisely who developed them. The *1907 Board of Superintendents Reports* made references as to what the reviews should cover and who was eligible to take them. What remains today at the City of Boston Archives are copies of exams starting in 1926 through 1962. The volume containing examinations from 1894-1924 is missing. What fun it would have been to read through those early tests. It would make us more acutely aware of all of the maladies of the time, plus realize the medical and technological advances that have entered nursing practice in the interim.

As early as May 17, 1907, in the *Records, Board of Superintendents*[109], several other requirements for nurses were enumerated. Any provisions concerning the appointment and the policies of employment that were related to teachers, including their marital status, were to apply to nurses. To clarify, the Board did not employ female teachers after marriage. In the same way, this rule would apply to nurses. Only under the following circumstances, would a nurse be granted a leave of absence: for her own illness, the death or serious illness of an immediate family member, the funeral of school staff, teachers conferences held by state boards of education, and or to join teachers associations, visit other schools; and be required by the Board of Superintendents on the recommendation of the Superintendent to attend another type of conference, or visit a school. These rules on attendance at conferences would become an issue over the years.

The Superintendent designated the Director of Physical Training and Athletics, in addition to control of the playgrounds, and management of school athletics, to be in charge of the school nursing service, including hiring. This person, always referred to as "he," was not educated in the medical field. However, we will note that, and again, move on.

Finally, the nursing supervisor, under the direction of the director of physical training and athletics, managed the school nurses. In her position, always referred

---

[109] *Records, Board of Superintendents*, Vol. 22, 1907, 122.

to as "she," the nursing supervisor was responsible for how they did their work, the time spent in their districts, documentation of their work, requisitioning of supplies, and completing any reports requested by the Superintendent.

Likewise, the school nurses, referred to as the district nurses, were to assist the doctors, known as medical inspectors, and carry out their orders. Their supervisor developed their assignments, including the number of hours spent at school and to whom to report, upon their arrival. As soon as the school nurse arrived at school, they reported to the principal or teacher in charge and obtained a list of all excluded students. In return, the school provided the school nurse with a place to accomplish their assignment.

Record-keeping was important. School nurses had to maintain a schedule for the visiting school doctor of students needing to be seen and treated, keep a record for the Superintendent of every child examined in the school, with their name, age, address, disease, treatment received in school, a record of all excluded pupils, and pupils to be visited. They had to keep proof of their own arrival and departure from each school.

Here is an example of the clinical record card[110] as it was called.

DATE
PUPIL'S CLINICAL RECORD CARD
Name
Residence
School
Teacher
Nurse
Physician
Age
Sex
Grade
Diagnosis
Treatment

Home visits were spelled out in detail. It was expected that the nurse should visit the homes of excluded students, but not when the student was excluded for

---

110   *Superintendent's Report, Special Report*: 173

smallpox, scarlet fever, diphtheria, measles, whooping cough, or mumps, which were all contagious diseases. A record must be kept of the visit and the aftermath of each case visit. The nurse should make a repeat home visit whenever necessary. During these visits, the nurse should demonstrate the details of a treatment, for instance, the treatment of pediculosis, when needed, just as Annie McKay did. If the student had a condition that could not be treated at home by the parents or the nurse, the nurse should strongly encourage the parent to seek treatment by their private doctor or go to a dispensary.

Interestingly, nurses were not allowed to treat, a then prevalent eye disease called trachoma, which was added to the exclusion list. Caused by *Chlamydia trachomatis*, trachoma still remains the second leading cause of blindness in many developing countries where there is poor personal hygiene. The condition is marked by numerous and repeated episodes of an inflammatory eye condition, with the risk of blindness occurring in middle-aged and older adults. Today, the treatment of choice is a single dose of the antibiotic, azithromycin.[111] To return to school, a student with a history of trachoma had to present a certificate from the medical inspector that he/she was free of contagion.

To digress, an article in *The New York Times* in 1903 described the battle against trachoma, "the eye disease which has come to be recognized as the great juvenile danger of the crowded districts" in other words, the tenements (Emergency Hospital). I maintain that similar incidents occurred in Boston. Since the school nurses in New York City started testing children's' vision, they ultimately found that 15 percent to 18 percent had well-advanced trachoma, which amounted to 6,000 to 7,000 children. The story continued that if the school nurse found that the child excluded for trachoma has not been treated, she would immediately refer the child to one of the hospitals set up to care for these cases. Children and parents deluged the nurse with requests for treatment. The "easy" cases would have needed to comply with "a little treatment a good eye washing, a trifle of bandaging, a few *drops* to take away, and the injunction to come the day after tomorrow." However,

---

111 Frick, Kevin D., Lietman, Thomas M., Holm, Susan Osaki, Jha, Hem C., Chaudhary, J.S.P., & Bhatta, Ramesh C. (2001). Eficacia con relación al costo de las medidas de lucha contra el tracoma: comparación del tratamiento de hogares determinados y el tratamiento masivo de niños. *Bulletin of the World Health Organization, 79*(3), 201-207. Retrieved March 11, 2015, from http://www.scielosp.org/scielo.php?script=sci_arttext&pid=S0042-96862001000300007&lng=en&tlng=es. 10.1590/S0042-96862001000300007.

for those who did not see that treatment through or even start it, an operation was required to save their sight.[112]

As *The New York Times* account progresses, the Russo-Polish parents brought their child to the hospital, not seeming to understand what was going on, although the child seemed to take it all in. If the children arrived in the afternoon, they were kept overnight, because invariably if sent home, the parents would allow them to eat, which would cause some very upset stomach's when they received ether the next morning. The children would climb up on the operating room table, with no complaints whatsoever, knowing that the doctors and nurses were helping them. When the child was put under with either, the eye surgeon, "turns back the eyelid and scrapes away at its underside. As if by magic, the granulations disappear," related the newspaper account. The surgeon followed by applying a paste to the eyes and then wrapped the area with bandages. The surgeon dipped his hands in a basin of water containing antiseptic, after he finished the operation, and went on to his next patient (Emergency Hospital). Obviously, this occurred before the development of hand scrubbing, and sterile gloves. In the late 1800s, thanks to Joseph Lister, the medical community became convinced that unseen germs can cause infection. They promoted aseptic technique of instruments, dressings, etc. and the simple act of hand washing when going between patients.

On another note, these passages give us insight into the children of poor immigrants who, on the one hand, were so grateful for these interventions on their behalf. At the same time, they were caught at a young age in a loyalty conflict with their parents because of the different practices and new culture in America. Hopefully, they would grow up to have a sense of pride in being an American.

The last part of the instructions in the *Superintendent's Notes* dealt with being absent from duty. If absent, the nurse must immediately notify the supervising nurse or the superintendent by telephone, telegraph, or by special messenger. Within five hours, if she had no plans to return the following day, she must complete and deliver a written application for a leave of absence. When returning to duty, after being out of work for more than one day for any reason, she must first report to the

---

112 Emergency Hospital for Treatment of Trachoma: Scenes in the Institution Organized for The Relief of Those Children Who Have Been Withdrawn from the Public Schools Recently. *New York Times (1857-Current file)*. ProQuest LLC. New York, N.Y.: Jan. 25, 1903. p. 25 (1 pp.)

supervising nurse and present a certificate of care from her doctor, if she was seen by one. Each district nurse would be entitled to four weeks of vacation, taken at a time that had been approved by the supervising nurse and superintendent, or at the same time that the supervising nurse would be taking her vacation.

These were stringent rules to live by in comparison to our standards today. Surprisingly, I found no mention of a five-and-a-half-day workweek. It is reassuring to note that regulations have been relaxed substantially, thanks in part to unionization.

As has been noted earlier in Chapter 5, the Board of Health employed the medical inspectors, and they were paid an annual salary of $200. The School Department had no jurisdiction over them. The Board of Health required them to visit the schools in their district every day or make special arrangements with the teachers and principals as to what worked best for their particular school.[113]

School Nurse Exams

In the meantime, Boston forged on with its plans for the school nurse exams, the first planned for Saturday, June 15, 1907. The nursing exam included questions on health problems and appraisal, nursing management, health promotion and disease prevention, special health issues, and professional concerns.

However, controversy never ceased, and a young woman named Anna Henderson requested to take the exam saying she was eligible because she had worked at a children's hospital under the supervision of doctors for one and a half years. She continued to say in her poignant letter: "I am very fond of children, like the work and know all the parents. As I am the only nurse in the schools who took the exam-surely, some exception should be taken in my case. I have no pull or influence, so direct this to you-enclosing some of the credentials for you to see. Please reconsider your decision."

A doctor's recommendation letter saying that her training at the Massachusetts Infant Asylum, and at the Boston Lying-In Hospital was more than the equivalent of the regular course of study for nurses accompanied her request. "I wish to testify

---

113 *Superintendent's Reports*: Special Report-170

too to her remarkable success as a nurse in the Washington District." J.B. Fitzgerald, MD, Director of Physical Training.[114] Accordingly, no record exists of Anna Henderson working as a nurse in the Washington District. If she was employed there, I speculate she worked there in another capacity other than a nurse, perhaps as a matron, or assistant matron as she had previously at the Massachusetts Infant Asylum.

Be that as it may, despite the letter and recommendations, the Board of Superintendents decided that under the evidence she submitted, Henderson was not admissible to the exam held June 15, 1907. As has been pointed out, Henderson had not taken a course in and graduated from a two-year hospital or training school.[115] Therefore, whether she took the exam is unclear, but if she did take the exam, she did so under false pretenses.

The Board of Superintendents continued on to those nurses outside of IDNA who did take the June exam and were accepted as Boston school nurses: Margaret E. Carley, Supervising Nurse, and Assistant Nurses – Sarah M. Cahoon, Mary Callaghan, Mary E. Canarie, Elizabeth R. R. Card, Edith S. Cooke, Miriam H. Crowell, Mary A. Didham, Jennie R. Dix, Mary S. Doherty, Annie I. Hollings, Mabel A. Hunter, Ellen C. MacAdam, Mary Martin, Helen F. McCaffrey, Katherine A. Moynihan, Katherine O'Callaghan, Sadie G. Reynolds, Emily A. Snow, Alice M. Sweeney, and Alma Taylor, totaling one supervisor and twenty nurses.[116] Are any of these names familiar, a cousin, aunt, or former neighbor?

Enter the Board of Registration in Nursing

In light of the controversies as to what truly represented a nurse, concerned nurses founded the Massachusetts Nurses Association[117] as early as 1903. Its purpose was to protect the nursing profession for the benefit of the public, the doctor, and the nurse, and create a law that would require the registration of nurses. They worked with

---

114 *Superintendent's Reports* 1907 September 13, 1907, p 205-206.

115 *Boston School Committee Reports September 30, 1907.* p 133.

116 *Boston School Committee Reports September 5, 1907.* p. 113-114.

117 Massachusetts Nurses Association. *History. 1903-2003: 100 Years of Caring for the Commonwealth.* Retrieved from http://www.massnurses.org/about-mna/history

legislators to create the Massachusetts Board of Registration in Nursing (BORN) in 1910.[115] The mission of BORN was, "to protect the health, safety, and welfare of the citizens of the Commonwealth through the fair and consistent application of the statutes and regulations governing nursing practice and nursing education." The charter notes that among other things, BORN "approves and monitors nursing education programs which lead to initial licensure, issues nursing licenses to qualified individuals, and investigates and takes action on complaints concerning the performance and conduct of licensed nurses.[118]" As a result of this law, the term "registered nurse" was born, the shortened form cited as RN to follow a nurse's name. The President of MNA, Mary Riddle, became the first RN in Massachusetts in 1910, and the first chairperson of BORN.

The new Boston school nurses set out into unchartered waters, as they worked with new laws and regulations, facing frustrations, challenges, unforeseen twists and turns. In time though, they will develop their mission based on Annie McKay's legacy and the ability to deliver evidence-based care that will, in turn, promote the health and academic success of their students. We will be carried into a new period in the history of this country, as the Boston school nurses become part of the American experience.

---

[118] Massachusetts Health and Human Services. (2015). About the Board. In *Mission Statement*. Retrieved from http://www.massnurses.org/about-mna/history

Chapter 7

Boston Public School Nurses: The Early Years

In the beginning, they were a quiet group, efficient, cooperative, empathetic, and by the same token, passionate about getting the job done. It would take them a while to validate what they were about, give them a perspective on what they were meant to do, and needing time for their story to develop and mature. Consider, in 1907, other than a few supervisors, student nurses mainly staffed the hospitals. The job opportunities open to graduate nurses were limited to private duty and district nursing. Thus, the original twenty-one nurses hired by the Boston School Committee were ecstatic just to have a responsible job. In a world that was changing, this position gave their lives some stability, predictability, and order.

The Boston School Committee delved into renovation and improvement projects across buildings to accommodate new technologies, such as electricity, and at the same time, enhancing the education of Boston's children and their safety. After the 1908 Collinwood School fire in Cleveland, where 172 children and two teachers died, schools across the country reviewed their buildings for better protection against fire.[119] Boston was no exception. Both the Chairman of the School Committee, James J. Storrow, and Superintendent Stratton Brooks, toured the school buildings to see if they left anything undone that would contribute further to the safety of the children and staff in the event of a fire.

---

119 Fearing, H. "Collinwood School Fire," *Cleveland Historical*, accessed May 30, 2015. Retrieved from http://clevelandhistorical.org/items/show/394

Meanwhile, Superintendent Brooks, as required by new regulations in 1902, signed licenses for minors to be hawkers, peddlers or bootblacks, in other words, sell newspapers and shine shoes. The minimum age for these trades was ten years, but by 1908, they raised it to eleven years. However, these trades caused some hardship for the students, since many of them were falling asleep in class, being exhausted. To increase their earnings, they needed to leave their house by 5:00 AM. When many of these exhausted boys arrived at school, they fell asleep on their desk. New regulations declared that licensed minors under the age of 14 could not sell newspapers until 6:30 in the morning. These new laws sought to give the boys more sleep and rest.[120]

As mentioned in Chapter 6, legislators established a new law in 1910 for working papers. It required an examination by a medical doctor saying that a minor was physically fit to do the work. This law led to the placement of a school physician and school nurse in the certificating office in Boston.

Robert Woods, Director of the South End Settlement House, raised the issue of schools again in 1909 when he spoke about "industrial education." He made the point that 80-95 percent of the students terminated their education at the end of elementary school. The reason for this was due to the meager financial predicament of the family. Parents simply could not afford to keep their children in school longer than the age of 14. He suggested implementing a program of "industrial education," what we now call vocational education. This curriculum, in the long term, would give the workingman a higher standard of living. People objected to this practice because it would train everyone to have a skill thus leaving no one to perform unskilled labor. Mr. Wood came back with his own arguments declaring that the chances of having no unskilled laborers were remote. "But supposing it to be real, this would stimulate intention to take the place of unskilled labor. A rise in the price of unskilled labor is a thing to be desired."[121]

In response to these problems in 1912, the School Committee established six prevocational centers in different parts of the city to steer boys to vocational schools

---

120 *Annual School Report School Document No.16*:8,9 (1907) Retrieved from https://archive.org/details/annualreport19051909bost/page Page 71-73.

121 Points to its Benefits: Robert A. Woods Speaks on "Industrial Education" before the Y.M.C.U. (1909, January 25). *Boston Daily Globe* (1872-1922). p.9. Retrieved December 28, 2007 from ProQuest Historical Newspapers Boston Globe (1872-1924) database (Document ID: 711648542.

and to give better preparation to boys who would be leaving the school system at 14 years of age.[122] They could attend the Boston Industrial School for Boys, located on Common Street near Washington Street. Notice this was only for boys.

Where did the girls go? The girls' vocational school, called the Trade School for Girls resided at 618-620 Massachusetts Avenue, between Shawmut Avenue and Washington Street in the South End. The redevelopment of the South End during the post-WWII era caused the eventual destruction of the building. Now it is the home of a Dunkin' Donuts, and a large parking lot.

As you recall, Chapter 5 relates how Annie McKay, Massachusetts first school nurse, assisted a girl in her vocational school application to study millinery design. At this school, students had a choice of two courses, each a year in length, one for girls who were under 15 years of age, and another for girls over 15 years of age. In addition to academic work related to the trades, they were offered dressmaking, and millinery, and learned how to operate straw and clothing machines. In addition, teachers taught how to buy clothes and prepare nutritious food. *"Although the special aim of the schoolwork is to fit girls to earn a living, the chief end of woman as the maker and keeper of a home is always considered."* See the image below - Picture of girls in dressmaking class.[123]

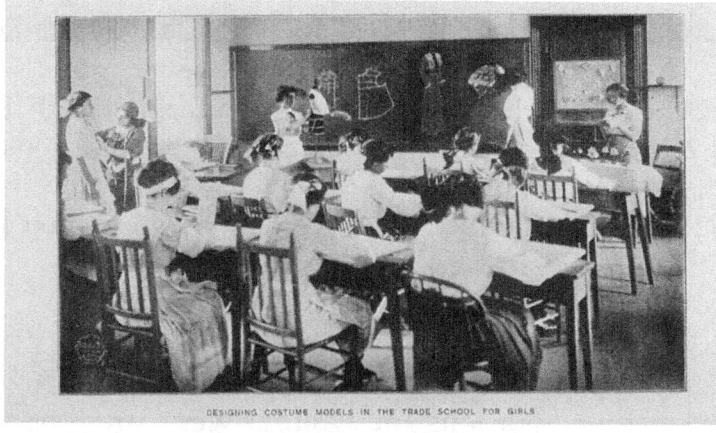

Girls in Dressmaking Class

122 *Annual School Report School Document No. 10.* (1912) Retrieved from https://ia700409.us.archive.org/35/items/annualreport1912bost/annualreport1912bost.pdf. Page 70.

123 *Annual School Report School Document No. 10.* (1912) Retrieved from https://ia700409.us.archive.org/35/items/annualreport1912bost/annualreport1912bost.pdf. Page 38-40.

As early as 1885, Clara Barton, founder of the American Red Cross, who regretted her own lack of educational opportunity, espoused higher aspirations for women. She encouraged numerous young women, "to put by your embroideries and your laundry... and commence your studies," and was delighted when they followed her advice.[124] These passages encapsulate the struggles that women had in obtaining an education and gaining equal privileges as men.

At the same time, the school nurses pushed forward, doing their work, and collecting data as did their predecessors. They dealt with diseases of the ear, eye, nose mouth, throat, skin, specific infectious diseases, and miscellaneous. The *Superintendent's Annual Report* contained a glowing account of their activities summarizing their first three months on the job in 1907.

The following abstract of the work done by the nursing division for the period from September 11, 1907, to December 31, 1907, speaks for itself, and it should be remembered that nurses are not permitted to visit homes where there are cases of contagious disease.

- Diseases of Ear, 1,137 cases cared for,
- Eye, 4528 cases were diagnosed and cared for, including 2,720 suffering from defective vision- of these 852 cases were treated by oculists,
- Nose, 2,020 cases of which 1,059 had adenoids, and 309 had the obstruction removed,
- Mouth, 1,241 cases, including 1,199 who had carious teeth,
- Throat, 1,258 cases, consisting of enlarged tonsils, tonsillitis, abscess, pharyngitis, and laryngitis,
- Skin, 8,602 cases, all of which cases were followed to their homes, and the parent or guardian instructed how to care for the same.

In addition to the above,

- 1,792 pupils having abrasions and wounds were cared for,
- 705 septic conditions cured,
- 244 cases of kidney disease recognized and treated and relieved,
- 121 cases rachitis (rickets) put on the correct line of treatment,

---

124 Pryor, E.B. *Clara Barton Professional Angel.* (1987). Philadelphia: University of Pennsylvania Press. Page 253.

- 213 cases of malnutrition advised as to diet and treatment,
- 221 cases of epilepsy found and advised,
- 96 cases of chorea (an abnormal, involuntary movement disorder),
- 47 cases of cardiac disease,
- 87 cases bronchitis, and
- 299 cases of anemia, all assisted.

Of the less common afflictions of childhood, 105 cases of deformity (spinal and extremities) were seen.[125]

Despite their workloads, their annual salaries remained the same in 1908 as outlined in Chapter 6: $648 annually for the nurses with a maximum of $840, and $924 for the nursing supervisor with a maximum of $1,116.[126] In comparison, a school janitor at Brighton High School earned $1,788, increased from $1,620 in 1907.[127] A first-year elementary school teacher received a salary of $972, with an annual increase of $48 to a maximum of $1,212.

Aid in Chelsea Fire

On April 12, 1908, Palm Sunday, a fire during a 40-mile (64 km) gale-force wind engulfed the neighboring city of Chelsea. The massive conflagration killed 19 people, rendered 12,000 people homeless, and destroyed a total of 1,500 buildings. At that time, there were no fire hydrants, no gas masks, and no fire trucks. The fire engine of the day was a horse-drawn steamer. Boston established relief committees and a receiving station for donated items.[128] The catastrophe brought a group of Boston school nurses to aid in relief work.

Picture the scene of long lines of hungry, displaced people, simultaneously

---

125 *Annual School Report School Document No.16*:8,9 (1907) Retrieved from https://archive.org/details/annualreport19051909bost/page Page 8-9.

126 *Proceedings of the School Committee, City of Boston* (1908, February 20). Retrieved from https://archive.org/stream/proceedingsofsch1908bost#page/34/mode/2up

127 *Proceedings of the School Committee, City of Boston* (1907, March 19). Retrieved from https://archive.org/stream/proceedingsofsch1907bost#page/37/mode/2up

128 Herwick III, E. (2014, April 11). Chelsea on Fire, 1908. *WGBH News*. Retrieved from http://wgbhnews.org/post/chelsea-fire-1908.

feeling destitute. When they realized they had lost everything, many citizens just threw themselves into the street and cried aloud in their suffering. All they had were the clothes on their backs. Hundreds of frantic parents could be heard sobbing as they searched for their children, while the soldiers who were called in, pitched tents for the homeless.[129] In addition to their nursing care, the Boston school nurses gave encouragement, a caring smile, a friendly voice, and an extended hand.

The Boston School Committee took notice also, and on June 1, 1908, received a communication from Superintendent Brooks detailing the services rendered by Supervising Nurse Carley and her Assistant Nurses to the suffering people of Chelsea. Their assistance was summarized as follows:

- Number of hours service 386
- Number of meals procured, prepared and served 1,920
- Number of dressings and cases requiring special nursing 295
- Number of maternity cases assisted 14
- Number of contagious cases discovered and isolated, including membranous croup, scarlet fever, diphtheria, measles 15
- Number of pneumonia and influenza cases 8
- Number of persons interviewed and registered 2,000
- Number of packages of clothing and supplies procured and disposed of 1,200
- Number of cases investigated 900

Boston School Committee Minutes June 1, 1908:

The Board expressed to Supervising Nurse Carley and to assistant nurses Buckley, Cahoon, Crowell, Daly, Dwyer, Felton, Fitzgerald, Hollings, Hunter, McCaffrey, Quirk, Reynolds, and Snow, its "appreciation and approval of the efficient service which they cheerfully and voluntarily rendered to persons needing medical attention during and after the recent Chelsea fire, and extends to them individually its sincere thanks for their valuable public service.[130]" Hopefully, the City of Chelsea

---

129   Pratt, W.M. *The Burning of Chelsea* (1908). Retrieved from https://books.google.com/books?hl=en&lr=&id=jjUpAAAAYAAJ&oi=fnd&pg=PA11&dq=Chelsea+fire+1908&ots=9zkKt7xir1&sig=kEmFJZnBfnalibJozqrDHoQsvXA#v=onepage&q=Chelsea%20fire%201908&f=false

130   *Boston School Committee Minutes* (1908, June 1): Boston, MA: p. 92. Boston Municipal Printing Office. Page 92.

appreciated the compassion, energy, and resourcefulness demonstrated by the school nurses. Approximately half of the Boston school nurses participated in this outstanding effort as they worked together toward the shared goal of recovery for the Chelsea community.

School Nurses and School Physicians

By 1909, a controversy erupted at a Boston School Physicians Association meeting when Dr. David Scannell MD, a Boston School Committee member, said the school physicians and the school nurses should show more cooperation with each other. In his opinion, they should all be working under the same management, the Board of Health. Instead, the Board of Health managed physicians, while school nurses reported to the Boston School Committee. He recommended that the Board of Health rules and School Committee regulations be uniform. Such contradictory regulations included, among other things, the period of exclusion for the various contagious diseases. Other recommendations asked whether Boston's parochial school children, one-fifth of Boston's children, should receive the services of a school nurse and whether they should increase the school physician's salary from $200 annually to $600.[131]

Rumblings of discontent appeared again in newspaper reports during 1911 and 1912, criticized by among others, Dr. Samuel Durgin, Chairman of the Board of Health, who, early on, supported school nurses. Comments ranged from too much interference from politicians who asked for favors to appoint their doctor friends, to inadequate examination rooms in the schools.

Dr. Ayer, a former school physician who resigned because of the small salary, maintained that school physicians should be appointed by competitive exam, as were house officers of Boston City Hospital. He noted that although Boston was the first in the nation to give medical examinations in the schools, other cities surpassed them. Boston school doctors performed exams, he argued, in the same way as they did when they started, 16 years ago. Interestingly, he didn't mention the practice of appointing school nurses by competitive exam. Was that not relevant?

131 To Promote Efficiency: Medical Inspection of Schools Discussed. Set of Rules Reported to Be Sent to Health Board. Dr. Scannell Addresses School Physicians. No Extravagance in Fenway. Rules for Physicians. Dr Durgin in Favor. (1909, February 27) *Boston Daily Globe* (1872-1922) p. 8. Retrieved from ProQuest Historical Newspapers Boston Globe (1872-1926). (Document ID: 706456002)

Dr. Durgin continued in the same newspaper article that the Boston School Committee supervised the school nurses. "It is extremely unfortunate that such an arrangement should ever have been allowed.[132]" On the other hand, he noted that since he could not acquire nurses for his own unit, he gladly supported the school department's need for more school nurses. He added whatever work the school nurses did, they did it well. This, in turn, made the doctor's work more valuable. He felt sure that in the future, the two departments would work together in harmony.[133]

Another newspaper article contained comments made by The Boston Association for the Relief and Control of Tuberculosis in an open letter to Dr. Durgin, Chairman of the Board of Health. This letter related that in the city's campaign against tuberculosis, it was most important the school children received a thorough medical inspection to safeguard them from disease, and especially tuberculosis. It emphasized these medical checkups should include teachers and janitors as well as a thorough cleanup of the school buildings. The school physicians should be of the highest quality. All of these undertakings would benefit the entire community, and "we know that it is your desire to make them so," the letter read.[134]

This controversy came to a climax at the Boston School Committee's meeting of December 18, 1911. The Boston Association for the Relief and Control of Tuberculosis sent a letter asking about the present employment arrangement of the school physicians and school nurses. Referring to that arrangement, they asked if it, "works to the best advantage for the health of the children, and if not, which department should control both sets of offices?"

After receiving that searing letter, the Boston School Committee (BSC), at

---

132 School Health Work Is Scored Experts Blame the Politicians. (1911, February 21) p. 1. *Boston Daily Globe (*1872-1922) p. 8. Retrieved from ProQuest Historical Newspapers Boston Globe (1872-1926). (Document ID: 698068152)

133 School Health Work Is Scored Experts Blame the Politicians. (1911, Feb. 21) p. 1. *Boston Daily Globe (*1872-1922) p. 8. Retrieved from ProQuest Historical Newspapers Boston Globe (1872-1926). (Doc. ID: 698068152)

134 Urges Work to Save Children: Appeal to Dr Durgin on Tuberculosis. Association Wants Doctors of High Ability for Schools. Public Help to Resist Political Pressure. (1911, March 14). *Boston Daily Globe (*1872-1922) p. 9. Retrieved October 31, 2009, from ProQuest Historical Newspapers Boston Globe (1872-1926). (Document ID: 698125322).

the very same meeting, ordered the preparation of a bill to develop appropriate legislation to "extend the authority of the School Committee to include the appointment and direction of school physicians, and to authorize the School Committee to make a sufficient appropriation to cover this additional expense." The BSC promptly notified the Boston Association for the Relief and Control of Tuberculosis of the action.[135] At last, they were getting their priorities straight. This dichotomy compromised the health of the school children. As will be seen, it takes time for legislation to move through the Massachusetts Statehouse.

The working arrangement of the school doctor and the school nurse continued to be a cause for concern, as was the lack of follow-up of the children's physical defects. Mayor Fitzgerald brought this concern to light at a conference. They needed more nurses for follow-up work, and they proposed giving charge to the Board of Health (*Would Increase Nurses' Force*). They finally agreed upon a compromise. Since there were 80 doctors and only about 30 nurses, the nurses should try to accompany the school doctor on his school visits, but when this was not possible, the school doctor should leave written instructions for the school nurse regarding the follow-up care needed.[136]

As outlined in Chapter 6, the school nurses were to assist the school doctors and carry out their orders. It made sense for the school doctor to leave a note for the school nurse if she was not there. That takes time, and apparently, was not done consistently. In all likelihood, the school doctor still considered the nurse a handmaiden. The doctors had to change their habits.

There continued to be a call for more school nurses so there would be at least one for each elementary school district. The BSC gave some thought to raising real estate taxes, but they filed this motion in the bottom drawer. Then the Director of School Hygiene and the Business Manager came up with a bright idea. They considered a transfer of expenditures from "Fuel and Light" for the salaries and expenses of nurses. The BSC accepted this and consequently, increased the number

---

135 *Proceedings of the School Committee of the City of Boston* (1911, December 18). p. 184, 212. Retrieved from https://archive.org/stream/proceedingsofsch1911bost#page/n3/mode/2up

136 Agree to Cooperate on School Hygiene. School Nurses Work with Health Board Doctors (1912, May 17) *Boston Daily Globe (*1872-1922) p.13. Retrieved from ProQuest Historical Newspapers Boston Globe (1872-1926). (Document ID:698479532).

of nurses to forty.[137] I hope that no one suffered from a lack of heat and insufficient light as a result of this action.

Duties of the School Nurse

The Annual Report of 1912 reported that each school district had a school nurse. Boston had an enrollment of approximately 110,000 elementary school children. These forty school nurses worked with the medical inspectors who were employed by the Board of Health. The duties of the school nurse were described as mostly educational, as they did not make a diagnosis or treat disease unless they received instructions from the school doctor. During the school day, they offered first aid for accidents and emergencies.[138]

Summary of School Nurses' Reports
For the year September 1912 to June 30, 1913

- Number of new pupils under care of school nurses 16,986
- Number of old pupils under care of school nurses 10,303
- Total number of pupils under care of school nurses 23,379
- Number of new homes visited by school nurses 14,409
- Number of old homes visited by school nurses   12,696
- Total number of homes visited by school nurses 27,105
- Hygiene talks and demonstrations given by nurses 24,975
  - In classrooms 14,869
  - In homes 10,106
- Vision corrected through school nurses 2,160 children
- Hearing corrected through school nurses 335 children
- Teeth corrected through school nurses 9,938 children
- Teeth corrected by family through instruction by school nurses 16,501 children
- Total number having dental defects remedied 26,439 children
- Removal of adenoids secured by school nurses:

---

137 *Proceedings of the School Committee of the City of Boston* (1911, December 18). Page 212. Retrieved from https://archive.org/stream/proceedingsofsch1911bost#page/n3/mode/2up

138 *Annual School Report School Document No. 10.* (1912) Retrieved from https://ia700409.us.archive.org/35/items/annualreport1912bost/annualreport1912bost.pdf.

- At hospital 449
- By family physician 30
- Total adenoid operations 479
- Examination of alleged defective vision secured by nurses:
  - At hospital 2,320 children
  - By family physician 246 children
- Total number having vision tested by medical experts 2,566 children
- Examination of alleged defective hearing secured by nurses:
- At hospital 666 children
- By family physician 19 children
- Total number of defective hearing examined by specialists 685 children
- Medical treatment at hospitals secured for 547 children
- Medical treatment secured from family physicians for 189 children
- Surgical treatment secured at hospitals for 415 children
- Surgical treatment secured from family physicians for 129 children
- Treatment for skin affections secured at hospitals 298 children
- Treatment for skin affections secured from family physicians for 154 children

The report continued praising the nurses for discovering a number of cases of contagious diseases in school and during home visits.

Disease	School	Home
Measles	25	31
Mumps	85	6
Scarlet fever	5	3
Chickenpox	40	5
Diphtheria	15	1
Whooping cough	25	10
Total	**195**	**56**

When a child was sick, the school nurse encouraged the family to take the child to the family doctor. If unable to do this, she urged the family to take the child to a public clinic. At times, the family circumstances, because of other commitments, did not facilitate taking the child themselves to see a medical doctor during the day. When this occurred, if the parent signed a written consent form, the school nurse would accompany the child to the dentist, oculist, clinic, or family doctor, for their appointment. The nurse could continue with any treatments that the child needed in school with written instructions from the doctor and parental permission.

Frequently the nurse visited the classrooms and talked to the children about personal hygiene, the importance of clean air in their homes, and performed toothbrush drills. She was also available to speak at parents' meetings and to visit their homes to demonstrate any special treatments needed for their children's health.[139] We must observe that in the intervening years, the school nurse's responsibilities had not changed since Annie McKay began in 1905, whereas the number of school nurses had increased, and there was more cooperation between the school doctor and the school nurse.

Position Changes

Another individual familiar to us from Chapters 4 and 5 returned to the headlines and came to our attention again. Martha Stark, the Superintendent at IDNA (Instructive District Nursing Association), Annie McKay's former boss, applied in 1911 for the position of head nurse with the Bureau of School Hygiene. The Board of Health chose her for this position one month ago. Dr. Durgin, Chairman of the Board of Health, had selected her for this position said, "He considered Miss Stark an exceptional woman for the position.[140]" Regardless, Mayor John Francis "Honey-Fitz" Fitzgerald refused to approve her selection. Perhaps her reputation, as mentioned in Chapter 5 had followed her (Mayor Fitzgerald was the father of Rose Kennedy and the grandfather of President John F. Kennedy. Years later, as President, John F Kennedy would name the presidential yacht "Honey-Fitz" after his grandfather).

Margaret Carley MD served as the supervising nurse of the Boston school nurses since their inception in 1907 by the Boston School Committee. It is interesting to note that a female doctor became the first supervisor of school nurses. She stepped down in 1911, and Helen McCaffrey, one of the first nurse hires by the Boston School Committee, became the supervising nurse.[141]

Perhaps Carley's presence opened the door for the first female school doctor.

---

139 *Annual School Report School Document No. 10.* (1912) Retrieved from https://ia700409.us.archive.org/35/items/annualreport1912bost/annualreport1912bost.pdf. P. 75-6

140 Rejects Name of Miss Stark. (1911, October 21). *Boston Daily Globe* (1872-1922) p.10. Retrieved from ProQuest Historical Newspapers Boston Globe (1872-1926). (Document ID: 709572252)

141 *Manual of the Public Schools of the City of Boston 1913.* Retrieved from https://archive.org/stream/manualofpublicsc1913bost#page/150/mode/2up Page 50.

The Board of Health offered Elizabeth J. Dadmun, a former Spanish War nurse and a graduate of Tufts Medical School, the position of school doctor. She then became the first woman named to that position. Score one for gender diversity in this male-dominated industry. Surprisingly, she received the same salary as a man in that position, $500 per year.[142] We can also see some progress in pay equity here.

Open Air Classrooms

The practice of having open air classrooms developed in response to the continuing threat of tuberculosis (TB), as mentioned in Chapter 4. In the early 20th century, researchers knew the cause of tuberculosis, but the cure still eluded them. Since 1853, when the death rate from consumption in Boston was at its highest at 48.16 per 10,000 of the population, the death rate had decreased to 17.73 per 10,000, resulting in about 1,122 deaths in 1907. By comparison, the death rate from diphtheria and croup was 3.31, about 144 deaths, and scarlet fever was 1.69, about 49 deaths.[143] At a time when there were no immunizations for these diseases and no cures, parents spent long nights watching over their feverish children, bringing down high fevers, holding their children close as they gasped for breath, keeping their airways clear, and encouraging them to drink water. If some of today's parents, who for several reasons refuse to immunize their children would spend just one night with their child suffering from diphtheria, they might change their mind regarding the need for immunizations.

The best advice the medical establishment could give the public about TB was to avoid germs. They did know that under laboratory conditions, ultra-violet light killed the tuberculosis bacillus. Therefore, they assumed that the combination of sunlight and fresh air would be helpful to tuberculosis patients, and consequently, developed this as a treatment. "The medical and nursing literature of the time is replete with calls for light, fresh air – the colder, the better – and a war against dust.[144]" Germany started this treatment in 1904, and it became popular all over Europe. At times it was carried to the extreme.

---

142 Woman Named School Doctor (1911, November 30). *Boston Daily Globe (1872-1922).* p. 1. Retrieved from ProQuest Historical Newspapers Boston Globe (1872-1926). (Document ID:709662252).

143 *Health Department City of Boston* (1907) Boston, MA. Page 44, 51. Boston Municipal Printing Office.

144 Penney, S. (1996). *A Century of Caring the History of the Victorian Order of Nurses for Canada.* Ontario, Canada. VON. Page 31.

In the early winter of 1908, Dr. James J. Minot, President of the Boston Association for the Relief and Control of Tuberculosis, presented the issue of open-air schools to the Boston School Committee (BSC).[145] Not known for making brash decisions, the Boston School Committee responded by establishing a commission of eminent Boston physicians to study this concept further. They used the same tactic as they did when considering employing school nurses in 1906. Thinking ahead, they called upon the Park Commission to work with them on the use of a building in Franklin Park for the experimental class that was now being conducted by the Association in partnership with the Boston School Committee at Parker Hill. That building would no longer be available, and they would be compelled to hold the class in a tent.

Questions arose, however, regarding the use of the building in the park for pre-tubercular children. How would that affect people using that public park for recreational purposes given that part of the building was a library? Was this the purpose envisioned by the city when it developed the parks? The response from the BSC was, "No definition made at any one time is a safe rule for the future.[146]" They were treading in new territory.

An example of proceeding with this innovative thinking was to review the primary responsibility of the Boston School Committee, which was to educate children. Now it was being asked to extend itself to many more responsibilities beyond the three r's. In like manner, the tasks of the Parks Department originally had nothing to do with playgrounds, but now it did.

To sustain this new interpretation, the Boston School Committee stated that any city department should do whatever it could to benefit the community. In this particular case, children's health would be the benefactor, and that would be, of course, a number one priority. As a result of these exchanges, the Parks Department made the necessary changes to the area around the structure, and the Boston School Committee renovated the building in Franklin Park which they would use as a classroom.

The open-air classes were for anemic and delicate children, those who were

---

[145] *Annual School Report School Document No. 8*. (1908) Boston, MA: Pages 56-59, Boston Municipal Printing Office.

[146] *Annual School Report School Document No. 8*. (1908) Boston, MA: Page 58, Boston Municipal Printing Office.

undersized, had nervous disorders, chronic bronchitis, those children returning to school after a long convalescence, or who they considered might develop tuberculosis. The schools would provide medical supervision, dental exams and treatment, and a regular course of study best adapted to students with pre-tuberculosis. The school physician chose them via a referral by the school nurse and teachers. Additionally, the School Committee emphasized to teachers and parents that fresh air in classrooms meant better health for their children because they would be less likely to catch a cold than in an overheated, airless classroom. See the image below - Open Air School in Franklin Park from School Health Department Report, 1921.

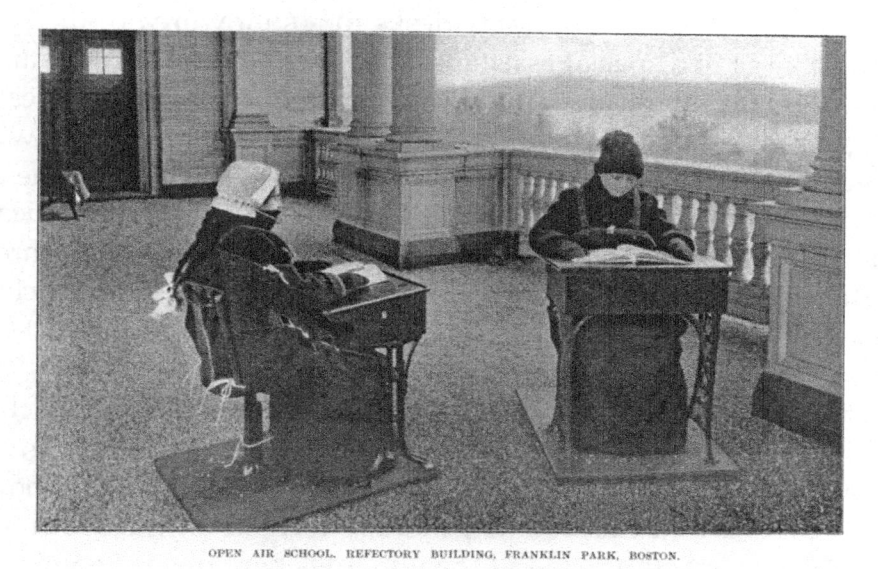

OPEN AIR SCHOOL, REFECTORY BUILDING, FRANKLIN PARK, BOSTON.

Open Air School in Franklin Park

The new open-air classroom opened in sunny Boston on January 18, 1909, the coldest month in the year. When you walked into the school, you saw children seated at desks and seats on moveable platforms. This arrangement allowed children to be moved around ensuring that each child receive the greatest amount of sunshine throughout the day. They divided the daily school program into periods covering rest, physical exercises, breathing exercises, and academics. Each child received from one to five meals of nourishing food per day, costing the child a meager five cents a day, the remainder paid for by the Boston Association for Relief and Control of Tuberculosis.

If you visited the classroom during their academic exercises, you would find the children encased in a canvas bag. Their rest time was from noon to 2 PM, and at that time, they would still be in their canvas bag, rolled in a blanket, on the roof of the building. You could climb up to the roof to say hi where a special shack was built to expose them to more sun. It could accommodate 25 pupils.[147]

Superintendent Stratton D. Brooks gave an example of creating open-air classes from existing schools. The principal of the Prescott Elementary School District experimented in 1909 around the instruction of children who were thin, pale, anemic, and repeatedly absent. He assembled a class of about 20 such children, with the advice and assistance of the school doctor and nurse. During pleasant weather, he seated the class in portable desks in a sunny area of the schoolyard, and under the charge of a special assistant. They carried on their regular academic work in this outdoor class setting. This arrangement showed excellent results as the average weight gain per child in a month was over three pounds for the whole class, some showing a gain of 10 and 11 pounds. Teachers expressed how the children's mental alertness, interest, and voluntary effort had increased dramatically. Also, their attendance improved from 58.3 absentee sessions in the previous three months to only 39 during the experiment. The Superintendent said that much could be accomplished in this regard in the readily available school facilities.[148]

The Boston School Committee yet wanted to renovate existing schools with more open-air plans, having windows that reached from floor to ceiling, and which occupied practically all of the space of one or more of the walls. The *Journal of Outdoor Life* observed that classrooms generally located on the south side of the buildings received more sunlight, and the windows kept open. Though the rooms were to be held at 67 degrees F (19 C), on frigid days the windows had to be closed to maintain that temperature. About five percent of the school population would attend these classes, amounting to around 5,000 pupils.[149]

The class size included about 36 students, about the same as the regular

---

147 *Annual School Report School Document No. 8*. (1908) Boston, MA: Pages 59-60, Boston Municipal Printing Office.

148 *Annual School Report School Document No. 15* (1909) Retrieved from https://ia800205.us.archive.org/6/items/annualreport1909bost/annualreport1909bost.pdf. Page 28-30.

149 *Annual School Report School Document No. 15* (1911) Retrieved from https://archive.org/stream/annualreport1911bost#page/4/mode/2up, Page 15.

classes. The students came from all of the elementary grades. Each day the school nurse performed assessments of clinical measurements, as height, weight, and temperature. They immediately investigated any changes. Results showed the children's appetite improved, they gained weight and slept better at night. It demonstrated that the anemic or pre-tubercular child made as satisfactory school progress on a study program of three hours per day as healthy children ordinarily made on a five-hour program. School nurses visited every home of students enrolled in these classes to give the parents instruction on the best home care for their children.

By 1915, however, they stopped using bags to wrap around the children. These did have some advantages, one being the ease with which the children could get in and out of them. They required no special fittings and were low cost. The disadvantages were the bag deprived the child of freedom of movement, which resulted in not allowing the child to leave his desk unless he got out of the bag. Another drawback was the bag exposed the neck and shoulders to the cold. See the image below - Indoor open-air classroom. The Cotting School, Industrial School for Crippled and Deformed Children.

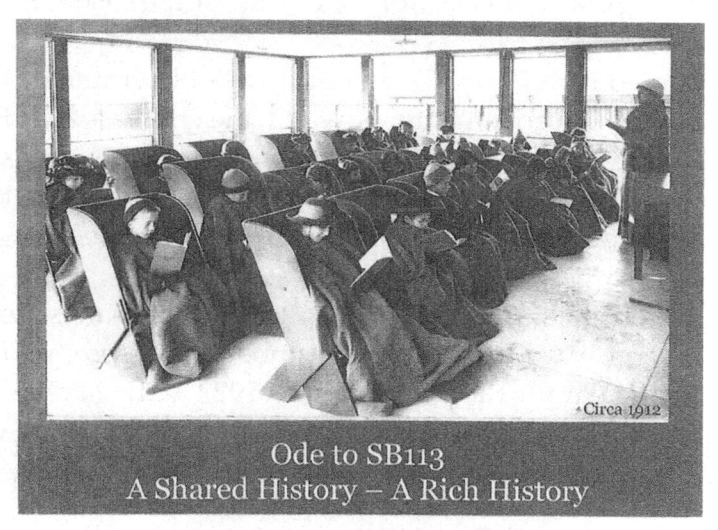

Indoor Open-Air Classroom

Dr. Ayres, whose comments were shared with us earlier in this chapter, said the children collected their special treasures and food in them. Consequently, the Boston schools had stopped using them because they were unable to clean them properly after continuous use. They replaced them with an "Eskimo coat" made of heavy woolen blankets with a hood. Manufacturer's cut the coat large enough to go on over a sweater or heavy jacket.

As readers know, children adapt to new situations more quickly than adults, so students took a certain amount of pride in being able to tolerate the cold environment. The staff just wanted them to be comfortable. When the teachers saw their students sitting in front of them with their teeth chattering, their lips blue, and their knees trembling, they knew they needed to close the windows or give the child another hat. Administrators encouraged teachers to walk up and down the aisles and grasp the students' hands to see how warm or cold they were, and to inquire if they were wearing warm underwear and dry socks.[150]

Boston's Course of Treatment

The child's parents or designate took the student every two weeks to the clinic at the Municipal Tuberculosis Hospital in Mattapan. When the doctor at the clinic declared that the child no longer had the disease, the child then returned to his regular school. At that time, the child would be followed by the school nurse and taken to the clinic at regular intervals for follow-up of the disease.[151]

Not everyone agreed with Boston's strategy. In a book written by Dr. Ernest Hoag, he points out that despite improvements shown by the children, it did not justify, "the return of the child to the indoor class. Relapse may occur," he wrote. "The mere fact that a tubercular tendency exists gives such a child an undeniable right to that type of school which will accomplish most to strengthen his physical defenses.[152]"

The BSC continued its staunch approach to the open-air schools concept for almost 20 years. Between 1914 and 1916 the number of classes stood at 15, servicing 470 students. The peak year for the program was 1922, with 24 classes servicing 690 students. From then on, the number decreased, until 1928, their last year, when they had 12 classes assisting 339 students. However, with the system-wide approach to

---

150   Kingsley, S.C. & Dresslar, F (1916). Open-Air Schools. In Department of the Interior Bureau of Education Bulletin, 1916 No. 23. Retrieved from http://books.google.com

151   *Annual School Report School Doc. No. 8*. (1908) Boston, MA: Page 59, Boston Municipal Printing Office.

152   Hoag, E., & Terman, L. (1914). *Health Work in The Schools*. Retrieved from https://books.google.com/books?id=4Bj9f5T4WnIC&pg=PA198&lpg=PA198&dq

improve the environment in all schools, Superintendent Franklin Dyer admitted as early as 1915, that the future would see the need for these special classes probably eliminated.

In the end, a combination of better health and medical inspections, and improved environmental controls in the schools led officials to conclude they no longer needed the open-air classes. At the same time, they denied admission to school to those students in hospitals and sanitariums who had tuberculosis and kept their hospital classes open. The later advent of antibiotics in 1943 brought cures for tuberculosis. However, the influence on architecture continued as the education community wanted an experience open to the outdoors.

School Nursing Makes the News

"**Guarding the Health** of 110,000 Children. Stupendous Task of 34 School Nurses of Boston-Patience, Tact, and Fortitude Required, and Much of Their Work is at the Children's Homes," shouted the headlines in an article in the *Boston Sunday Globe*, November 2, 1913. We see a swirl of images depicting the various roles the school nurse played- attending to first aid needs in school; taking students to the dentist; escorting a sick child home and instructing parents on health conditions during a home visit. The article tells us a little bit more about the school nurse such as she did not wear a uniform, as did the nurses from the Instructive District Nursing Association (IDNA). She wore street clothes so she would be more accepting to the children and parents. See the image below – School Nurse with Children.

The article gave no school nurse's name, but they do name their supervisor, Miss Helen McCaffey. The reporter relates the story of a seven-year-old girl, Angelina Rocca of the North End who was born with rickets, the result of a lack of vitamin D. If readers are of a certain age, you would remember swallowing two teaspoons of cod liver oil

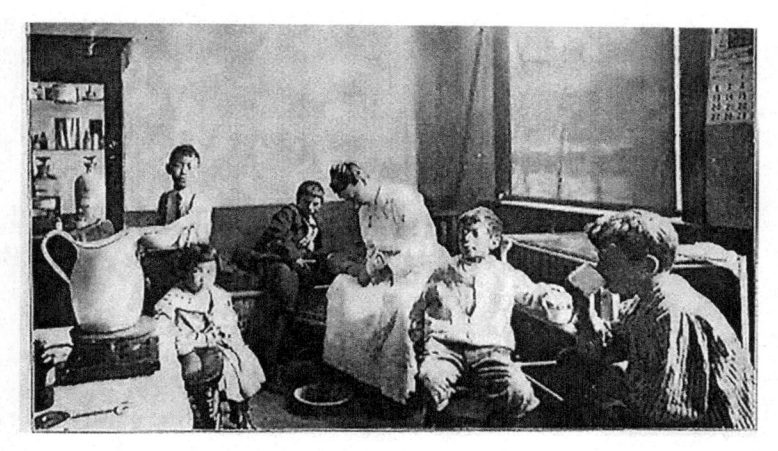

School Nurse with Children

every day as a vitamin D supplement. You would not forget the disagreeable, fishy smell. Angelina could barely walk to school every day because of her deformed and disabled legs. Her small face with her dark Sicilian eyes showed her pain.

The school nurse spoke with her immigrant parents, the father, a hard-working man, about surgery to treat Angelina's condition. She visited the house every day, but Angelina's parents were terrified of their child undergoing an operation in a hospital. After much persistence, and over a period of time, both parents consented. Shortly thereafter, Children's Hospital, admitted Angelina after the nurse brought her there. Fortunately, this story has a marvelous ending. Angelina returned home and within four months walked to school with straight legs and a happy smile as a result of the school nurse's interventions.

The scope of the home visits, the article continues, in addition to good hygiene and preventive health practices, catches one by surprise because it was fundamental to the survival of the family. Techniques taught by school nurses ranged on subjects such as how to operate a stove or range in the kitchen. Many of these mothers from Italy, Russia, Poland, or wherever, were accustomed to cooking for the family in an open fireplace. As a consequence, the school nurse instructed them in the use of a damper on a stove or range so that all of their food was not smoked.

Another part of this article was puzzling. It related that the school nurses were all trained nurses and teachers having passed both exams and were on equal footing with the teachers. Oh, if only that were true. Sadly, it wasn't. There are no documents that claim Boston school nurses took exams to be teachers. The following is a comparison of wages paid[153] to teachers, nurses, and janitors in 1913.

- Janitor $39.29 per week x 52 = $2,043.08 per year.
- Nurse $840.00 per year
- Teachers $1,176.00 per year

This difference in salaries would persist as the Boston school nurses grappled with a cornucopia of issues.

---

153 *City Officials and Employees* 1913 (1914) Boston, MA: p. 243,245,327,328. Boston Municipal Printing Office

The newspaper story continued to say there were not enough of these nurses, and they were overworked. Every school nurse worked with school doctors, visited the schools either in the morning or afternoon to conduct their collective responsibilities, and afterward, still had time to do charity work for the families. These 34 nurses provided Christmas dinners for 983 families, furnished shoes for 74 children, furnished free eyeglasses for 85 children, artificial eyes for 5, and distributed 7,740 toothbrushes to children. That, "work springs wholly from the heart," the article stated. The positive commentary clearly depicted the labors of school nurses but ended saying that despite all of their accomplishments, their account comprises barely two pages in the *Superintendent's Annual Report*. If that had been a private, charitable organization, they would have put out a report, "that would take a week to read.[154]"

Boston School Committee Appoints School Doctors

To form a more perfect relationship between school nurses and school physicians, and better serve the children of Boston, the Boston School Committee appointed their own physicians from a civil service list of doctors as of 1915.

As a result, the new department became more agreeable to everyone, because now a medical director was in charge instead of a layperson. William H. Devine, MD held office hours at the School Committee Building on Monday and Thursday, 11:00 AM to 12:00 noon. Generally, medical director was a part-time position.[155] This unit also included a supervising nurse, one medical inspector of special classes, forty-three school physicians, and forty assistant nurses.[156]

Doctors who worked in the school system fundamentally came from three sectors: the young doctor first starting in practice who needed the extra income,

---

154 Philpott, A. J. Guarding the Health of 110,000 Children. Stupendous Task of 34 School Nurses of Boston Patience, Tact and Fortitude Required, and Much of Their Work is at the Children's Homes. (1913, November 2) *Boston Daily Globe* (1872-1922) p. 61. Retrieved from ProQuest Historical Newspapers Boston Globe (1872-1926). (Document ID: 714248052

155 *Manual of the Public Schools of the City of Boston 1917*. Retrieved from https://archive.org/stream/manualofpublicsc1917bost#page/n5/mode/2u Page 174.

156 *Annual School Report of the Superintendent 1917*. Retrieved from https://archive.org/stream/report1917bost" \l "page/54/mode/2up. Page 51-52.

and hoped he would gain a few patients; the middle-aged doctor who was still struggling to make ends meet in his practice; and the successful doctor who, at an earlier time had needed the money. However, this doctor stayed on as a medical inspector because of the love of the work and did all he could do to help the school. Some sectors had a different perspective on what the school doctor did, saying that given the financial rewards were slim, the physicians ran into a school for a few minutes, asked if any children needed an exam, checked them, and then ran out again.[157]

"Hats off to the old, and coats off to the new," Boston School Superintendent Stratton Brooks said at the end of the year. Meanwhile, the school nurses press on, knowing that they must anticipate and prepare for every eventuality fate throws in their path.

---

157 Kefauver, C.R. (1909, August). Obstacles in the Path of the School Nurse. *The American Journal of Nursing*. P. 815-822. Lippincott Williams & Wilkins. Retrieved from http://www.jstor.org/stable/3403647

Chapter 8

School Nurse State Law 1921

On Tuesday afternoon, May 3, 1921, on the fourth floor of the Massachusetts State House in Boston, Governor Channing H. Cox, surrounded by supporters, signed *An Act Providing for the Appointment of School Nurses in the Public Schools*, called Chapter 357 of the Acts of 1921. Although it would undergo several changes, this critical bill would ultimately affect all the children in the Commonwealth by promoting their health and academic success. Surrounded by supporters, Governor Channing Cox signs school nurse law. See the image of the signing below -Photo from *Boston Globe*.

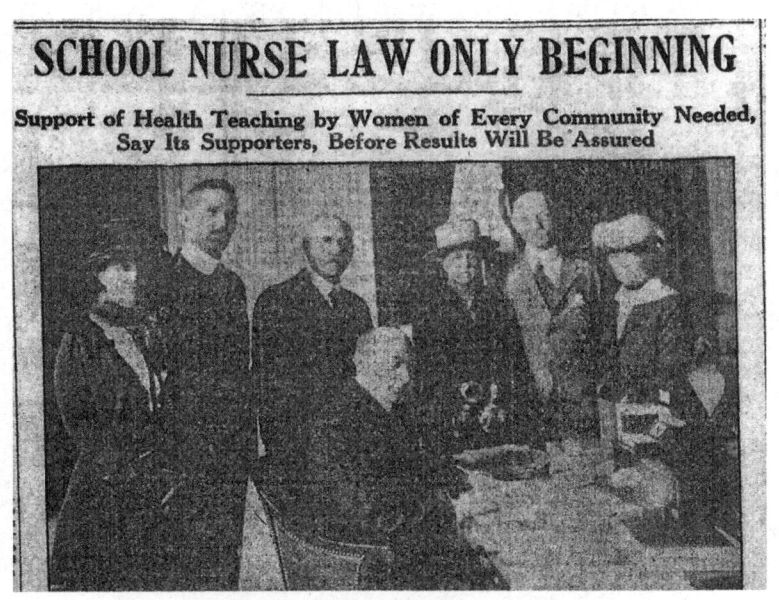

SCHOOL NURSE LAW ONLY BEGINNING

Support of Health Teaching by Women of Every Community Needed, Say Its Supporters, Before Results Will Be Assured

Governor Channing Cox Signs School Nurse Law

On hearing the bills regarding school nurses and physical training were signed, Miss Lucy B. Crain, secretary of the Committee on Physical Training, said it was a five-year battle to get legislation passed for school nurses and physical training. "What we are working for is an adequate health promotion program for our public-school children." Miss Crain continued, "A good physical education law consists of four parts-1. Medical examination, 2. Teaching of simple health habits, 3. Physical training, 4. School nurses." She added, "Now is the time for every woman's club, every Parent-Teacher Association, every child welfare society, to form a school health promotion committee and to see that physical education reaches its maturity in every town.[158]"

Crain then told the story of a school nurse in the city of Cambridge who reported that she had a group of undernourished children. After some research, the nurse found that these children were recent immigrants from Southern Europe, where they kept a cute little goat in their backyard. They gave the children the milk that the goat produced. Now that the family had immigrated to Cambridge, they had nowhere to keep a goat. Goat's milk is full of vitamins A, C, and D, and contains calcium, potassium, and magnesium, which are vital for immunity, all needed to fight the contagious diseases of that time. It offered a bonanza of benefits for the children.

However, they found only cow's milk in Cambridge, which cost $.18 a quart, milk and too pricey for them. Besides, they thought milk was only a drink anyway, and not knowing the nutritional value, they stopped buying it. The school nurse made a home visit and taught the mother the nutritional value of milk. Almost immediately, they noted that when the children started to drink milk, their weight came within the normal range. This anecdote demonstrated the value of having a school nurse.[159]

The Massachusetts School Nurse Law

Massachusetts passed the following School Nurse Law in 1921.

---

158   School Nurse Law Only Beginning: Support of Health Teaching by Women (1921, May 8). *Boston Daily Globe* (1872-1922), p. E6. Retrieved from ProQuest Historical Newspapers Boston Globe (1872-1926). (Doc. ID: 719740152).

159   Ibid.

Be it enacted, etc., as follows:

SECTION 1.

The school committee shall appoint one or more school physicians and nurses, shall assign them to the public schools within its jurisdiction, shall provide them with all proper facilities for the performance of their duties and shall assign one or more physicians to the examination of children who apply for health certificates required by section eighty-seven of chapter one hundred and forty-nine, but in cities where the medical inspection hereinafter prescribed is substantially provided by the board of health, said board shall appoint and assign the school physicians and nurses. The department may exempt towns having a valuation of less than one million dollars from so much of this section as relates to school nurses.

SECTION 2.

A superintendency district formed and conducted under the provisions of section sixty or a superintendency union formed and conducted under the provisions of sections sixty-one to sixty-four, inclusive, may employ one or more school physicians and may employ one or more school nurses; determine the relative amount of service to be rendered by each in each town; fix the compensation of each person so employed; apportion the payment thereof among the several towns; and certify the respective shares to the several town treasurers. A school physician or nurse so employed may be removed by a two-thirds vote of the full membership of the joint committee.

Section 53B- The towns comprised in a superintendency district or union employing, to the satisfaction of the department, one or more school physicians and nurses in accordance with the provisions of section fifty-three A shall be exempt from the provisions of section fifty-three requiring the appointment of such persons.

Approved May 3, 1921.

Now, what are the benefits and drawbacks of this act? To begin with, it requires the appointment of *nurses*, but it does not define what a *nurse* is or what education she should have. As of 1910, trained nurses could use the designation *RN* after their name, and obviously, the legislation omitted this requirement. Because of this, some towns hired a less expensive nurse, namely a *practical nurse*. The program of study for practical nurses can run from three months to a year, as compared to a program for registered nurses, which at that time was two to three years. Another drawback to this law was that it was not mandatory; it was permissive.

Perhaps the most dramatic example of the shortcomings involved towns that had a valuation of less than one million dollars, probably corresponding to their real estate values. Massachusetts omitted these towns from the law. The state made a study of properties to establish the basis of apportionment of State and County taxes. It became House Document No. 1547.[160] Massachusetts did not require the following towns to appoint nurses. As you read through these names, I challenge you, that if you are familiar with one of the municipalities, you might have lived there at one time, worked there, resided a township away, visited relatives there, then try to recall when the town eventually started its school nurse program. Maybe you may want to do a little research!

In 1915, the population of Massachusetts was 3,693,310. There were 355 cities and towns in 1920. Currently, there are 351. The creation of the Quabbin Reservoir in 1938 caused the loss of four municipalities. The total number of towns that were exempted from hiring a school nurse totaled 66 or 5.37%.

In all probability, these were the rural towns in rural districts. Picture the white farmhouse with the attached red barn but whose population could benefit just as much as the city dweller from knowledge and protection of contagious diseases. During the early 20th century, scientists discovered that disease-bearing pathogens, such as found in fecal matter, could be in our drinking water supplies. As a result, communities sought ways to reduce microbial contaminants in water that were causing typhoid, dysentery, and cholera epidemics.[161]

See the list of towns exempted from hiring school nurses on the next page.

---

160   Massachusetts Legislative Documents. House 1401-1589, 1922. p. 2-12.

161   Environmental Protection Agency. (2000, February). *The History of Drinking Water Treatment*. Office of Water (4606). Retrieved from http://www.http://www.epa.gov/ogwdw/consumer/pdf/hist.pdf

TOWNS EXEMPTED FROM HIRING SCHOOL NURSES

COUNTY	NUMBER OF TOWNS	TOWNS EXEMPTED
Barnstable County	3	Eastham, Mashpee, Truro.
Berkshire County	16	Alford, Clarksburg, Egremont, Hancock, Hinsdale, Monterey, Mt. Washington, New Ashford, Otis, Peru, Richmond Sandisfield, Savoy, Tyringham, Washington, Windsor.
Bristol County	1	Berkley.
Dukes County	2	Gay Head, West Tisbury.
Essex County	0	
Franklin County	12	Bernardston, Charlemont, Gill, Hawley, Heath, Leverett, Leyden, Monroe, New Salem, Rowe, Shutesbury, Warwick
Hampden County	6	Granville, Hampden, Holland, Montgomery, Tolland, Wales.
Hampshire County	12	Chesterfield, Cummington, Enfield, Goshen, Greenwich, Middlefield, Pelham, Plainfield, Prescott, Southampton, Westhampton, Werthington
Middlesex County	3	Boxborough, Carlisle, Dunstable.
Nantucket County	0	
Norfolk County	0	
Plymouth County	2	Halifax, Plympton.
Suffolk County	0	
Worcester County	9	Berlin, Bolton, Dana, East Brookfield, Mendon, New Braintree, Oakham, Paxton, Phillipston.

Having school nurses may have led to reduced pollution of streams, produce, and a decontaminated milk supply. Consider the innocent pollution of our streams, the infection of city dwellers through the milk supply, by their fruits and vegetables all washed with polluted water. The water supply of farms from surface wells becomes easily polluted from human excretions. As a result, the contamination of wells became a source of disease. This pollution found its way into milk affecting the lives and health of people many miles away from the source of contamination.

The dangers from bacteria in milk arose from unsanitary collection and storage, which was corrected by pasteurization. It took the licensing by health authorities including inspection and testing of dairies, milk dealers and vendors of milk, for example, milk wagons, to guarantee a clean and safe supply of milk for consumers.

Obtaining Support for the Bill

Characteristically, some supported the legislation, and others did not. A new movement afoot emerged among women, which was changing the face of sports and recreation in Boston. The physical culture movement coincided with societal changes occurring in immigration, industrialization, the development of the modern concept of public health, and the fight for women's suffrage. The last was won in 1920 when Congress passed the 19th Amendment giving women the right to vote. At this moment in time, people began to realize the correlation between their health and diet, which led them to support school nursing. Ellen Richards, the first woman to graduate from MIT in this country, said the food you ate, the air you breathed, and the water you drank, all affected your health.[162]

Another example, of school nursing supporters, was women who in the early 20th century began riding bikes for their recreation and health. A bicycle cost $125, a lot of money at that time. With their restrictive clothing and elaborate hairstyles, it was a challenge for women to ride a bike. They wore long, heavy skirts, tight shoes, and whalebone corsets that displaced vital organs. To join the bicycle craze, they abandoned their old-style clothing and replaced it with clothing adapted for these activities. This new fashion carried over into everyday attire.

Several of the groups who advocated for legislation providing for school nurses, a director of health education, and teaching simple health habits, became allies on a host of other issues. The State Education Committee announced they had obtained the support of 15 organizations. To name a few, the Massachusetts Federation of Teachers, not surprising, the Federation of Women's Church Societies of Somerville, Women's Trade Union League, Massachusetts League of Women Voters, Instructive District Nursing Association (IDNA), and the New England Women's Press Association.[163] It

---

162 Rowbotham, S. (2011). *Dreamers of a New Day: Women Who Invented the Twentieth Century*, 125. Retrieved from https://books.google.com/books?isbn=1844678075

163 Fifteen Organizations to Aid Health Campaign. (1919, November 15). *Boston Daily Globe (1872-1922)*, p. 4. Retrieved November 1, 2009 from ProQuest Historical Newspapers Boston Globe (1872-1926). (Document ID: 720026112).

was heartening to see that our previously mentioned and still relevant IDNA remained interested in the school nursing program through this time.

The Debate

The sharp debate took place in the Senate. Senator Beck of Chelsea said instead of the bill they should give the State Board of Education authorization to establish standards and courses of instruction for teaching of physical training in the public schools. He contended our existing laws could accomplish these changes. On the other hand, Senator Churchill of Amherst spoke in favor of the bill, saying that the original proposal was rather weak, referring to the 1906 law appointing school physicians, and gave no provision for follow up of health problems.

At this point in 1921, schools notified parents of their child's defect or illness, but required no further action. Senator Chamberfield of Springfield, who spoke of the employment of school nurses, said, "If every Senator were to give individual instances of benefits arising through their work, not all would be said in its favor." He did not elaborate. At one point, he said he feared that the inspection of children in the schools might go to the extreme. Then again, Senator Kearney of Boston opposed one portion of the bill that required a child to obtain the permission of the school if he wanted to work. He felt this might present a hardship for the family. Senator Loring of Beverly emphasized, however, that portion of the bill was inserted to protect a child with a heart defect or other serious ailment from engaging in work that would further harm him.[164]

In the House, Representative Webster of Boxford moved to amend the bill to make it mandatory instead of permissive and not applicable to towns with a valuation of less than $3,000,000, instead of the $1,000,000. At the same time, Representative Hinckley of Barnstable declared the bill "unfair, unjust and unnecessary." He added it was "designed to fool women," because it didn't force towns to have a school nurse, but only permitted them to do so.[165]

---

[164] Senate Wrangles on Child Health. (1919, Jun 27). *Boston Daily Globe* (1872-1922), Page 13. Retrieved from http://search.proquest.com/docview/50374747491?

[165] School Nurse Bill Through the House (1921, April 27). *Boston Daily Globe* (1872-1922), p.18. Retrieved from ProQuest Historical Newspapers Boston Globe (1872-1926). (Document ID: 718661972).

Never to be outmaneuvered, the Schoolmasters Club of Massachusetts invited three prominent physicians to speak at their meeting on a blustery winter night, seeking professional advice about the proposed changes in the school health laws. They were Dr. Thomas Harrington, Director of the Department of Hygiene of the Boston Public Schools, Dr. Richard Cabot of Harvard Medical School, and Dr. Thomas Storey, Director of the Department of Hygiene of the College of the City of New York. All agreed that teachers, rather than school doctors or school nurses, should teach the pedagogy of good health habits in school. Dr. Cabot added, "Janitors also have a vital part to play in the problem."

Cabot declared that the school nurses, if you can call them that, for he felt that a better name was needed, demanded a different type of training for schoolwork, which they didn't receive in the hospitals. Commenting on the medical inspections in schools, he went on to say that the follow up of diagnosed conditions should be treated in school clinics, adding, "If this is not unpleasantly socialistic." He continued that the parents through local hospitals could do the follow-up work, but, "there is a great waste of time and energy in thus following up cases needing treatment.[166]" He had a unique perspective on this issue.

Dr. Cabot suggested that more scientific tests be done to evaluate their better health campaigns, for example, dental treatment for students. What kind of effect would this have on students? Would they be better students as a result of having had that treatment? He wanted answers to these questions.

Commissioner David Snedden, another physician in attendance, agreed that the name "school nurses," should not be used, but something like "health assistants." The State Normal Schools, he thought, should offer a course to give them special instruction (So-called Normal Schools were then used primarily to train teachers). He followed this saying that the State Normal Schools should offer this program shortly, and, undoubtedly, the medical community would oppose it. The article then describes Dr. Cabot looking at him, nodding his head, and smiling. Together, they praised the development of more playgrounds and physical education activities for children to incorporate the teachings of hygiene and preventive medicine.[167]

166   Health of Pupils. Three Physicians Address Schoolmasters' Club. (1915. Feb. 14). *Boston Daily Globe (1872-1922)*. p.13. ProQuest Historical Newspapers Boston Globe (1872-1926). (Doc. ID: 502882686).

167   Ibid.

That exchange of comments was very disheartening, especially since it included Dr. Harrington, who was the Director of the Department of Hygiene, the school nurses' boss. Did the panel take questions afterward? If they did, I would have raised my hand, waved it wildly to be noticed, stood up and asked some pointed questions (One hopes I would be wearing comfortable clothes and not one of those hideous hats).

"Gentleman, is it better for a student to receive in school some dental treatments and education about the proper care of the teeth than hold his jaw in pain during class time because of untreated dental caries, which would eventually lead to the extraction of the tooth? The first school nurse, Annie McKay used the nursing process as school nurses do today: assessment of the health condition, intervention, meaning rendering treatment or medicine, plus importantly follow up, to evaluate the results."

"How would you consider a health assistant, who has had only a course in teaching healthy habits to be able to screen a student with a rash and possible chickenpox? Would the health assistant know how to evaluate the rash? Wouldn't a registered nurse be better qualified to accomplish these tasks?"

"It ought to pass," reported the Ways and Means Committee on the bill, "to safeguard the health of schoolchildren.[168]" (Favor Bill to Safeguard School Children's Health). Today we know that it did, despite the divergent points of view. Over the years, we will witness the changes that are made. Now, let us pick up where we left off, and again follow the early Boston school nurses as they continue their epic journey.

---

[168] Favor Bill to Safeguard School Children's Health. (1919, June 22). *Boston Daily Globe (1872-1922)*, p 7. Retrieved from ProQuest Historical Newspapers Boston Globe (1872-1926). (Document ID: 503734717).

Twentieth Century Milestones

1912 - Children's Bureau established; promotes welfare of children, addresses child labor issues.

1920 - The 19th Amendment to the Constitution was passed, giving women the right to vote.
- Boston Dispensary establishes the "nation's first or nutrition clinic."
- Prohibition Begins

1921 - Massachusetts School Nurse Law passed.
- Boston law requires that milk be pasteurized, decreasing the occurrences of summer diarrhea and dysentery.
- Insulin discovered by Dr. Fredrick Banting.

1923 - "Goldmark Report," Nursing and Nursing Education in the U.S.; criticized the low standards, inadequate financing, and lack of separation of education from service in nursing education; Advocated financial support of university-based schools of nursing.

1924 - Chadwick Clinics for detection of childhood tuberculosis began, became recognized as a world model.

1927 - Hinton serologic test for syphilis, supplants Wasserman test.
- Italian anarchist immigrants Sacco and Vanzetti were sent to the electric chair after a seven-year trial in Boston. Their execution sparked riots in London, Paris, and Germany, helped to reinforce the image of Boston as a hotbed of intolerance and discipline.

1928 - Alexander Fleming discovers penicillin.
- Massachusetts Nurses Association drafts and publishes a code of ethic for nurses in Massachusetts.

Chapter 9

The Beginnings of the Boston Public School Nurses Club

Part One

I am gazing at the eight-foot square painting titled *The Daughters of Edward Darley Boit* by John Singer Sargent. This impressionist portrait can be found in the Art of the Americas Wing, at Boston's Museum of Fine Arts. Painted in 1882, the composition depicts four young girls in the foyer of their elegant Paris apartment: the daughters of American Edward Darley Boit and his wife Mary Louisa Cushing Boit, friends of Mr. Sargent.[169]

At the time, audiences interpreted that the girls had just completed playing a game. Modern interpretations have varied, but I think the portrait depicts the girls, all wearing the same white pinafores, growing in different stages from childhood to adolescence and there are some similarities to the development of the Boston school nurses. The spacing of the subjects indicates some isolation, suggesting the separation of the school nurse from other medical personnel, entirely on her own in the school. The youngest child, four-year-old Julia, sits on the floor, intent on playing with her doll, perhaps interrupted when someone walked into the room, similar to the beginning of school nursing, as they were singularly focused on what they were doing. Eight-year-old Mary Louisa stands to her left, poised, more grown-up, looking straight ahead, seeming to know and understand what her responsibilities are in the 1920s of school nursing. Twelve-year old Jane, and fourteen-year-old Florence stand in the background,

---

169   *Sister Wendy's American Collection*. The Daughters of Edward Darley Boit. Retrieved from: http://www.pbs.org/wgbh/sisterwendy/works/dau.htm

teenagers, much taller, and looking more mature, independent, and self-reliant. They seem to say, "We have it down pat now, though we may not like all of the current aspects of school nursing, and it may not be smooth sailing, we will work to move forward making positive changes for our students and ourselves."

The Boston Public School Nurses Club

The Boston Public School Nurses did move forward, and just like the other school disciplines, formed a club with the permission of the Superintendent of Schools. It would eventually become the *Nurse Faculty Senate*. Early on, it was mostly a social gathering with exchanges about nurses' charity work in the schools. They also sent flowers to their members in cases of illness and bereavement. As time passed, however, they became a dynamic group focusing on promoting student health and academic success, nurse practices, and continuing education.

Polio Epidemic - 1916

As if a harbinger of things to come, an infantile paralysis (polio) epidemic hit the city during the summer of 1916. The question arose whether to open the schools as planned in September. Mayor James Michael Curley declared in *The Globe* he would not be sending his children because of the fear of contagion. Chapter 13 follows the polio epidemics in more detail.

Flu Epidemic 1918

A commentary in the Boston School Committee Minutes for November 1918, gave school nurses Saturdays off "nursing service excused" during November. At first glance, I thought they were giving them a five-day work week, instead of their five-and-one-half day work week, but further perusing proved otherwise. The Boston School Committee had received a communication from the Instructive District Nursing Association (precursor to the Visiting Nurse Association, remember them from Chapters 1, 4, and 5) thanking them for their "public-spirited action shown … In releasing nurses and teachers *to serve the city in fighting the influenza epidemic.*" They noted, "the school nurses were invaluable in rendering skilled care to the very sick patients." They further related the teachers aided in clerical work, and some went into the homes offering care.[170]

---

170 *Proceedings of the School Committee, City of Boston 1918.* p. 128 Retrieved from https://archive.org/details/proceedingsofsch1918bost Page 203.

The *Spanish flu*, as it was sometimes referred to, killed an estimated 50 million people worldwide, more than the 16 million lives lost in WWI. It originally started at an army base at Fort Riley, Kansas the previous spring in March 1918. From there it followed troops across the Atlantic and then arrived back in Boston to incubate in the large sailors' barracks known as the Receiving Ship at Commonwealth Pier on August 27, 1918. Sick sailors first started reporting to sickbay, presenting symptoms of fever, sore throat, and headache. Young stalwart sailors who probably would have preferred to be out carousing said they felt like they "had been beaten all over with a club." Scientists believe the flu triggered an overreaction by the immune system, thus causing the immune system to turn against itself.

As a result, the patient's lungs filled up with fluid, and their skin, deprived of oxygen became mottled and discolored. Many of the afflicted came down with severe nosebleeds. The blood discharged out of their nostrils with such force that the nurses had to skedaddle to avoid the spew of blood. The flu was the primary or first phase of the disease. Many who died expired as a result of secondary infections such as pneumonia, rather than influenza itself.

Quickly, the flu spread among the neighboring military bases. By early September, 63 men had succumbed to the disease. The Massachusetts Department of Health reported to newspapers that an epidemic was on its way and in all likelihood would spread to the civilian population.[171]

Do you remember the Spanish flu affecting the family in the British period drama television series *Downton Abbey*? They did away with one of their characters, sweet, kind, selfless Lavinia Swire, the fiancée of Matthew Crawley, heir to Downton Abbey. Matthew was on the rebound from icy, imperiously delightful, arrogant Lady Mary, who at first rejected him. Lavinia was sitting up in bed talking with her fiancée, and 24 hours later, she was dead. Was that the way it happened or did PBS (Public Broadcasting System) fictionalize the details of the contagion? Doctors have said that some patients did succumb to the disease very quickly. "When a doctor would see a patient really blue, they knew they had this very severe pulmonary disease, and that it predicted death within 24 to 48 hours," explained Michael Osterholm, Director of the University of Minnesota's Center of Infectious Disease Research and Policy.

---

171   *Timeline: Influenza Across America in 1918*. American Experience WGBH. Retrieved from http://www.pbs.org/wgbh/americanexperience/features/timeline/influenza/

The incubation period was one to three days. At the same time, it is highly unlikely that Lavinia would have been the only inhabitant at Downton Abbey to fall victim to the disease since people knew at that time that it was highly contagious and were generally fearful of contracting the Spanish flu.[172]

The Director of Medical Inspection for the Boston Public Schools, Dr. Devine, in 1918, sent no report. In his report to the Superintendent in 1919, he apologized and said he did not have the time. Similarly, there was no *Annual Report of the Superintendent 1918*. It makes sense that this missing account was the first time since 1847 that a statement was absent or misplaced. In times of duress, such as during the flu epidemic, other duties superseded their importance, and they were not composed at all.

Dr. Devine was in charge of the Emergency Hospital at St. John's Seminary in Brighton during the epidemic and remained on duty there for 22 exhausting days. Fourteen Boston school nurses worked right along with him. The school nurses at the hospital gave 223 days of nursing services. Reporting on their work, he said they were "faithful and efficient" and was much indebted to them. (*Annual School Report of the Superintendent 1919*: 95-96). The remaining nurses were said to be either ill themselves or caring for their family members.[173]

School nursing supervisor, Helen McCaffey's report, ending on June 1919, provided more details about the work of the school nurses during the flu epidemic. Fifteen school nurses volunteered their services to the Instructive District Nursing Association (IDNA). While they were working for IDNA, these 15 school nurses made 2,375 home visits to care for the flu victims. Of all the nurses working for IDNA during the pandemic, over 60 percent of them contracted influenza during the epidemic. Sadly, one died.[174]

Imagine these nurses receiving their assignments for the day, hitting the streets with their nurses' bags in hand, donning their masks and stepping into the pestilent

---

172 Stern, M.J. The Worst Pandemic in America. Retrieved from "http://www.washingtonpost.com/dyn/content/article/2007/01/17/AR2007011701113.|

173 *Annual School Report of the Superintendent 1919*. Retrieved from https://archive.org/stream/report1919bost. Page 103.

174 Boston, Massachusetts and the 1918-1919 Influenza Epidemic/The American Influenza Epidemic of 1918: *A digital Encyclopedia* – Google Chrome. Retrieved from www.influenzaarchives.org.

ridden homes. From available records of the time, one of these nurses recalls making nearly 100 home visits and caring for 500 patients. Another nurse cites visiting a home where both the husband and wife were stricken. When, unfortunately, the husband died, a kind doctor treating them brought the wife to his own home to recuperate. "One never to be forgotten day at the height of the epidemic," this same nurse remembered, "it seemed as if all the city was dying, in the homes serious illness, on the streets funeral processions.[175]"

We can all salute these school nurses and doctors who put their own lives at risk for the sake of others. See the image below - Cars lined up on Chester Square to drive nurses to homes during flu epidemic. Photo from the Howard Gotlieb Archival Center, Boston University, IDNA Collection.

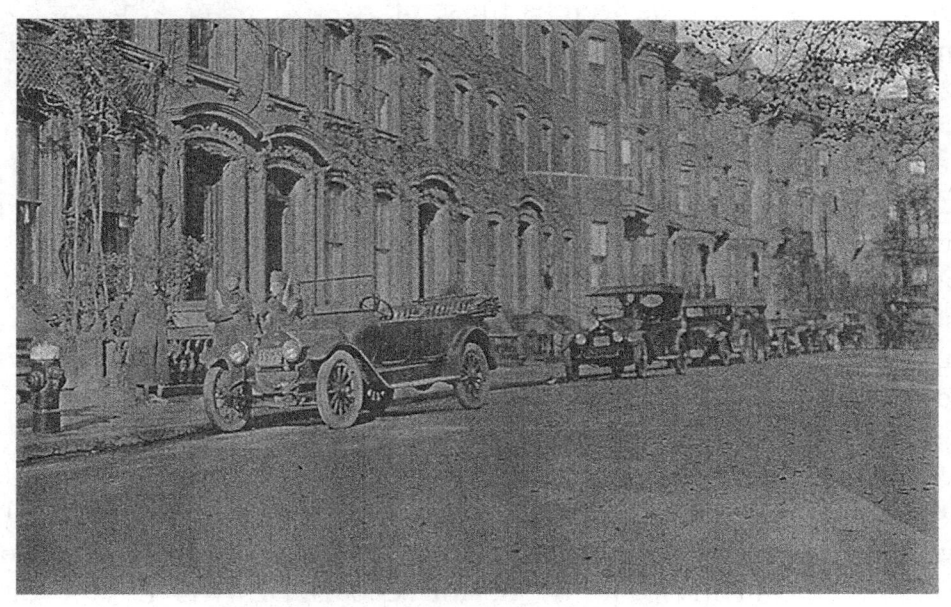

Cars lined up on Chester Square to drive nurses to homes during the flu epidemic

---

175   Boston, Massachusetts and the 1918-1919 Influenza Epidemic/The American Influenza Epidemic of 1918: *A digital Encyclopedia* – Google Chrome. Retrieved from www.influenzaarchives.org.

Shortages of Everything

At this time, shortages became the most significant issue. The First World War, noted earlier in Chapter 2, drained Massachusetts of doctors and nurses called into military service. As an example, there was a scarcity of coal to heat the schools, causing many disruptions.[176] There were bond drives and draft calls for young men as well as doctors. See the image to the right - The Red Cross calls for volunteers. Boston struggled to meet the demands of war as well as those of the community. Dr. Devine referred to the influenza epidemic in September and October of 1918 as the greatest calamity that had hit the city. The Boston Health Department reported on October 3rd that 175 people died within 24 hours, a decrease of 27 deaths from the previous day.[177] During those months 4,023 persons died from the disease. Children did not escape, as 211 children died between the ages of five and fifteen. Newspapers declared the urgent call for nurses.

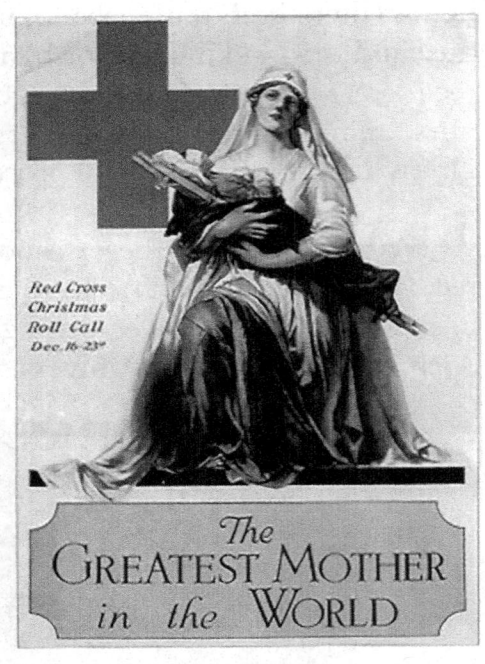

Red Cross Roll Call

Since the epidemic affected so many teachers, staff, children, and their families, Superintendent Frank V. Thompson decided to close the schools on September 25th, two days before Governor Samuel McCall's declaration to close all schools and theatres. The Medical Director for the Boston schools, Dr. W.H. Devine, disagreed. He argued that Boston's 100,00 students were safer in school, where trained nurses could examine them if they fell ill. The Boston schools would remain closed until October 21, 1918. The city permitted Boston's 265 school buildings to be converted to temporary emergency hospitals if needed. School nurses, including other staff,

---

176 See Small Hope of Coal for Schools (1918, February 19). *Boston Daily Globe* (1872-1922) p. 8. Retrieved from ProQuest Historical Newspapers Boston Globe (1872-1926).

177 Grippe Toll Drops to 170 in Boston (1918, October 8). *Boston Daily Globe* (1872-1922). Page 1. Retrieved from ProQuest Historical Newspapers Boston Globe (1872-1926). (Document ID: 719336222)

were paid their regular salary if they engaged in relief work to aid the city's nurses in combating the epidemic.[178]

As with all questions about the Spanish flu, we should not come to a quick and easy answer but should mull over the issue of school closings. Not all cities followed the example of Boston by closing the schools. For instance, New York City's Health Commissioner, Dr. Royal S. Copeland, found that following the practice of quarantine and isolation during the influenza pandemic kept it under control. The New York City Board of Health deemed it a "reportable disease," thus requiring physicians to isolate and home quarantine infected individuals. With the help of the teachers referring children with suspicious symptoms, the New York City school doctors and nurses then carried out their thorough, routine medical inspections. Doctors and nurses sent feverish children home with someone from the health department who could check the status of the students' family. Nevertheless, New York City considered it wiser to keep the children in school, under supervision, than have them playing in the streets. However, people were still fearful of sending their children to school because they were afraid of acquiring an infection.

In the long run, near the beginning of October, to gain a better handle on just how bad the epidemic situation was, the Massachusetts Department of Health made influenza a reportable disease, effective Oct 2, 1918.[179]

We can draw some similarities to the 2020 coronavirus pandemic where Boston as of April 9, 2020 has 1,877 total cases and 15 coronavirus related deaths. The schools are closed, as well as all non-essential businesses; all residents are to stay at home, wear a cloth mask when while they are outside their homes, observe social distancing, hand washing, and a curfew. We hope these measures will see the virus decline.

Nurses Club in the News

They must have had mixed emotions to find their name in the newspapers, but this is the first mention of the Boston Public School Nurses Club in the news. School nurses asked for a raise in salary, which they would do time and again. In their

---

[178] Boston, Massachusetts and the 1918-1919 Influenza Epidemic/The American Influenza Epidemic of 1918: *A digital Encyclopedia* – Google Chrome. Retrieved from www.influenzaarchives.org.

[179] Ibid.

petition put before the Boston School Committee (BSC) in October 1919, President of the Club Alma Taylor cited the current starting salary of Boston school nurses as $804 and the maximum salary as $1,092. Taylor compared that to the starting wages for school nurses in neighboring Brookline at $1,638 and Brockton at $1,200. Did the BSC feel that school nurses should receive only emotional gratification when they provided service caring for students and the school community?

At the same time, the teachers also asked for an increase in salary, citing the current feelings of unrest and discouragement in their ranks. In their remarks, they requested, "a salary schedule that would provide a decent living.[180]"

In the meantime, the Boston police, a mostly Irish American force fostered economic problems of their own. They alleged their salaries had not kept up with the inflation after WWI. Additionally, they demanded shorter hours, higher pay, and better working conditions. New phrases like collective bargaining appeared, and after seeing the results of the workers' revolution in Russia, Americans were suspicious of unions. As a result, Boston's Police Commissioner Edwin U. Curtis refused to support a police union acting on behalf of the policemen and suspended the leaders from the force in August 1919.

Subsequently, 1,100 policemen declared a strike in September 1919, resulting in street riots. This strike proved to be a critical juncture for Governor Calvin Coolidge. Immediately, he sprang into action and deployed the Massachusetts Guard that dissipated the striking police action. Coolidge did not rehire the striking policemen. They lost their jobs. Instead, he gave the jobs to returning veterans, granting them higher pay, additional holidays, and free uniforms. He commented to the head of the American Federation of Labor, Samuel Gompers, "There is no right to strike against the public safety by anybody, anywhere, any time."

Coolidge's strong response to the striking policemen brought about a decline in union membership, and most work stoppages across the country after the war were unsuccessful.[181] His reaction to the strike enhanced John Calvin Coolidge's

---

180 Teachers Ask Quick Action on Salaries; Want Money Authorized at Special Session School Nurses Also Come Forward with Request for Raise. (1919, October 21). *Boston Daily Globe (*1872-1922) p. 3. Retrieved from ProQuest Historical Newspapers Boston Globe (1872-1926). (Doc. ID: 719890102).

181 United States History Boston Police Strike.

political career as he rose to become the 30th President of the United States in 1923.

I wonder what effect this event had on the school nurses. Would they retreat from their endeavors to gain professional recognition and a five-day workweek for themselves? No write-ups appeared in the newspapers or journals, but it would be understandable at this point if some nurses were filled with mixed emotions: how to reconcile the ideal of selfless service with the necessity of making a living. The nurses did continue on. Earlier in the year, they asked for a pension privilege upon honorably retiring. The school nurses called attention to the fact they were "engaged in supervising the health of the school children in teaching proper methods of cleanliness, health, and hygiene every day and they feel that they may be looked upon as teachers of a kind." The Boston School Committee placed it on file. However, the Boston Teachers Club sent a letter endorsing their request for a pension, which the teachers acquired in 1908.

It is interesting to note the initial educational requirement for teachers. The Boston School Committee appointed inexperienced teachers directly after graduation from a two-year Normal School course giving them a minimum salary of $696. They supplemented this salary by one full year of training in classroom teaching under the supervision of the Department of Practice and Training.[182] Is that so different from the requirements for a school nurse, which were graduation from a hospital or similar institution after studying nursing for at least two years? As will be noted in future chapters, the nurses will request changes in the educational requirements that will more closely follow those of schoolteachers.

Part Two - The Roaring 1920s

As the War to End All Wars came to a close, a new American era emerged, known as the Roaring 20s. Flappers danced to music dominated by jazz and the blues. Traveling dance bands played all over the U.S. The economy boomed, and parties were plentiful despite prohibition. The 1924 Immigration Act halted European immigration and increased migration from the South and the Caribbean. Toward the end of the decade, the 1929 stock market crash marked the beginning of the

---

182 Osgood, R.L. (1989). *History of Special Education in The Boston Public Schools to 1945* (Doctoral dissertation). Claremont, CA: Claremont Graduate School Press

Great Depression, covering a period till 1941, inflicting massive unemployment, bank failures, and hardship on the American people.

Amidst these ongoing events, the school nurses carved their path. Another flu epidemic hit the city in 1920, calling again on the school nurses to augment the ranks of the Instructive District Nursing Association (IDNA). Twelve public school nurses came to the rescue and volunteered their time. Mayor Peters, citing the shortage of nurses, called all city departments to release their automobiles to health officials to transport nurses visiting the sick. In Roslindale, school nurses were transported through the snow using two sleigh barges.[183]

Equal Pay for Equal Work

The new decade heralded an anticipated raise for the schoolteachers of Boston in January 1920. For the first time, salary increases included the school nurses. *The Boston Daily Globe* reported that three-fourths of the teachers would receive $384 more than they did in 1919 or an addition of $32 per month.[184] The Boston School Committee appointed teachers of various ranks on what was called a graduated salary scale, which began at a fixed minimum wage and progressed by annual increments of different amounts for different levels until they reached the fixed maximum salary.

Another article later in the year compared the salaries of New York City 7th and 8th- grade teachers, who received $3,250 a year as compared to the maximum of $1,750 for Boston schoolteachers (Boston Has 115,000 School Children[185]). Apparently, the comparison with New York City teacher salaries made a difference because the teachers, doctors, and nurses would receive another raise in September 1921.

---

183 Decrease Reported in Influenza Deaths: Mayor Asks Use of all Possible City Autos Shortage of Nurses Brings Appeal for Release from Private Work. (1920, February 6). *Boston Daily Globe (1872-1922)*, p.3. Retrieved from ProQuest Historical Newspapers Boston Globe (1872-1926). (Document ID: 720155142).

184 Fix Teachers' Pay Under New Schedule: School Nurses' Pensions Plan Laid Over Corcoran Tells Committee Action Bars Bill for This Year. (1920, January 6). *Boston Daily Globe* (1872-1922), p. 16. Retrieved from ProQuest Historical Newspapers Boston Globe (1872-1926). (Document ID: 720123562).

185 Boston Has 115,000 School Children (1920, September 9). *Boston Daily Globe* (1872-1922), p 12. Retrieved from http://search.proquest.com/docview/

New Salary Schedule[186] for Teachers, Nurses, and Doctors in 1920 and 1921

First Year		Annual Increment		Maximum	
1920	1921	1920	1921	1920	1921
Salaries Supervising nurse					
$1,740	$1,956	$120	$120	$1,980	$2,096
School Nurses					
$1,080	$1,296	$96	$96	$1,368	$1,584
Teachers: Asst. to Masters					
$1,980		$120		$2,820	
Grammar school					
$1,080	$1,788	$96	$96	$1,752	$1,980
Medical Director					
$3,300	$3,516				
School Physicians					
$804	$900				
School Physicians Assigned to Certificating Office					
$1,200	$1,296				

Unfortunately, the Boston School Committee denied the request for school nurse pensions later in the year, but they received support for their application from the Boston Teachers Club, which lifted their spirits. Another new problem unfolded, that of equal pay for equal work, becoming a contentious, hot issue sadly, over decades. As has been pointed out, all the rules and regulations that affected Boston female teachers similarly applied to school nurses, as ordered by

---

186 *Proceedings of the School Committee, City of Boston 1920* p. 122. Retrieved from https://archive.org/stream/proceedingsofsch1920bost#page/n3/mode/2up *Proceedings of the School Committee, City of Boston 1921* p. 263. Retrieved from https://archive.org/stream/proceedingsofsch1921bost#page/n3/mode/2up

Superintendent Stratton D. Brooks in 1907. Not that men were waiting in line to be school nurses in the 1920s, but for school nurses, this practice was more a matter of discrimination against women.

The Boston School Committee (BSC) received several letters of support from various school clubs wishing to go on record as endorsing the petition of the Boston Women High School Teachers for equal pay for equal work. The Teachers' Club reported that they voted unanimously to approve the appeal of the women high schoolteachers, which requested the abolition of sex discrimination to the apportionment of salaries.[187] There were 91 different categories of teaching positions, 35 different salary grades, and 50 different administrative titles and salary grades. All of these categories resulted in an incredibly complex school personnel structure. However, considering Boston during this era, the female schoolteachers were ahead of their time. Bridging the salary gap never occurred to the BSC, and additionally, they were not visionaries. As a result, the BSC filed it in their bottom drawer.

They had many reasons for this. The Schoolmen's Economic Association exerted a powerful force to maintain high salaries for men. Their arguments reflected those of their New York City counterparts that men commanded more money in the marketplace than women. They asserted that boys required male role models. Also, if women were paid the same as men, it might dissuade them from getting married and raising a family. Yet, California female teachers won equal pay in 1870, eighty years before Boston. Following that, New York City teachers won salary equality in 1911 after only two decades of promoting their cause with local politicians. By 1925, most American cities paid the same salaries to men and women teachers who performed comparable jobs.

The obstacle against equalized pay in Boston for female teachers arose from a coalition of Yankee and Irish Catholic conservatives. They believed that men should receive a higher salary than women. Hence, they held the traditional Catholic view of the time that women should marry, stay home, and raise children.[188] Accordingly, this view also applied to school nurses.

---

187   *Proceedings of the School Committee, City of Boston 1920* Pages 35,69. Retrieved from https://archive.org/stream/proceedingsofsch1920bost#page/n3/mode/2up

188   Cronin, JM. (2008). *Reforming Boston Schools, 1930-2006: Overcoming Corruption and Racial Segregation*. New York: Palgrave Macmillan, Page 42.

Often, one individual steps forward, despite opposition and becomes a champion of the downtrodden. In this instance, a member of the Boston School Committee, physical education enthusiast Joseph Lee argued, "it was bad policy to force young women to make an absolute choice between teaching and marriage.[189]" Lee, a longtime supporter of school nurses and physical education, appeared in the photo at the signing of the bill appointing nurses in the Massachusetts schools in 1921 (See Chapter 8). Recall, whatever applied to teachers, correlated to school nurses.

Recently, I met a former Boston high school teacher at a Framingham State University alumni event. Despite being from the class of 1944, this spirited 90 plus gal, Virginia W. arrived at the event using the MBTA, even changing lines at the Park Street station. She had taught home economics at the old Jamaica Plain High School, now condominiums, and recalls making a choice for a career rather than marriage. However, after teaching for 26 years, she decided she had enough, choosing then to retire and get married.

Boston has a mixed history in its approach to the fairer sex. Though Boston opened America's first free public school, the Mather, located in Dorchester in 1639, it only served boys. The town elders voted against allowing girls to attend school. Almost a century and a half transpired before they permitted girls to attend the Mather in 1784, and then only from June to October. The Mather School, its descendent, continues to this day. To illustrate another example, the city first elected women to the Boston School Committee in 1874, but the Board voted not to seat them. Furthermore, the court sustained the Board. It was not until the legislature passed a law that year declaring a woman eligible to sit on the Board, that they accepted them.[190]

In Massachusetts, this issue of equal rights would march through numerous statewide referendums, even allegations of a corrupt school committee, but finally, in 1953, Boston passed a new statewide teacher tenure law allowing women to continue teaching after marriage. Not until 1957, did Massachusetts, however, authorize a single salary scale for all teachers, regardless of sex, years behind

---

189   Ibid. Page 40.

190   Review of Boston Schools. Past and present, with some reflections on their characters and characteristics. (1924). [Review of *BOSTON SCHOOLS. Past and present, with some reflections on their characters and characteristics*]. *The Journal of Education*, 99(9) (2469), 248–248. Retrieved from http://www.jstor.org/stable/42749793

other states. This simmering dispute, pitting female schoolteachers against male schoolteachers and their supporters, and how it involved school nurses will be followed more closely in future chapters.

Nursing Shortage

The newspapers in the 1920s post war era ran stories disclosing that never had there been such a shortage of nurses in America. Some of the smaller hospitals were forced to close down because of the lack of nurses. Miss M. L. Wakefield, who was in charge of nurses at Children's Hospital, Boston, said during the war, patriotism sparked an interest in the profession. However, she said, "people during the past dozen months have grown intensely weary of everything connected with war. They have become more pleasure seeking, and they do not turn to a line of work, which makes such demands when other work is available, which offers them more freedom." The Nursing Division of the American Red Cross and other nursing organizations planned a campaign to demonstrate all the opportunities open to women who became professional nurses.[191]

Symptomatic of the nursing shortage, to encourage more applicants, Boston school nurses requested a change in the qualifications for the school nurse exam. They wanted to add wording to the effect of: *Nurse or at least six months experience in school nursing*, removing from the qualifications they would be required to take a course in public school nursing. Then it would read: *Evidence of graduation from a hospital or similar institution giving a course of instruction in nursing at least two years in length; and completion of a course in public school nursing conducted under the direction of the board of superintendents or at least six months experience in school nursing*. In response, the Boston School Committee agreed to make the changes.[192]

School Nurses Work with Diphtheria Prevention

School nurses again participated in conquering communicable diseases. The year 1922

---

191   Thousands of Nurses Needed (1920, August 15). *Boston Daily Globe (*1872-1922) p.33 Retrieved from ProQuest Historical Newspapers Boston Globe (1872-1926). (Document ID:504006211?accountid=9675)

192   *Proceedings of the School Committee, City of Boston 1920* p. 122. Retrieved from https://archive.org/stream/proceedingsofsch1920bost#page/n3/mode/2up Page 205.

brought an invigorating fight against diphtheria, with the use of the Schick test, a new tool of preventative medicine. Diphtheria is a contagious disease caused by bacteria and characterized by fever, swollen glands, and the formation of a false membrane in the air passages, especially the throat, where it causes breathing difficulty. It is communicated to others by coughing or sneezing. Death occurs in 5-10 percent of people infected with diphtheria. In children under 5 years of age and adults over 40 years of age, the fatality rate rose to a whopping 20 percent.

In 1913, Dr. Bela Schick, a Vienna, Austrian scientist, developed a test to determine if a person had acquired some immunity to diphtheria after being exposed to those bacteria. When the patient developed a reddening and slight swelling at the site of the Schick injection test, it indicated the person had not been exposed to diphtheria and was called a positive reaction. On the other hand, a negative response to the Schick test indicated that the person had previously been exposed to diphtheria and had developed immunity to the disease. Those children and adults that had a positive Schick test were immunized with a safe antitoxin.

Dr. Schick arrived in Boston for a week's visit on February 7, 1923. [193]" Dr. Schick spoke to the assembled doctors and nurses at a dinner given in his honor, providing a detailed explanation of the steps leading to his discovery. However, the newspaper reported "his pronunciation of English is so imperfect that little of it could be understood.[194]" In today's politically correct climate, would that commentary have been made about a distinguished, internationally respected scientist?

Health officials reported in February 1923, about half of the children receiving the Schick test were found to be immune, and not one child who was previously declared immune subsequently caught the disease. In the past 68 working days, Boston Health officials had treated 30,000 children who showed a positive Schick test with the three injections of the toxin-antitoxin mixture. They reduced the diphtheria mortality rate from 25 deaths per 100,000 to 13 in that short amount of time.[195]

---

193 Austrian Pasteur Tendered Banquet. (1923, Feb 09). *Boston Daily Globe (1923-1927)*, p.9. Retrieved from http://search.proquest.com/docview/497137924?accountid=9675

194 Ibid.

195 Schick Tests Whole School. (1923, Feb 07). *Boston Daily Globe (1923-1927)*, p.12. Retrieved from http://search.proquest.com/docview/497183494?accountid=9675
https://archive.org/stream/proceedingsofsch1924bost#page/n5/mode/2up

As time progressed, many more children received the Schick tests, and by February 1924, the Boston School Committee opened a campaign offering Schick tests in the Boston schools with the written consent of parents, backed by the Boston Health Department and the assistance of school nurses. Because of an interesting chain of circumstances along the way, it became challenging for the school nurses to obtain parental signed consents. Newspapers shouted in huge headlines that 19 students at Concord Academy and 25 students at McElwain School in Bridgewater became ill after receiving the diphtheria vaccine. The students experienced high fevers and swollen arms that turned a dark color. Waiting for an explanation, some deeper complicated reason, doctors who rushed up to see the students revealed that after placing the diphtheria vaccine in an ice chest it became frozen. This altered the previously unknown properties of the serum. Experts had already decided to make changes in the serum.

Dr. Schick, who happened to be visiting New York City, swiftly came to Massachusetts and visited the Concord Academy students. Thankful that the students were not seriously ill, the physicians still ordered the students to remain in bed for several weeks. (Medical treatment has changed since that time. Now a patient is sent home within a week after open-heart surgery and the installation of a pacemaker).

Despite the incident with the frozen serum, Boston Health Commissioner Dr. F. X. Mahoney announced they would go ahead with their Schick test plans in the Boston Public Schools, saying the serum they would use would be absolutely perfect.[196] Without a doubt, I am confident the school nurses made many home visits to give information, reassurance, and put to rest the fears of parents about the serum. Subsequently, after they completed their campaign in the Boston Public Schools, the Boston School Committee (BSC) reported in 1925 that of the 12,004 children who were formerly susceptible to diphtheria, 83 percent now showed immunity to this disease. Both the Boston Health Department and the Boston School Committee expressed their grateful appreciation to the school physicians, the school nurses and the teachers for their assistance and cooperation.[197]

---

196 25 More Victims of Frozen Serum. (1924, Feb 07). *Boston Daily Globe (1923-1927)*, p.1. Retrieved from http://search.proquest.com/docview/497658209?accountid=9675

197 *Proceedings of the School Committee, City of Boston 1925* p. 39. Retrieved from https://archive.org/stream/proceedingsofsch1925bost#page/n43/mode/2up/search/nurses. Page 39.

In addition to their regular salary, the BSC paid seven school physicians an extra $500 for additional services rendered in connection with Schick testing in the Boston Public Schools.[198] They did not mention any other staff who received a bonus.

At a talk in 1928, Dr. Ceconi, Director of the Hygiene Department of the Boston Public Schools, declared that in the future they would omit using the Schick test and from then on would use the diphtheria toxin-antitoxin for all kindergarten and first graders. In the past year and a half, he related, the Boston Public Schools (BPS) had immunized 20,000 children in the primary grades. They planned to continue this arrangement annually so that in eight to ten years, 100 percent of the children would be immunized against diphtheria.

The School Nurse, the Working Child, and the Certificating Office 1920

The year 1920 found Boston Superintendent Frank V. Thompson, with a reputation as a very thoughtful man. With a total school population of 115,000, the number of students exceeded their expectations. Boston experienced a surge in immigration of Italian and Jewish immigrants, and these people settled in Dorchester and East Boston. The school populace consisted of 93,000 elementary pupils, 18,000 high school pupils, and 4,000 in continuation schools, for students who were employed part-time. They had 19 open-air classes with five additional ones planned, and 172 portable schools.[199] Thompson reported the Department of Medical Inspection consisted of one director, one supervising nurse, one medical inspector of special classes, 47 school physicians, and 47 school nurses.

The Superintendent demonstrated concern about the issue of working children, the protection of the working child, and the many entangling regulations and laws. The law that required a physical exam by a doctor for working papers originated in 1910, as mentioned earlier in this chapter, and Chapter 7. This significant law would involve both the school physician and school nurse, because it required establishing the certificating office or what we call today, the working paper clinic, making them a vital part of the school program. However, educational authorities

---

198 *Proceedings of the School Committee, City of Boston 1924*. P. 87. Retrieved from https://archive.org/stream/proceedingsofsch1924bost#page/n5/mode/2up

199 Boston Has 115,000 School Children (1920, September 9). *Boston Daily Globe* (1872-1922), p12. Retrieved from http://search.proquest.com/docview/

proposed these child labor laws because of their concern for the child's loss of an education. In contrast, the health care establishment argued about industries deleterious effect on a child's growth and development.

Doctors' Perspectives on Working Children

As early as 1910, Dr. Thomas F. Harrington, Boston's Director of Hygiene wrote in *The Journal of Education*, "Out of school continued work defeats often the good accomplished in schoolwork and is a positive factor of ill health." He continued to describe the results of an investigation involving 34 Boston school nurses visiting 22,292 homes, where they found many circumstances that could cause ill health among school children. They found a more significant amount of anemic and nervous children among working school children, especially those that toiled inside, as opposed to newsboys who worked outside. One common denominator in all these findings was the presence of tea drinking children, which, in his opinion, caused much of the children's ill health.[200] Remember, Annie McKay talking about the poor dietary habits of the school children in Chapter 5?

He concluded that children were much more prone than adults to suffer ill effects from overwork. He believed children should not be allowed to work under the age of 12 and children attending full sessions in school should not work more than five hours a day, or eight hours on Saturday.

Add to this, the shock of the public to find 29.1 percent of those young men between the ages of 21 and 30 years of age called up by the draft during World War I were rejected on medical grounds. Some of these were correctible defects which if found earlier, could have been treated.[201] These facts brought home to the community the importance of medical inspections in schools, treatment, and the need for follow-up of defects found, all done by the school nurse.

Another Boston physician, Dr. William R. P. Emerson, of Tufts Medical School, expressed his thoughts on growing children as noted in a 1926 article in *The Boston*

---

200 Harrington, T. (1910). Health and Education: Health Indispensable. *The Journal of Education*, 71(11(1771), 300. Retrieved from http://www.jstor/stable/42814402

201 Kort, M. (1984, December) The Delivery of Primary Health Care in American Public Schools. *Journal of School Health*, 54(11), 453-456.

Daily Globe. He believed the five causes that interfered with the growth of children were physical defects, lack of control at home, over fatigue, faulty food habits, and poor health habits.[202] The reader can recall that in Chapter 5, Annie McKay took her students for follow-up exams to the Boston Dispensary associated with Tufts Medical School.

We can summarize from these points of view that the children did not drink milk, which is packed with vitamin D and calcium. As mentioned earlier in this chapter, the law required the pasteurization of milk in 1921. A deficiency of vitamin D in growing children led to rickets. Among other things, the shafts of the long bones eventually become soft from lack of the mineral. They may bend according to the direction in which stress is put on them, thus the curvature of the bone.

Frequently, the family did not serve quality food and had unhealthy eating habits. Cheap fish and beans were the primary proteins of their diet, but they did not get enough of it because it was the most expensive. Green vegetables predominated in the warm months, but in the winter their chief vegetable was the potato. The poor Italians consumed bananas in various stages of decay. The coarsest and cheapest flour baked their bread. Children drank coffee, which contains no nutrients.[203]

The newsboys were in better health than the boys who worked indoors, probably because of poorly ventilated workrooms, and the inhalation of dangerous particles. Children worked long hours, not getting enough sleep that was prejudicial to their health and physical development. It would take several years of health education in the schools and the community before these changes in behaviors became realized.

For these reasons, the school nurse in the certificating office found herself in a unique position, not only due to her technical skills and knowledge. Because of her human insight and empathy, she had the opportunity to advocate and protect those students, perhaps not all physically fit, and provide resources for their families. The school nurse needed to know the critical rules and regulations regarding working children and have a clear understanding of the law. For the first time these children were venturing off from their protected classrooms into the working world.

---

202   Emerson, W. If Your Children Are Growing. (1926, March 28). *Boston Daily Globe* (1923-1927), pp 1. Retrieved from http://search.proquest.com/docview/86078585

203   Cornell, W. (1913). *Health and Medical Inspection of School Children.* Retrieved from Full text of "Health and medical inspection of school children" Page 485.

The History of Child Labor Laws

The United States modeled its child labor laws after those of England's Elizabethan Poor Laws of 1594 and 1601. Specifically, to banish idleness, during the reign of Queen Elizabeth I, they passed laws requiring the children of vagrants to become apprentices, as early as five years of age. Subsequent acts confirmed that children should begin working at 12 unless they had affluent parents. Colonial America patterned their laws for the care of the impoverished after these Elizabethan laws.

On a visit to a Boston factory, George Washington, in the late 1700s, our first president, reported in his diary, "They have 28 looms at work, and 14 girls spinning-children turn the wheels for them.[204]" This passage provides exclusive insight into the factory's workforce where the children functioned in a group, not as apprentices. Another side to the child labor debate declared that it allocated fewer hours to grown men because the children underbid them. This same argument would crop up again during the Depression.

Elizabeth Barrett Browning wrote a powerful and moving poem[205] called *The Cry of the Children* protesting the terrible conditions and exploitation of child labor in England. When *Blackwood's Edinburgh* magazine published it in August 1843, the English people read it extensively. It aroused a cry of protest across the country against the harshness and injustice of the child labor system. Here are a few lines.

> *For, all day, we drag our burden tiring, Through the coal-dark, underground -*
> *Or, all day, we drive the wheels of iron*
> *In the factories, round and round.*
>
> **- Elizabeth Barrett Browning**

Among the states, Massachusetts pioneered the development of child labor

---

204 D'Olier, K. (1914). The School Nurse's Relation to the Child Applying for Working Papers. *The American Journal of Nursing*, 15(2), 106-109. Retrieved from http://www.jstor.org/stable/3404526.

205 Barrett Browning. (1843, August). The Cry of the Children. In *Blackwood's Edinburgh*. Retrieved from http://www.bl.uk/collection-items/elizabeth-barrett-in-blackwoods-edinburgh-magazine#sthash.Y6rjlBpy.dpuf

laws protecting children from exploitation. The earliest law, written in 1836, stated that all children had to attend school at least three months of the year until age 15. In 1860, the General Statutes included an educational requirement for employment that children under 12 working in manufacturing businesses had to attend school 18 weeks in the 12 months preceding the job and the same for the current year. Hours of work for children under 12 were limited to 10 hours a day. The labor laws sought to clarify their definitions in 1909. They defined a "child" or "minor" as a person under 18 years of age, a "young person" one between the ages of 14 and 18, and a "woman" 18 years of age or older.

Over the years the legislature fine-tuned the laws adding in 1914 gold employment certificates for literate minors and gray certificates for illiterate minors, those young people over the age of 14 who were unable to read and write. The latter were required to attend evening school. Employers had to keep copies of these certificates on file.[206]

The Massachusetts Legislature in 1913 empowered the school committee in any city having a population of over 50,000 people to regulate the street trades and their uses by minors between the ages of 12 and 16, 12 for boys and 18 for girls. The law required minors to wear a badge issued by the city, in a conspicuous place while working at their trade. The so-called street trades included selling newspapers on the streets and blacking boots, (shoeshine boys), and as such required the school committee to grant a license to those minors. The regulations prohibited night work, and only permitted work during school hours if the minor possessed an employment certificate.

The Legislature continued to adjust the laws, making school attendance compulsory, and making it mandatory for children under the age of 16, if not employed, to attend school. If the minor between the ages of 16-21 could not read and write, they had to attend an evening school. Working conditions for minors under the age of 16 were limited to an eight-hour day, and a six-day, 48-hour week. For those older, boys under 18 and girls under 21, their job hours were extended to a ten-hour day, a six-day week, and a 54-hour week. Night work was forbidden for children under 16, and between 10:00 PM and 5:00 AM for boys under 18 and girls under 21.

---

206   Union, Women's Educational and Industrial. (2013) p. 116-117. *Training for Store Service*. London: Forgotten Books. (Original work published 1920) United States History, *Boston Police Strike*. Retrieved from http://www.u-s-history.com/

During summer vacations, by 1916, children could be granted employment certificates even though they had not completed the fourth grade if they met other requirements. Once a young woman married, she was exempt from provisions requiring illiterate minors to attend evening school. How would that benefit them?.[207] Though these labor laws protected minors at the time, they had repercussions for Massachusetts' economy later down the road.

Working Minors

Superintendent Thompson, troubled about the welfare and future of these working children, looked at their earnings. A boy of 12 to 14 could earn as much as $8-10 a week as a newsboy while still attending elementary school. A *Boston Globe* at that time cost $.02 per paper. On the other hand, a young man of high school age could earn from $10-15 a week plus his high school education working as an errand or office boy. Young adults whose sole occupations were selling newspapers and magazines could earn from $25-50 a week. Sometimes these hawkers would "own" a corner and supply the pedestrian traffic with daily newspapers and various magazines at busy city intersections. A weekly income of $25 would amount to $1,300 annually, which was equal to the maximum earnings of the school nurse.

These earnings became a wicked enticement for young boys eager to become young men. They contributed their wages to the family income, gained independence at home, and sought the same at school. However, school authorities, before permitting them to leave, required that they follow all the state's educational requirements and school attendance laws. These cases would come to the nurse in the certification office, the student's last stop before leaving school.

The following is one such case reported by Timothy F. Regan, Supervisor of Licensed Minors.[208]

"John S___, age 12, residence Silver St, South Boston, was found on Boston Common, 10 a.m., October 14, 1919, not attending school. He had been selling newspapers together

---

207 *Annual School Report of the Superintendent* 1920. p. 79-80. Retrieved from https://archive.org/stream/report1920bost#page/79/mode/2up.

208 *Annual School Report of the Superintendent 1919.* Retrieved from https://archive.org/stream/report1919bost. Page 82-83.

with John C, and they had in their mutual possession $1.83 received from the selling of newspapers. John S. had not been home to eat or sleep since October 7, and had, during that time, been truant from school and "bunking out," sleeping under stairs in an alley running from Washington St."

To continue this 12-year-old student's story, the reader's flashback is needed to the time when he was first found to be truant. The Boston Public Schools placed John S. in the Disciplinary Day School class on January 30, 1919. Then, because of other complaints, he stood before the Boston Juvenile Court four more times. As a result, he was placed under the care of the State Board of Charities until March 7, 1919, just one week. He appeared in court again in May 1919 and the Court once more placed him under the care of the State Board of Charities. By September 8th, he was assigned to the Disciplinary Day School class only to be absent and truant during eight sessions.[209]

Imagine being the nurse seeing this minor in your office. What thoughts come to you? Through what interesting chain of circumstances did the influence of tradition and family cultures collide as the world changed play its part in this boy's behavior?

Certificating Office

The certification office, a beckoning opportunity for students, became their last stop before leaving their full-time school career. Initially, the office in 1915 was located at 218 Tremont St, but by 1932 it moved to the Continuation School, 25 Warrenton Street, in the area now called Bay Village. Tall, modern apartment buildings have replaced the old brick building. The certification office issued Educational and Employment Certificates and Licenses to minors under 14 years of age, eager to become newsboys, bootblacks, messengers or peddlers. The office performed physical exams daily between the hours of 9 and 11 AM. The school nurse there worked at both the certificating office and the Continuation School.

Once there, the student would meet the school physician and school nurse for a physical exam to determine if he had the strength and ability to do the job for which

---

[209] *Annual School Report of the Superintendent 1919.* Retrieved from https://archive.org/stream/report1919bost. Page 82.

he was applying. Would such a boy, anxious to obtain a certificate, tell the doctor or the nurse about ailments like chest pains when he runs around the park? Given human nature, that remains questionable.

A visit to the certificating office would have run something similar to this example and looking back, this is what could have transpired.

The school nurse, Miss MacN., opens the door to the waiting room. She is a middle-aged woman in her early thirties, with blue-gray eyes, fair, freckled skin, thick, brown, shiny hair styled into a bun, and dressed in a simple, comfortable, below the knee dress. Outside, the snow falls quietly, cold, soft, lacy flakes. She glances upward and exhales as she gazes across at the full room, where every chair is taken, and people lining the walls. They brush the snow off their coats. It is 9:00 A.M. She thinks that we have only two hours to examine all of these students. How can we do a thorough job? There is no use complaining, so I better get started.

Students line up on a first-come, first served bases, removing a number from the spindle with instructions in English, "Take a number from the spindle and please have a seat." Willy C. and family hold the number "1." Consequently, they are the first patients to be seen this day, and we will follow Willy C. through his journey at the certificating office. I wonder if Willy C. considers what the outcome will be when opening the door to the examination room. Will it resemble that of the character Eilis Lacey in John Crowley's romantic drama movie, *Brooklyn*? After departing the ship, and successfully passing through immigration, Eilis opens the door and glimpses a brilliant, radiant light shining around her. She imagines these shafts of light as symbols of a window of opportunity awaiting her. Perhaps he feels the same way.

The student arrives, a school record in hand, showing his age and grade at school. His mother, holding the inevitable baby over her arm, walks in with him. The pastel day dress she is wearing is better than her usual housedress. She seems a little nervous sitting in the folding chair opposite the desk, her ankles crossed demurely. The fashion trend of the day means Willy C. is wearing the obligatory knee-length trousers, heavy knee socks, and a knitted pullover.[210] His school health

---

210   Love to Know. Retrieved from http://childrens-clothing.lovetoknow.com/1920-childrens-fashion-facts.

record lists all of his physical exams, as well as his history of communicable diseases and any particular treatments or operations that he has received. Also, regarding his childhood diseases, the date he contracted them, and whether he suffered from a mild or severe case.[211]

Miss MacN. has witnessed this same scenario over and over again. She speculates if Willy C. realizes he will be working every day for the rest of his life. The combined $20.00 per week from Willy C. and his brother will add handsomely to the family income. She quickly thinks of her salary that includes a $96.00 stipend for working at the certificating office, totaling $1,344.00.[212] The combined income of the two brothers working part-time will amount to a little less than the school nurse's salary. Where is the justice in that? Now stop thinking these radical thoughts and get back to the task at hand, she reminds herself.

Miss MacN. begins Willy C.'s physical exam by verifying his age and grade with his school. She asks him about his schedule, the number of hours he plans to work, reminding all in the room that he could only work until 9:00 PM each night. Following this, she weighs and measures him, checks his eyes with the Snellen eye test card, and tests his hearing with the accumeter. The Snellen eye test chart is used to assess visual acuity. Can the readers remember the letters? While Miss MacN is examining Willy C., she notices his mother squinting at the letters from where she is sitting. She will say something to his mother about that before they leave.

If nurse MacN. finds a problem with his hearing, she could retest his hearing with an Audiometer. An electric audiometer was developed in 1923. (However, the *Superintendents Report of 1929* refers to the new audiometer used for hearing testing. Compared to the results of the previous method used by the teachers, which found that one and a half percent of the students had a hearing defect, the audiometer found eight percent had defective hearing, a far more accurate test. The school nurse receives the referrals for students with defective hearing,

---

211 D'Olier, K. (1914). The School Nurse's Relation to the Child Applying for Working Papers. *The American Journal of Nursing*, 15(2), Page 108. Retrieved from http://www.jstor.org/stable/3404526.

212 *Proceedings of the School Committee, City of Boston 1926* p.153. Retrieved from https://archive.org/stream/proceedingsofsch1926bost#page/152/mode/2up/search/nurse+salaries

rechecks them, and then arranges for their examination by either the school otologist or the family physician if needed.)[213]

There were several well-known methods of testing the hearing by air conduction. For instance, sometimes they used the hearing distance for whispering, finding a big difference between the hearing distance for numbers and that for other words. Also, they contrasted the hearing distance for whispered sounds with that for whispered speech and used tuning forks and a whistle.[214]

Nurse MacN. continues the exam by checking the child's teeth to see if he has decayed first or second teeth and reddened or inflamed gums. "Open your mouth and say 'Ah,' " she says, so that she can observe his pharynx, tonsils, adenoids, and teeth, with the help of a wooden tongue depressor, looking especially for defective nasal breathing, mouth breathing, enlarged lymph glands, and enlarged tonsils. "Do you have any trouble swallowing?" she asks, about the size of the tonsils and the adenoids. "Please say 'l, m, n, o, p.'" Willy C. pronounced the letters clearly without thickness in his speech, ruling out problems with enlarged adenoids and mouth breathing.[215]

After she uses the wooden tongue depressor, she breaks it and places it in a receptacle where at the end of the day the custodians will burn it. This is done for sanitary reasons. She forges ahead checking for goiter, an enlargement of the thyroid gland at the base of the neck, hernia-bulging areas, orthopedic defects, as a curvature of the spine, flat-footedness, and then lastly if he has a scar left from a smallpox vaccination, making the nurse's exam almost complete. Willy C.'s face breaks into a slow smile, and though he enjoys the extra attention, he is glad that this is over.[216]

Unfortunately, it is not over. As Miss MacN. pulls out a book in the desk drawer and smiles kindheartedly, she sits the boy down at the side of her desk. The school

---

213 *Annual School Report of the Superintendent 1929.* Page 273. Retrieved from https://archive.org/stream/report1929bost#page/4/mode/1up

214 Mackenzie, G. (1922) Mixed Forms of Deafness. *Eye, Ear Nose & Throat Monthly Vol. 1&2*, 449. Retrieved from https://books.google.com/books?id=h0IbAQAAMAAJ

215 Ayres, L.P., Ayres-Burgess, M. (1915). *Health Work in the Public Schools Vol. 2*. Cleveland Found. P. 38.

216 Clark, T. (1922, September 8). The School Nurse: Her Duties and Responsibilities. *Public Health Reports* 37(36), 2193-2205. Retrieved from http://www.jstor.org/stable/3404526. Page 2199.

nurse asks him to read some sentences aloud and write some sentences she then reads aloud to him. With rapt, positive attention, Willy C. picks up the pencil, and guides his hand in the swirls of cursive penmanship, completing the task. Another workbook comes out of the drawer, and in this workbook, she asks him to solve some simple math problems. She looks directly at his blue eyes, and says, "Do the best you can, lad."

Nodding his head, and picking up the yellow pencil again, he proceeds with the assignment: $9 \times 6 = \underline{}$; $193 \times 54 = \underline{}$; and so on. As has been pointed out earlier, the student should be capable of reading and writing at the fourth-grade level. One of the teachers generously advised the school nurse what workbooks to use. Thankfully, Willy C. passes these portions of the exam and manages to dart a gaze to his mother, seated in the room.

Next follows an interview with his parent, Mrs. C., as to how she fed Willy C. as an infant, the income and occupations of the family, any older children, and their rent or mortgage. Nurse MacN. mentions to Mrs. C. that she noticed her squinting at the eye chart. Would she have time for an eye test? With her head dipping to her chest, and the baby on her lap starting to fuss, she replies she has no time. The nurse records everything.

Now, it was the doctor's turn, and he must examine the child's heart and lungs using a stethoscope on bare skin. Looking at the boy, he asks, "Now what is it that you want to do?"

The boy replies, "I'm 12 years old. I want to be a newsboy, Sir."

The doctor continues, "Do you feel up to doing this work?"

"Yes, Sir," is the response.

He reviews the child's health record, and if warranted, would have explored other conditions as needed. Since the physician finds no gross defects, Willy C. is well on his way to obtaining his gold educational certificate.

Miss MacN. bids farewell to Willy C. and his family, receiving a big, irresistible smile from the young man. For a fleeting moment, she wonders if in her personal life, she will regret not being on the receiving end of these tender moments.

However, large families with endless work had not been an attraction for her. She envisioned a different life for herself and perhaps would be following the Irish "single blessedness" for a while longer. Nurse MacN. encourages Willy C. to continue with his studies after reaching 16, to see the school nurse if he has any problems and to mind his parents. She looks at Mrs. C. compulsively nodding her head, eager to leave, and walking out of the office. Miss MacN. gazes at the full waiting room, walks over to the desk, and calls number two.

Report of School Nurse Assigned to Certificating Office[217] 1928-1929

Assisted school physician with
   Physical examinations 4,236
   Inspections 6,372
Certificates granted 9,555
   refused 1,053
Inspections of hair 4,236
Consultations with pupils 3,587
Consultations with teachers 771
Hours assisting school physician 559 ½
Treatments given 399
Consultations with parents in office 957
Visits to homes 733

Consultations with
- school nurses 20
- social workers 18
- employers 24
- social agencies 12

Consultations on telephone with agencies 1,247

Assisting physicians of Department of Public Health
   with examination in connection with Ten Year
   Underweight Program 4

---

217 *Annual School Report of the Superintendent 1929.* Pages 144-145. Retrieved from https://archive.org/stream/report1929bost#page/4/mode/1up

Pupils remaining in school as result of follow-up work 52
Money expended from School Nurses' Fund $42
Cases reported to Attendance Department 110
Dental appointments made (approximate) 900
Number having dental work completed 120
Defective vision cases corrected 220
Malnutrition cases under treatment 120
Skin cases under treatment 63
Thyroid cases under treatment 4
Organic heart cases under treatment 24
Tonsil and adenoid operations 61

Pupils escorted to clinics:

Clinic	Number Pupils
Eye	2
Medical	1
Surgical	1
Dental	3
Total	**7**

Following Up on Defects

Dental caries remained the most significant single defect found during the physical exam, according to the report from the Certificating Office. Generally, the nurse referred the student to his dentist or to the Forsyth Dental Infirmary in Boston, which ministered to underserved children. School nurses referred underweight children to the new rest and nutrition classes, started as a result of the Massachusetts State Department of Health "underweight program."

Supervising nurse Miss Helen F. McCaffrey detailed some of the follow-up work of the nurse in the certification office. For instance, the certification office issued eight certificates certifying to the unfitness of a child to work, forwarding them to the Overseers of the Public Welfare. They advised these children to remain in school, and their mothers continued to receive aid. Charitable organizations received referrals from the school nurse in the certification office to place three boys under better living conditions. Another case referral to a benevolent organization requested immediate help, and three other cases applied for clothes from helpful organizations.[218] As noted, the school nurse found it necessary to report these children to charitable organizations to improve their home conditions and provide nourishing food.

In a 1928 address given by Dr. John A. Ceconi, Director of the Hygiene Department of the Boston Public Schools, sponsored by the Boston Health League, Dr. Ceconi said the BPS medical personnel consisted of a director (Dr. Ceconi), 56 school physicians, six supervising school physicians, one sanitary inspector (inspects the school buildings), one otologist, one nutrition specialist, one supervising nurse, three assistant nursing supervisors, and 56 school nurses. He described the school nurses as a "capable and efficient nursing staff" and competent to protect the children in the advent of an explosive outbreak of a communicable disease.[219] He praised the family doctors and dentists who had corrected the many health problems of the students in the city. Though the city provided clinics for the indigent, "in the past two years, more than 50 percent of the physical and dental defects of our children have been corrected by the family physician. The Department of School Hygiene does not advocate nor patronize State medicine.[220]" Apparently, he desired to clarify their position on the treatment component of school health services.

The Roaring 1920s Comes to a Close

The school nurses received an increase in salary in 1926, which undoubtedly lifted their spirits since the Boston School Committee had bypassed them during the last set of increases five years ago.[221]

---

218   *Annual School Report of the Superintendent 1924*.p. 110. Retrieved from https://archive.org/stream/report1924bost#page/110/mode/2up

219   Dr. Ceconi Praises Family Doctors and Dentists. (1928, Jan 31). *Daily Boston Globe (1928-1960)*, p. 25. Retrieved from http://search.proquest.com/docview/747449783?accountid=9675

220   Dr. Ceconi Praises Family Doctors and Dentists. (1928, Jan 31). *Daily Boston Globe (1928-1960)*, p. 25. Retrieved from http://search.proquest.com/docview/747449783?accountid=9675

221   School Nurses Get Pay Boost: Physicians Receive Rise with Flat Salary Minor Adjustments in List Are Made by Committee Several Promotions and Transfers Effected. (1926, June 22). *Boston Daily Globe (1923-1960)*, p.14. Retrieved November 1, 2009, ProQuest Historical Newspapers Boston Globe (1872-1926). (Document ID:1651545802).

New Salary Schedule for Nurses, Teachers, and Physicians in 1926[222]

	First Year	Annual Increment	Maximum
Salaries			
Supervising Nurse	$2,040	$120	$3,000
Asst. Sprvsg. Nurse	$1,824	$96	$2,208
School Nurses	$1,248	$96	$1,920
School Nurse Assigned to Certificating Office	$1,248	$96	$2,112
Teachers:			
Sub Masters: Elementary	$2,016	$144	$3,600
Assistants: Elementary	$1,248	$96	$2,304
Medical Director	$6,060		
School Physicians	$960	$120	$1,200
School Physicians Assigned to Certificating Office			$1,800

Note that the school nurses and teachers had the same salary base, but the teachers had a higher maximum salary.

The Boston school nurses in the early 20th century participated in many historical medical and public health events, including societal changes such as the infantile paralysis epidemic of 1916, the flu epidemics of 1918 and 1920, the nursing

---

[222] *Proceedings of the School Committee, City of Boston 1926* p.153. Retrieved from https://archive.org/stream/proceedingsofsch1926bost#page/152/mode/2up/search/nurse+salaries

shortage, the fight for equal pay for equal work, the battle against exploitation of children, the 1924 war on diphtheria, and all along the way advocating for better health for their students and their families. The school nurses demonstrated not only strong assessment skills and knowledge, but showed excellent communication skills, and had a deep personal understanding of parents and teachers. A new chapter will show how the Boston school nurses and the city itself weathered the Great Depression.

Chapter 10

The Boston Public School Nurses Endure the Depression

The Great Depression and the 1930s

The Depression was a time of financial struggles and hardship. Franklin Delano Roosevelt became the new United States President in 1933, replacing Herbert Hoover. Roosevelt's New Deal brought some relief to Massachusetts in the form of the National Recovery Act of 1933, funding 700 jobs to build three bridges across the Cape Cod Canal. Another example of the New Deal was the Civilian Conservation Corps (CCC), which functioned from 1933 to 1942, providing many jobs for young unemployed, unmarried men from families on relief, to build roads, plant trees, and work on segments of the Appalachian Trail. However, long-established patterns of Yankee self-reliance existed. Mayor James M. Curley of Boston welcomed the public works projects but resisted direct financial relief to impoverished families.

A child film star arrived on the scene, Shirley Temple, with 56 golden ringlets, whose films generated hope and optimism. "It is a splendid thing," said President Franklin D. Roosevelt, "that for just 15 cents an American can go to a movie and look at the smiling face of a baby and forget his troubles."[223] Songs from the Great Depression provided people the opportunity to complain of their lost jobs and

---

223 Brumfield, B. (2014, February 11). Famed former child actress Shirley Temple dies. *CNN Entertainment*. Retrieved from http://www.cnn.com/2014/02/11/showbiz/hollywood-shirley-temple-death/

invisible and unknown future. E.Y. Harberg wrote perhaps one of the most famous songs, "Brother Can You Spare a Dime?"[224]

Boston suffered with the rest of the nation during the Great Depression. Bankruptcies, bank closings, cutbacks, and unemployment besieged the city. "Boston's industrial labor force earned 37 percent less in 1939 than in 1929, and the city lost 25 percent of its jobs as well," stated historians, Richard D. Brown and Jack Tager in their book, *Massachusetts: A Concise History*. By 1939, Boston had an unemployment rate of 19.9 percent.[225] The city's clothing industry alone fired 30% of its employees. Many leather, shoe, and furniture factories relocated to less expensive areas of the country. It was especially hard on those at the bottom levels of society, particularly the immigrants. The unemployment rate of South Boston's Irish population jumped to 33 percent. By 1934, in the North End, with its high concentration of Italians, unemployment had reached 40 percent. The estimate of unemployed people in Boston by October 1932 was 98,000 people, rising to 108,000 by July 1932. Factory shutdowns deprived entire families of jobs and tore the family unit apart.

During the 1930s, manufacturing employees earned about $17.00 per week, averaging $3.40 a day. Doctors earned $61.00 per week.[226] The number of families seeking welfare assistance during 1929-1932 jumped from 7,463 to 40,672.[227] Welfare payments started at $4.00 per week for single men and women and rose to a maximum of $15.00 for a family of seven. A city councilor in 1937 asked to introduce new sarcastic instructions that welfare families receive more than the $40.00 allotted each month for the care and feeding of each Park Department horse.[228]

Children's Hospital reported that many families were unable to pay their bills because of numerous unemployed heads of families. They treated 4,904 ward patients

---

224   *Songs of the Great Depression and the Dust Bowl Migrants*. Retrieved from https://www.loc.gov/item/ihas.200197402/

225   Brown, R., & Tager, J. (2000). *Massachusetts: A Concise History*. Amherst: UMass Press.

226   *Great Depression - The Depression Facts*. Retrieved from http://great-depression-

227   Trout, C. (1977). *Boston: The Great Depression and the New Deal*. New York: Oxford Univ. Press. P. 175.

228   Ibid. P. 361.

in 1933, charging 56 percent substantially reduced rates or no charge at all.[229]

During the 2020 COVID-19 pandemic, more than 22 million Americans lost their jobs in a three-week period. Will 1929 repeat itself?

Nurses During the Great Depression

Boston school nurses were not the only nurses affected by the Depression. Private duty nurses were among the earliest to suffer, simply because people could not afford to hire a nurse for a family member. Therefore, large numbers of private duty nurses were unemployed. As noted earlier, people found they could not pay for the services of physicians, private duty nurses, or hospitals. Officials estimated in 1932, at the height of the depression, between 8,000 and 10,000 nurses of the 230,482 people who identified themselves as professional nurses in the United States searched for work.[230] It came to the point that nurses traveled to other states looking for jobs. However, the employment situation became so intense, concerned nursing organizations placed notices in the *American Journal of Nursing* warning fellow nurses not to come to their state for a job.[231]

Amidst all of the belt-tightening, Boston decided in no way could it increase taxes on an already overburdened populace. They developed a cutback plan for all city and county departments. This plan asked city employees to voluntarily contribute monthly to the Public Welfare Department for the unemployment fund, depending on their salary. If they made $1,600 a year or less, they were asked to contribute one day's wages. Employees receiving from $1,600 to $3,000 a year would contribute two days' pay per month, and all city and county employees who received more than $3,000 per year would contribute three days' salary per month. These voluntary contributions extended over a time period covering five months from November 1931 to June 30, 1932, and raised $237,019.38, and thus, they extended it again to December 31, 1932.

---

229 Children's Hospital Names Abbott Again. (1933, Feb 28). *Daily Boston Globe (1928-1960)*. p. 22. Retrieved from http://search.proquest.com/docview/758523824?accountid=9675

230 *Great Depression - The Depression Facts*. Retrieved from http://great-depression-

231 Brodie, B. (2012). Nurses' Struggles During the Great Depression: Prelude to Professional Status. *Windows in Time* 2(1) 8. Retrieved from Snippets from the past http://go.galegroup.com/ps/i.do?id=GALE%7CA301556280&v=2.1&u=mlin_b_bpublic&it=r&p=AONE&sw=w

This program detracted from the school nurse's salary in the following way. The annual base salary of the school nurse started at $1,248, with a maximum of $1,920. Her contribution, depending on her salary, would be $6 – 8 per month.[232] Should we be surprised that 11 nurses refused to make voluntary contributions? The Boston School Committee found that unacceptable and docked their salaries equal to the amount given by others on that day or days (Welfare Fund Gifts Total $237,019.38).[233] What would the reader do?

Additionally, later in 1932, the school department suspended all annual increments. The nurse's increase amounted to $96[234] In 1932, the poverty level consisted of families and individuals earning $1,500 per year, and the subsistence level comprised those earning $750 per year. However, that included 41% of the population. Those families earning over $10,000 a year and single individuals earning over $5,000 annually, involved only 2.4% of Americans[235] in 1935. The school nurses barely escaped the poverty designation. After a while, the city restored the salary increments[236] in July 1934. At the same time, the Boston School nurses had a lot to be thankful for, i.e., they had a job. Some of them may have supported their extended family.

BPS Nurses Activities During the Great Depression

The Superintendent's Report in 1932 contained another commentary by A. Isabelle Timmons, President, Boston Teachers Club, referring in Biblical terms to the welfare work performed by the school nurses, teachers, and other school staff. To illustrate, "For I was hungry, and you gave me something to eat, I was thirsty, and you gave me something to drink, I was a stranger, and you invited me in, naked, and you

---

232 *Proceedings of the School Committee, City of Boston 1932*. Retrieved from https://archive.org/stream/proceedingsofsch1932bost#page/148/mode/2up/search/teachers p. 117

233 Welfare Fund Gifts Total $237,019.38. (1932, Jul 23). *Daily Boston Globe (1928-1960)* Retrieved from http://search.proquest.com/docview/758433864?accountid=9675

234 Ibid. Page 147-149.

235 Stull, A. A. (2013*). Stories of the children of the Great Depression: What I learned from my parents.* Retrieved from http://lib.dr.iastate.edu/cgi/viewcontent.cgi?article=4589&context=etd

236 *Proceedings of the School Committee, City of Boston 1934*. Retrieved from https://archive.org/stream/proceedingsofsch1934bost#page/200/mode/2up p. 142.

clothed me, I was sick, and you visited me." Matthew 25: 35,36. In no short time, the overriding goal of the school staff became that no child in their care would miss school time as a result of a lack of food or insufficient clothing. The Boston City Council noted every year when the schools opened, the welfare department workers visiting the schools would find children kept home because of inadequate clothing and shoes.

Many schools developed school funds to meet the classrooms situations where children arrived wearing no rain boots in a heavy rainstorm, or as they referred to them as rubbers, or another appeared without wearing a coat on the coldest days, a third one walked in wearing threadbare clothing, a fourth skinny and haggard, and a fifth worried about a home situation. Athletic Associations contributed to the funds as well, while some districts held food sales, movie nights, or asked philanthropic organizations to donate.

The school nurses established the nurses' fund that donated to all elementary and intermediate schools. Every year the nurses held a bridge party where they sold tickets to teachers and friends. They gave the money realized at the event to the districts in proportion to the number of tickets sold from that school district. The money funded many needs of the schools.

The Headmasters from the various schools listed a variety of ways they used the money:

- milk at recess
- nutrition classes including lunch
- eyeglasses
- repair of eyeglasses
- shoes, rubbers, clothing
- medical and dental work including tonsil and adenoid operations
- car fares
- drill uniforms
- graduation outfits
- hair cuts
- derbac combs (a brand of metal comb used to remove head lice)
- coal
- wood
- furniture
- Thanksgiving and Christmas dinners

- rents paid
- gas and electric light bills paid
- loans to families
- weekly allowance to boy or girl so they would not have to leave school
- sewing, dressmaking, and milliner supplies provided in cases where pupils would otherwise have to drop the course
- violin lessons for talented children
- musical instruments purchased
- contributions to welfare organizations
- rented typewriters so pupils might work at home
- Christmas gifts to hospitals
- contributions to mothers unable to work

In 1932, the fund collected $2,612.08.[237] A little goes a long way.

The masters (principals) depended on the school nurses since the school nurses, and attendance officers as well visited the children's homes. Consequently, nurses could advise the principals regarding the proper disbursement of the various funds that came to the schools. All articles of clothing that arrived at the school went directly to the nurse. Before the nurse distributed the clothing to the needy, they cleaned and repaired them when necessary. Each child that received the clothes did not know where they came from, nor did anyone else know the child had received them.

Again, administration asked the principals how many articles they had received, although they counted about 12,000. A more accurate tally amounted to 200,000 articles accepted. Isabelle Timmons further commented, "Many masters have paid high tribute to the splendid work of the nurses within their respective districts. It should be known that we have a group of diligent nurses of whom we are justly proud."[238]

The Life of a Depression-Era Family

This narrative is an example of how one family, the Ahearn's, lived during the Great

---

[237] *Annual School Report of the Superintendent 1932.* Retrieved from https://archive.org/stream/report1932bost#page/14/mode/2up p. 21-22, 27.

[238] Ibid. p. 22.

Depression, as told through the eyes of a young boy in a book he wrote many years later. The family endures many hardships, such as unemployment, loss of self-respect, parental anxiety, and hunger. Food deprivation affected many children during the Depression. As has been noted, the Boston School Department offered several nutrition programs supported by private funds. Additionally, there were the Nurses Fund, free school lunches, and the food pantry. Sadly, for the most part, the benefits system abandoned this family, but other forces intervened and came to their rescue.

Aloysius J. Ahearn wrote the book *From Rags to Patches* about what his life was like growing up in a depression-era family in Boston. This chapter describes his father's unemployment, and the family's financial struggles feeding eight hungry kids. He admits that at times the family didn't eat, at other times they begged for food, and they never had enough money for the necessities of life, never mind the extravagances.[239] They called him Little Al. He grew up as the oldest of eight children living through the Great Depression with his father, Felix, mother, Anna, and seven siblings. Some of the details, of course, he didn't know, but over the years, his Mom and Dad elaborated on their comments.

Little Al recalls the one person who brought a smile to his father's face, a faraway look to his eye, followed by "Ah, that was a great man" was surprisingly not Franklin Delano Roosevelt, nor the revered Winston Churchill, but a Mayor of Boston, the legendary James Michael Curley. Curley rose in life from humble beginnings emerging as the mayor, a congressman, and governor of Massachusetts.

This incident in 1935 finds the family on welfare, living in a rented tenement on Moreland Street, Roxbury. Felix remained unemployed and trying to feed eight hungry kids. For the past three days, they had nothing

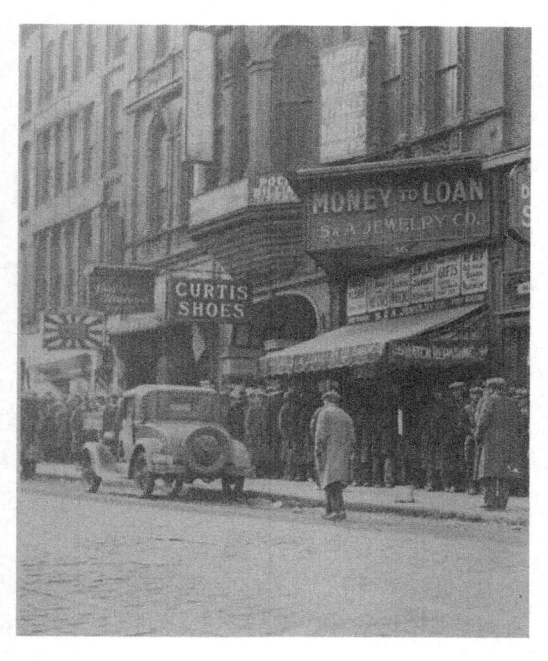

---

[239] Ahearn, A. (2007). *From Rags to Patches Growing up in Boston during the Great Depression.* U.S.A.: Booklocker.com Inc.

to eat but a concoction of boiled molasses and onions to fill their belly's, stoically waiting for the most important day of the week, Tuesday, welfare payment day. Even though they received welfare, Felix searched for work every day, but found no jobs for carpenters nor anything else.

Tuesday came, and Felix proceeded to the welfare office in Mission Hill on a cold, blustery, November day to collect his $12 a week. However, Felix arrived before the office opened at 9:00 AM, and already about 75 men queued up in line, jumping up and down, rubbing their arms together, and pulling their hats down over their ears. So, he decided to pop into the tavern across the street for a quick nickel beer to stay warm. Though Felix hocked his watch for cash some time ago, he estimated that he had enough time to return to the line after drinking his beverage, which he did. I don't understand how a cold beer can warm a person on a frosty winter's day, but somehow it did for Felix Ahearn. See the image above. A bread line in Boston's North End 1931 (Photo courtesy of Photo Library at Boston Public Library).

Finding the line moved at a moderate pace, Felix Ahearn advanced to the pay window in 30 minutes. However, when he arrived, the female city worker, Miss Jones, staunchly informed him that "Ahearn," since it started with an "A," meant that he should have been at the head of the line.

"Well, you missed your place in line…You are on the list…and you will have to come back next week." Felix Ahearn listened in stunned silence, his well-meaning look vanishing from his face. She continued saying she didn't make the rules, and she just enforced them.

Felix unleashed back at her, "But I've got eight hungry kids at home. They don't have anything to eat. I need that money."

"I'm sorry, you'll have to come back next week," was her reply (Ahearn: 138).

"By gosh, I need that money this week. I'm not leaving without my money- even if I have to tear the gosh darn place apart."

Unfortunately, that remark became the last straw for Miss Jones, as she immediately called the posted policeman casually drinking a hot cup of coffee. The policeman quickly came to the aid of Miss Jones, asking her why she called.

She remarked, "Mr. Ahearn has missed his place in line. The rules say if you miss your place in line, you have to come back next week. He's just out of luck. I'm sick of these loafers hanging out in the barroom, then wanting to get their money when they're good and ready."

Felix responded, "These guys are starving to death, and they're only trying to stay warm."[240]

Felix turned to the policeman and conveyed his plight of eight hungry kids who had not had a solid meal in three days, including a three-month-old baby at home who needed milk. The police officer, a big Irish cop with a ruddy complexion, took Felix aside and commiserated with him, understanding since he had five kids of his own. The cop came up with a solution. He directed Felix to see the only person who, at this point, could help him, in the policeman's view, Jimmy Curley in Jamaica Plain, the Mayor himself. So, Felix walked the two miles, still at 30, an able-bodied young man, to Mayor Curley's house at 350 Jamaicaway, now a city historical site.

Felix knocked on the front door, and after explaining his story was ushered in to see the Mayor seated at his desk, looking at the card. The Mayor's face conveyed a kindly look, with twinkling blue eyes and white hair that was combed flat in the fashion of the day.[241]

As Felix unfolded his dramatic family story, Mayor Curley listened intently, and at the same time, scrutinized him carefully. A tall, well-built Irish man stood in front of him, with large hands, dressed in working man's clothes, visibly a hard-working man, who clearly had run into hard times. Then he wrote something down on a paper and handed it to Felix.

"Here, take this note back to the welfare office. They'll give you the money." Felix thanked him profusely. Then the Mayor reached into his pocket and gave Felix a five-dollar bill, a little extra something he called it. The Mayor replied that

---

240   Ahearn, A. (2007). *From Rags to Patches Growing up in Boston during the Great Depression.* U.S.A.: Booklocker.com Inc. P. 138.

241   Ahearn, A. (2007). *From Rags to Patches Growing up in Boston during the Great Depression.* U.S.A.: Booklocker.com Inc. P. 140.

he enjoyed meeting him and hoped they would meet again.

Later that day at home, the baby Arlene had begun to cry. With no milk and not even the dreaded molasses and onion concoction to eat, hunger dominated the children's minds, and their stomachs gurgled and growled. That afternoon, Little Al was looking out the window, wondering where his dad was. Lo and behold, he saw his pa coming down the hill. Felix walked home fast, and both of his hands carried big bags, brimming with groceries. Little Al considered Dad as a family hero. Felix bolted up the stairs and into the house with a big smile on his face, hugging Anna, and placing bags of bread, milk, apples, hotdogs, canned beans, and green vegetables on the table. "We eat again," Felix said.[242]

Several months later, Felix Ahearn, at last, returned to work. Father and son had visited the Public Garden and were returning home via Tremont Street.. Much to his surprise, Felix spotted Jimmy Curley carrying a walking stick, alone, and as always, discriminately dressed in a suit and gray spats. The mayor stopped when he recognized Felix, shaking his hand. He even remembered his name, calling him Mr. Ahearn. They exchanged pleasantries. The mayor bent low from the waist and shook my hand, and then patted my head, said, Aloysius. Then Felix and the mayor smiled, shook hands again, and both parties continued walking their separate ways down the street. Young Aloysius remembered that chance encounter well. "It was one of the proudest moments of my life."[243]

There have been many newspaper stories written about the corruption during Jimmy Curley's time in office. However, he originated from the working class, was the son of poor immigrants, understood the working man, and the working people loved him. "Yet he dressed like a lord, spoke like a poet, had the heart of a Samaritan, and never forgot a face," related Aloysius many years later when he described Jimmy Curley. As noted in Ahearn's book, the mayor would take money out of his pocket to give to someone in need; such was his commitment to his people. We encountered Mayor Curley earlier in Chapter 9, working with Boston school nurses during the infantile paralysis and diphtheria outbreaks. This story from Aloysius J. Ahearn showed a kind and humble side of his larger-than-life personality.

242   Ahearn, A. (2007). *From Rags to Patches Growing up in Boston during the Great Depression.* U.S.A.: Booklocker.com Inc. P. 141.

243   Ibid. 143.

However, the bigger picture here demonstrates the food deprivation that the children were experiencing and the breakdown of the system. What could the school nurses have done to alleviate these circumstances? Mrs. Ahearn must have felt distraught by this situation. Nonetheless, the dreaded molasses and onion concoction provided the children with nutrients such as magnesium, copper, iron, potassium, as well as B Complex vitamins and Vitamin C. When they exhausted that supply, the children became so weak they couldn't make a noise.

What was their behavior in school? We ask again, did the family not know of the Nurses Fund or the food pantry, or would they be too proud to ask for help? Did the children attend a school that offered nutrition classes plus lunch? Actually, the Superintendent's Report of 1939 lists the school nutrition groups, but the list did not include schools that Aloysius attended.[244] Therefore, he did not receive the benefit of a free lunch. What about the milk fund for needy school children, which we will hear more about in Chapter 11, that Dr. Mackey, a member of the BSC, established?[245] As we said earlier, the nurses advised the principals regarding the proper disbursement of the various funds that came to the schools, then, what happened?[246]

Perhaps the school nurses' assignments, that is, the multiple schools they covered, were so overwhelming, hunger was so widespread, that the problem was recognized, but the school nurses could not rectify it. For example, one nurse in Roxbury had the Dearborn, covering 1,560 students. Another assignment included both the Dillaway and Dudley with a top-heavy total of 2,918, yet another's assignment consisted of the Boston Disciplinary Day School and the Henry L. Higginson totaling 1,768 students. A fourth comprised the Julia Ward Howe, one of the schools that Aloysius attended, and the Lewis Intermediate with a total of 2,438.[247] The assignments hardly seem equal. Perhaps the staffing levels met

---

244 *Annual School Report of the Superintendent 1939*. Retrieved from https:// archive.org/stream/report1939bost#page/n5/mode/2up P. 94

245 New School Board Men Give Ideas for Pupils' Welfare. (1932, Jan 04). *Daily Boston Globe (1928-1960)* Retrieved from http://search.proquest.com/docview/758442325?accountid=9675

246 *Annual School Report of the Superintendent 1932*. Retrieved from https://archive.org/stream/report1932bost#page/14/mode/2up P. 27.

247 *Manual of the Public Schools of the City of Boston 1935*. Retrieved from https://archive.org/stream/manualofpublicsc1935bost#page/272/mode/2up P. 269-272.

the health and safety needs of their student population, but as far as we know, at that time, the Boston School Committee's agenda did not include school nurse workloads. Regardless, the Ahearn case obviously fell through the social safety net.

As a further note, young Al grew into adulthood, graduated from college, and built an accomplished career. After obtaining his master's degree from Harvard, he taught English for many years. Aloysius has lived in Connecticut since 1960, after he retired as an Army Major, and then served as a state representative from Connecticut. In 2016, he was 90 years young. I contacted him to see if he could shed any light on his school nurse's memories during the Great Depression. Really not expecting to hear from him, within a week, I received a two-page, handwritten letter from Aloysius Ahearn with a Guardian Angel medal tucked inside. What a pleasant surprise.

Aloysius wrote that he vaguely remembers the school nurse, though he loves nurses, but can recall her intervention associated with an incident in 1938 or 1939 in gym class at the Patrick T. Campbell Jr. High School in Dorchester. Now known as the Martin Luther King School, it is the same school in the same place on Lawrence Avenue. In the gym class, taught by Miss Dailey, and he remembers her name, she requested them to stand at attention for several minutes.[248] He related that Army drill sergeants could learn a few things from her. As was frequently the case, he was suffering from hunger because of their shortage of food at home and looked forward to the lunch period after this class. The ten-cent lunch consisted of a one-half pint bottle of milk, usually a grilled cheese or egg salad sandwich, and a bowl of Scotch broth. He related that he got dizzy and started to stagger, and at the same time, asked to be excused from the class. Realizing that she had gone a little too far, Miss Dailey rushed to him, seeing how pale and weak he was, put her arm around him, and at the same time, shouting at the rest of the class "At ease. Class rest."

Miss Daily quickly rushed him to the school nurse's office. He doesn't remember her name, but that was Sally Givner's assignment.[249] The school nurse gave him some orange juice and let him lie on a cot in her office until lunchtime. He doesn't recall if Givner sent a letter home, but nonetheless, this incident more than likely raised a red

---

248 *Manual of the Public Schools of the City of Boston 1939*. Retrieved from https://archive.org/stream/manualofpublicsc1939bost#page/158/mode/2up P. 157.

249 Ibid. P. 158.

flag on her records, and she added this family to her list of those in need.[250]

In his book and in personal phone contact, he related in answer to my questions, that on Saturday mornings he and his mother would walk to the Howard Avenue School to receive their free allotment of surplus food given by the Public Works Administration (PWA), a part of Roosevelt's 1933 National Recovery Act. They stood in line to receive their weekly ration of milk and the staple of the week, such as 25 pounds of raisins or 25 pounds of cornmeal. Thus, the family's weekly menu was almost wholly dependent on the surplus food supply, and Anna Ahearn developed recipes accordingly.[251]

Regarding their clothes, he remembers his mother going to the St. Vincent De Paul Society for used clothing.[252] Feeding and clothing a large family was a monumental task during the Great Depression, but as Aloysius points out, the family survived with courage, hard work, perseverance, and an indomitable spirit, mixed with joy and laughter.[253]

The Great Depression Continues

Whenever a city's population changes, this effect can be felt in the schools, and therefore it filters down to the school nurses, sometimes in increased assignments due to school closings or openings. Consider the theory that stringent labor laws in Boston were partly responsible for the relocation and closing of the factories. When factories, eager to lower costs, took steps to hire younger employees to add on a late-night shift, they found that what they were doing was illegal. The laws prohibited night work for children under 16, and between 10 PM and 5 AM for boys under 18 and girls under 21. Therefore, as a result, employers looked elsewhere. They abandoned the old brick and mortar factories of Boston and built new factories in the warm south, with the bonus of less stringent child labor laws.

---

250   A. Ahearn, personal communications, June 24, 2016.

251   Ahearn, A. (2007). *From Rags to Patches Growing up in Boston during the Great Depression.* U.S.A.: Booklocker.com Inc. P. 89.

252   A. Ahearn, personal communications, June 24, 2016.

253   Ahearn, A. (2007). *From Rags to Patches Growing up in Boston during the Great Depression.* U.S.A.: Booklocker.com Inc.

A study published in the *Journal of Political Economy* in 1946 found that southern labor covering a variety of industries was equal in productivity and efficiency to northern labor doing the same work. The wage rates paid in the south to workers ranged from 10-25 percent lower than in the north. For many years the large, brick mills belonging to the wood furniture and textile industry, were a part of the New England landscape. Comparable wage rates in the new southern plants averaged 15-30 percent below northern wages, with no differences in labor efficiency or labor productivity.[254]

During the 1930s, immigration decreased to a much lesser rate due to the lingering effects of WWI and the more restrictive immigration laws. "Over half of all Bostonians," said Seymour Sarason and John Doris, "still in all likelihood were either born outside the United States, or their parents were, in a population of over three-quarters of a million."[255]

Boston's Population (1920 - 1940)[256]

Year	Total Population	School Enrollment
1920	748,060	113,000
1930	781,188	130,000
1940	770,000	120,000

Enrollment peaked in the Boston Public Schools in 1934 at 134,288 students. Reasons that contributed to the decline ranged from a lower birth rate during the Depression, an increase in parochial school enrollment, and changes in Federal housing policies that encouraged residents to flee to the suburbs, facts that will be covered later in more detail.

---

254 Lester, R. A. (1946). Effectiveness of Factory Labor: South-North Comparisons. *Journal of Political Economy*, 54(1), 60–75. Retrieved from http://www.jstor.org/stable/1824934, P. 73-74.

255 Sarason, S. & Doris, J. (1979). *Educational Handicap, Public Policy and Social History,* New York, New York: The Free Press.

256 Cronin, J. (2008). *Reforming Boston's Schools, 1930-2006. Overcoming Corruption and Racial Segregation.* New York: Palgrave Macmillan. P. 6.

Public School Enrollments (1935-60)[257]

Year	Public School Membership	Parochial School Enrollments
1935	134,288	28,000 (est.)
1940	110,448	29,090
1945	94,820	30,000 (est.)
1960	86,792	43,264

Change in School Nurse Certificate

The school nurses requested a change in the school nurse certificate required by the school department. Basically, they had RN (Registered Nurse) added to their name. We have no way of knowing if other than registered nurses applied for the position since there were no Boston Public School Nurses minutes at this time and no reports in area newspapers. Therefore, they added Massachusetts registration as a requirement for the school nurse certificate. By 1934, the requirements for the document would read:

> *Graduation from a high school approved by the board of superintendents, or evidence of an equivalent academic education; graduation from a hospital or similar institution giving a course of instruction in nursing <u>at least three years in length</u>; Massachusetts registration; and (a) completion <u>of an approved course in public school nursing</u> at least six months in length or (b) or at least six months in school nursing or (c) two years' nursing experience which shall include work with and/or training in communicable diseases which training may be a part of the regular hospital training course, or (d) completion of a course in public school nursing conducted under the direction of the superintendents.*[258]

At this time, Superintendent Patrick T. Campbell acted to grant teachers and members of the supervising staff, except the supervising nurse, assistant supervising nurses and supervising school physicians, a leave of absence for study and travel,

---

257 Ibid. P. 49.

258 *Proceedings of the School Committee of the City of Boston 1934.* Retrieved from https://archive.org/stream/proceedingsofsch1934bost#page/200/mode/2up

or for rest for one year. This plan would start at the beginning of the school year and be for one full year. Eligible teachers were required to have completed seven consecutive years of service. For a leave of absence for rest, teachers qualified after completing 20 consecutive years of service in the Boston schools.[259]

These leaves of absence developed into sabbaticals and extended professional development. There was no mention of the salary associated with it. The Boston Teachers Union contract in 2015 cites that the Superintendent, the School Committee, and the Center for Leadership Development decide whether and how many, if any, they award in a given year, and the salary attached to it. Now school nurses are included.[260]

From this point on, join me as we follow the Boston school nurses as the Great Depression winds down, and they continue their journey. We now move forward to a new chapter where we will hear from the school nurses themselves in the form of minutes from their meetings. Their story allows us to see what was lost as well as what was gained in the political, economic, and social transformation of the 20th century.

---

[259] Ibid. P. 200

[260] Boston Teachers Union Contract. Retrieved from http://btu.org/wp-content/uploads/2015/10/8_BTU-Contract-Article-VI.pd P. 83.

Chapter 11

The Boston Public School Nurses Club Presses On

How do you love those who oppress you? Over many decades in the 20th century, the Boston School Nurses found themselves in this bewildering predicament with the various mayors of Boston. This part of their history developed because the mayors sought to transfer them from the Boston Public Schools to the Department of Health and Hospitals or the Boston Public Health Commission. Recall a similar situation in Chapter 8, when school nurses and school physicians worked under two different city departments. The city, always on the lookout to lower costs, hoped that by consolidating city departments they would lower their expenses. However, I leave my readers to develop their own perspectives on these issues.

From this time, we will journey together along a railroad track full of unforeseen twists and turns. They continue to cope with the Great Depression by working hard to preserve their unity, learning new nursing practices, maintaining their education, pursuing a five-day work-week and pay equity, coping with role confusion, and at the same time, articulating what they do to eliminate or minimize health-related barriers to student success. We plan to accomplish this journey with the assistance of the *Boston School Committee Minutes*, the *Annual Reports of the Superintendent, School Health Reports* from the City of Boston Archives, newspaper and journal articles from this era, plus the addition of a new perspective; the only existing minutes from the Boston School Nurses Club. Now we will hear their voices and listen to their words concerning the issues they encountered.

Minutes of the Boston Public School Nurses Club

The story of the Boston Public School Nurses Club (BPSNC) starts out in October 25, 1935, the earliest recorded meeting. However, their Constitution and By-Laws were dated 1917, and the only surviving *Boston Public School Nurses Club Minutes* began on this date in 1935. Their opening statement begins:

> *The first meeting of the Boston Public School Nurses Club was held at the Hotel Bellevue on Friday, October 25, 1935, at half-past five o'clock. Miss Julia Cronin, President, called the meeting to order at six o'clock. Tea and cakes were served to members before the meeting. Miss Clifford made a motion that present officers remain in office for the coming year.*[261]

The present officers agreed to that motion. This account verifies that the club must have existed before this time, but either no minutes were taken, or no records survived, or the club became inactive at various times in its history. Furthermore, The *Boston Public School Annual Manual* lists the BPSNC as one of the school associations since 1910.

The Hotel Bellevue on Beacon and Somerset Streets was a convenient spot across from the Massachusetts State House. Several years later in 1946, a young, dashing, and handsome John F. Kennedy made the decision to run for the congressional seat once held by his grandfather, the colorful John "Honey Fitz" Fitzgerald, a two-term Mayor of Boston, State Senator, and State Representative. JFK moved to Boston and lived at the Hotel Bellevue briefly. Wanting to be close to 83-year-old "Honey Fitz" and receive some advice for his campaign, he rented a two-room suite down the hall. Do you recall "Honey Fitz" Fitzgerald from Chapter 8? Now the former Hotel Bellevue has transformed into an elegant, residential condo building. How exciting it would have been for the school nurses if they had caught a glimpse of the young JFK and cherished that memory for a lifetime as he progressed to the White House. However, that chance to meet would have been a fantasy because, by 1946, the nurses met in the Hotel Lenox, on Boylston Street, near Copley Square, which still remains in the same location.

They conducted their regular meetings similar to any other sessions at that

---

[261] *BPSNC Minutes*: 10/25/1935

time. The Hotel Bellevue always served tea and cakes to the members at the close of their meetings. We seem to have lost that elegant style. The members voted to meet on Fridays and to invite guests and speakers. Miss Julia G. Cronin, the President, had some foresight. Though the members wanted to have more social meetings, she suggested to club members to give careful thought and consideration to questions and problems which might require more keen analysis.[262] Cronin spoke for the need of cooperation and loyalty of every member to make the club an active and successful one. That short account tells us she was a forward-thinking nurse leader, knowing with a sense of shared purpose, it would enable the BPSNC to surmount all the odds. They could make a positive contribution to support student achievement and address the constantly changing demands of school health. Miss Cronin remained as their President for nine years, until 1944. Her assignment included four schools in West Roxbury, the area where she resided.[263]

At their meetings during the next several years, they discussed the issue of a five-day work week, a minimum starting salary, attendance at professional nurses' meetings, and lastly, pensions. Their president, however, told them to refrain from discussing their employment grievances outside of the club. One could speculate about her reasoning about this approach. Perhaps she did not want them to appear as suffragettes. Additionally, maybe she feared suspicions the public had about organized unions at the time, reminiscent of the Russian Revolution hoards.

In 1935, one of their guest speakers was the Chairman of the Boston School Committee (BSC), Frederick R. Sullivan. He relayed to the school nurses that he would be glad to help them, but in return, he expected loyalty to the BSC. While startling, the nurses desperately needed the BSC to maintain their jobs, amidst the city's proliferating cost-saving measures.[264] Recollect that the BSC initially hired them for a pilot program in 1905. Another BSC member, Henry Smith, visited their meeting in April 1936. He wished he might have an opportunity to meet them in their schools and observe their work.[265] Also, they discussed the five-day work

---

262   Ibid.

263   *Manual of the Boston Public Schools 1939*. P. 165. Retrieved from https://archive.org/stream/manualofpublicsc1939bost#page/164/mode/2up

264   *BPSNC Minutes*: 1/31/1936

265   *BPSNC Minutes*: 4/27/1936

week. He suggested sending this request to the BSC where they would take the subject under consideration as to its advantages and disadvantages. I wonder if Henry Smith visited a nurse in her school or if they quickly dispatched their request to the BSC. If that occurred, there was no further reference to it.

Cost Cutting Measures

Mayor Frederick W. Mansfield sent a letter in June 1935 to the BSC demanding that they trim the school budget. Since the school nurses were part of the School Department budget, it required vigilance on their part to see how it affected their position. Increases in the school budget emerged as a source of concern as far back as 1915, and many mayors tried in vain over the years to curtail the rising costs.

Earlier, when Mayor James M. Curley asked the Finance Commission to investigate the upsurge in expenses, this resulted in the development of the Survey of 1916.[266] The conclusions and recommendations from the earlier report were 1) the BSC adopt a plan of maintaining a ratio of one doctor to two nurses to provide medical inspections of the students; 2) add special hearing tests to discover students with defective hearing; 3) transfer students with hearing loss to the Horace Mann School for the Deaf, and 4) extend classes for children with speech defects. Over time, the School Department implemented all of these recommendations, except for the ratio of doctors to nurses.

The BSC attempted another round of cost-cutting by conducting another survey in 1929. This found the cost of industrial equipment for high schools exceeded the cost of equipment for all other departments combined. Yet, only 17 percent of the students used this equipment. Therefore, to condense expenses, the BSC decided all new shop construction should be of factory construction quality and located in the basement of the buildings.[267] Apparently, they did not think highly of tradesmen.

Mayor Frederick W. Mansfield's letter to the Boston School Committee advised them of a variety of ways to trim their budget. In regards, to the Department of School Hygiene, and this affected the nurses directly, he suggested they simply reduce their

---

266 *Annual School Report of the Superintendent 1930*. P. 19-20. Retrieved from https://archive.org/stream/report1930bost#page/18/mode/2up

267 Ibid. P. 23

numbers. In other words, reduce the number of supervisors, school physicians, and nurses, and eliminate the supervisors of health education and the sanitary inspector. In addition, since the doctors and nurses only worked 40 weeks a year, during that time they should strive to increase the number of medical inspections and home visits they do every day to permit the proposed decrease in their numbers.

As far as the cleanliness and sanitation of the schools, the mayor thought this should be the job of the School Buildings Department. Also, the Health Department provided building inspection as well. Why then, did the school department require another sanitary inspector?[268] Likewise, the Mayor also attacked the night watchmen, desiring to eliminate 25-night watchmen for 25 schools.

Other issues concerned the extended use of public schools after hours for non-necessities. Music departments were on the chopping block also, since the Mayor considered them overmanned. An additional department, the mechanical arts department, claimed the Mayor, was overmanned and overemphasized (Mechanical arts featured wood and metalworking, photography, and sewing).[269]

The vocational guidance department, in the Mayor's opinion, should be eliminated, since it was unnecessary. In different economic times than these, vocational guidance counselors might find their place, but not now when hundreds of applicants applied for each job.

The Physical Education Department also stood to lose supervisors, physical education teachers, playground teachers, custodians, supplies, and assistants, all of which the Mayor thought were over the top. He requested that the Parks Department of the City of Boston be allowed to provide these services which the Boston School Department frequently duplicated.[270]

Mayor Mansfield's letter contained a strong message about how to reduce city expenditures. It reminds one of a nature walk through the Bible's Revelation. That

---

268 *Proceedings of the School Committee of the City of Boston 1935*. P. 74. Retrieved from https://archive.org/stream/proceedingsofsch1935bost#page/66/mode/2up/search

269 *Proceedings of the School Committee of the City of Boston 1935*. P. 73. Retrieved from https://archive.org/stream/proceedingsofsch1935bost#page/66/mode/2up/search

270 Ibid. P. 74.

text has a reputation as the science fiction/horror story of the Bible. Frequently, the narrative sets out what horrible things could happen to induce fear. Would this soon take place? Was the time near?

In response, the Boston School Committee passed their own proposed budget despite the Mayor's veto and regretted their difference of opinion. Their reply to the Mayor's suggestions regarding decreases in the Department of School Hygiene designated strong support of maintaining the Boston School Committee's relationship with the Department of School Hygiene:

> "To curtail the activities of the Department of School Hygiene which has the duty of caring for the health of the school children of Boston, would necessarily result in a lower health average among the children, particularly since medical authorities inform us that malnutrition, consequent upon five years of depression, has lowered the powers of resistance of the children to disease and necessitates additional medical attention. The value of this Department to the children of Boston is best demonstrated by the decrease in the number of deaths caused by scarlet fever since the year 1920. In that year, 82 school children died of this dread disease. Last year but 24. Furthermore, the number of deaths caused by diphtheria in the year 1923 was 176 and in 1934 but 9. The practical elimination of deaths from scarlet fever and diphtheria is directly attributable to the immunization of the school children by the school physicians. Each school physician must now care for the health of over 2,000 school children. To reduce the number of school physicians will mean the lessening of this essential health activity."[271]

Once again, the BSC saved the school nurses and the Department of School Hygiene in this go around.

The BSC offered another persuasive counter argument in response to the other school departments threatened by reductions. They reasoned that to reduce the number of playgrounds would undermine the system, which Boston created as the first system of school playgrounds in the U.S. These playgrounds provided safe and supervised play areas for children. A critical factor in reducing deaths and accidents involving children from automobiles correlates to keeping the children

---

[271] *Proceedings of the School Committee of the City of Boston 1935*. P. 75. Retrieved from https://archive.org/stream/proceedingsofsch1935bost#page/66/mode/2up/search

in playgrounds and off streets that had an increasing number of cars. Raising the question of whether to restrict the extended use of school buildings, the BSC voiced their opinion that to curtail those activities and trainings would deny those benefits to those who did not have a high school or college education.

The BSC decided that all of these proposals fell into the everyday scope of educational problems. This decision affected these propositions: 1) downsize the Music Department, with all of its educational advantages, 2) cut back the Manual Arts Department, 3) dispose of the Department of Vocational Guidance, 4) resolve who should be guarding the schools at night against vandalism, and 5) determine what employees were needed most by the school system and what staff could be let go. They concluded that they possessed the experience, wisdom, and sound judgment to manage these problems, more so than the Mayor.[272] The roller coaster ride of ups and downs for school staff temporarily ended.

Jobs with the Boston School Committee

Amidst the discussions about finance, other disturbing issues cropped up during the Depression. I wonder if these allegations in the long term affected the school nurses in any way. *The Boston Globe* ran a story on December 11, 1935 about ten young teachers seeking permanent positions working with what they called a "bagman" or broker who promised them jobs for a $1,250 fee. Boston School Superintendent Patrick Campbell termed the charges ridiculous and called for an investigation. Of course, the five-day investigation, without hearings, revealed nothing, and the Superintendent reported "no truth to the charges." Suffolk County District Attorney William J. Foley became involved insisting the so-called "bagman" might be someone inside the Boston School Committee and requested a grand jury investigation.

Within the next few weeks, on December 21, another BSC member, Dr. Charles J. Mackey of South Boston revealed two of his closest friends, both from South Boston, were indicted on nine counts of "soliciting to gain a bribe." They proposed to candidates they would be able to assist them in acquiring the three votes on the BSC necessary for a teaching position. Dr. Mackey reported he felt "betrayed" by

---

272 *Proceedings of the School Committee of the City of Boston 1935.* P. 76. Retrieved from https://archive.org/stream/proceedingsofsch1935bost#page/66/mode/2up/search

this disloyalty to their friendship.[273] *The Boston Globe* interviewed Dr. Mackey in 1932 after his election to a four-year term. Dr. Mackey said that "the health and environment of the children attending the schools were of more importance even than their intellectual development," and he believed one member of that body should be a doctor. In the meantime, he revealed that he had already made plans to provide free milk for school children that needed it, at no cost to the School Department or taxpayers.[274] Different people see an event in different ways. The question here is, was Dr. Mackey involved?

Shortly after that, the Grand Jury heard from an unsuccessful candidate for a music director administrative position, saying he was coerced to pay $2,000 to guarantee his appointment.[275] The BSC ignored hiring teachers based on merit.

This, however, did not apply to school nurses. As reported in Chapter 6, the city passed a law to employ school nurses known as Chapter 357 of the Acts of 1907, *An Act Relative to the Appointment of Nurses by the School Committee of the City of Boston, May 3, 1907*. Strict guidelines from the BSC and Superintendent Stratton D. Brooks dictated the requirements of nurses in the Boston Public Schools. The BPSNC requested the BSC in 1934 to add the requirement of registered nurse, RN to the school nurse certificate, as noted in Chapter 10. Schools of nursing in the 1930s required applicants to be high school graduates, and the State Board of Nurse Examiners accredited all schools of nursing. In 1937, the BPSNC advised all school nurses to register at the State House, so no comment could be made they were not Registered Nurses. The nurses made a suggestion the following year to have RN placed after each nurse's name in the *School Committee Manual*.

Actions of the Boston Public School Nurses Club

During this stressful time, the BPSNC managed to accomplish two critical items on their agenda. One of these was the development of a strategy to deal with the

---

273 Cronin, J. *Reforming Boston School, 1930-2006. Page 37. Overcoming Corruption and Racial Segregation.* (2008). New York: Palgrave Mac-Millan.

274 New School Board Men Give Ideas for Pupils' Welfare. (1932, Jan 04). *Daily Boston Globe (1928-1960)* Retrieved from http://search.proquest.com/docview/758442325?accountid=9675

275 Cronin, J. *Reforming Boston School, 1930-2006. Page 37. Overcoming Corruption and Racial Segregation.* (2008). New York: Palgrave Mac-Millan.

consolidation of city departments, and the second was the transfer of school health services to the Board of Health. These ideas became possible laws in the form of two bills in the Massachusetts Legislature. House Bill 366 deemed to consolidate city departments. House Bill 1200, (Chapter 71, Appendix 6) permitted cities and towns to transfer their School Health Service to the local Boards of Health. This same threat of transferring school health services would come up again later in 1946.

At the same time, newspapers carried the story that the Boston Finance Commission declared Boston could easily reduce its 40 odd departments to 15 or 20, and simultaneously, reorganize city government. As recommended in the report, this meant incorporating the School Health departments into the Health Department.[276]

In response, Miss Cronin encouraged Boston Public School Nurses Club (BPSNC) members to write their senators opposing passage of HB 366. By February 1937, they engaged a lawyer to represent their interests, a Mr. Parker. He would confer with Miss Cronin, and she would follow his advice in all matters. The BPSNC held another meeting in March regarding HB1200 and to report on Miss Cronin's communication with Mr. Parker. He advised that nurses not contact their senators and representatives in their districts, as they would be regarded as a party to "political ring," what today we would call political maneuvers.

Now, let us explore Mr. Parker, a lawyer, and a professional man a little bit more. What was his attitude toward school nurses? He seemed to hold women in the manner of the time, believing that they should be home cooking, cleaning, and caring for children. He probably thought they were biding their time as school nurses until future marriage and motherhood. Why should they not contact their state representatives and senators to voice their concerns?

The BPSNC asked all members to contribute $5.00 toward Mr. Parker's fee. Miss Cronin reported Mr. Parker represented the nurses in the legislative hearings about HB 1200 "in a very able manner."[277] The club decided to register at the State House. This enabled them to receive bulletins of bills listed for hearings pertaining to school health.

276 "Fin Com" Asks City Council Kill Mayor's Mergers Plan. (1936, Nov 23). *Daily Boston Globe (1928-1960)*, pp. 1. Retrieved from http://search.proquest.com/docview/815098558?accountid=9675

277 *BPSNC Minutes*: 4/3037

Unfortunately, the treasurer of the BPSNC reported in May that not everyone had made a donation, as some had a different attitude towards their situation. No further explanation described what this "attitude" included. They considered asking the school physicians to join their protest of HB 366 since they would also be affected. However, they voted unanimously to have Mr. Parker pay attention to only nursing interests. "Primarily, the club was interested in the position, rating, and protection of the nurses."[278] Again, Miss Cronin requested the nurses be loyal to the club and unless members were united, it would be difficult to proceed in matters for future advancement and interests of nurses. She recognized that women, despite gaining the vote in 1920, were not united. The loss of the suffragettes' solidarity left women with very different priorities.[279]

School nurses also brought attention to another problem on their priority list. Up until then, this problem had been overlooked and accepted as routine, the five-day work week. School nurses worked until one o'clock on Saturday afternoon whereas all city departments closed at twelve o'clock. Initially, they asked Dr. Keenan, the supervising physician at the time, to grant the nurses Saturday morning off. He hesitated, saying home visits made that day meaningful. The nurses felt, however, that Saturday morning home visits did not work well for the family. The children were home, parents were busy with housework or shopping, and on the whole such visits were unsatisfactory. Nurses suggested that an afternoon be given for home calls. Dr. Keenan said he would consider the matter and confer with the Superintendent.

A half day's work on Saturday had been part of the work week for Boston school nurses since 1905, when the Boston School Committee and the Instructive District Nurse Association assigned the first school nurse, Annie McKay, to three schools. Annie McKay used the time on Saturdays to make home visits and to catch up on paperwork.

After a time, the BPSNC considered a petition should be drawn up and sent through their Supervising Nurse, Miss McCaffrey to Dr. Keenan and the School

---

278   *BPSNC Minutes*: 5/28/1937

279   Women in American Politics in the Twentieth Century - *The Gilder Lehrman Institute of American History*. Retrieved from http://www.gilderlehrman.org/history-by-era/womens-history/essays/women-american-politics-twentieth-century

Committee. However, the club voted nine to eight not to move forward in this manner. They discussed a plan suggested by Dr. Keenan in June that they work until 5:30 PM, and not on Saturday morning. Their response asserted it became very dark even at 5 PM during the winter months and this would make for a very long day. Therefore, this did not meet with their approval.

Why were the school nurses so timid about approaching the Boston School Committee? Everyone walks in the footsteps of others. Whose footsteps did they walk in? No footsteps materialized for them to follow. This was virgin territory for them.

Boston School Committee candidates running for office attended their meeting to introduce themselves to school nurses in October 1937. We must assume they were made aware of the school nurses desire for the five-day work week. One of them was Mr. Joseph Lee, the same person who appeared in the photograph at the signing of the 1921 bill appointing nurses to schools. Ultimately, the Boston School Committee responded to their urgings and granted them a five-day work week in June 1938.[280]

To celebrate this event, the school nurses decided to hold an informal dinner that cost about $1.50 each, and all agreed. It developed into something more substantial, and they began referring to it as a banquet. They held their dinner at Schrafft's on West Street and invited Mayor Tobin and his wife, members of the School Committee and their wives, and presidents of school organizations.

Charles' blog describes Schrafft's as the place to be for everyone, the "gold star" example of what eating out in Boston was all about, plus, it included function rooms available for rent. West Street is a historic district in Boston, one of the city's "ladder districts" that runs between Tremont Street and Washington Street in the Downtown Crossing area. The Schrafft's building at 16-24 West Street was built in 1922 and housed the flagship candy store and restaurant for more than 50 years. Founded in 1861, Schrafft's expanded from a candy company to include restaurants. See the image below. Where could you find those prices today? But as the years passed and the economy declined, Schrafft's couldn't keep up with the times, and all of their Boston restaurants closed by 1973. Only the ice cream line

---

[280] *Proceedings of the School Committee of the City of Boston 1938.* (96) Retrieved from https://archive.org/stream/proceedingsofsch1938bost#page/96/mode/2up/search/nurse

has survived.[281] In later years, the area underwent development to become Suffolk University dormitories. Recently, this neighborhood expanded to include a towering residential area.

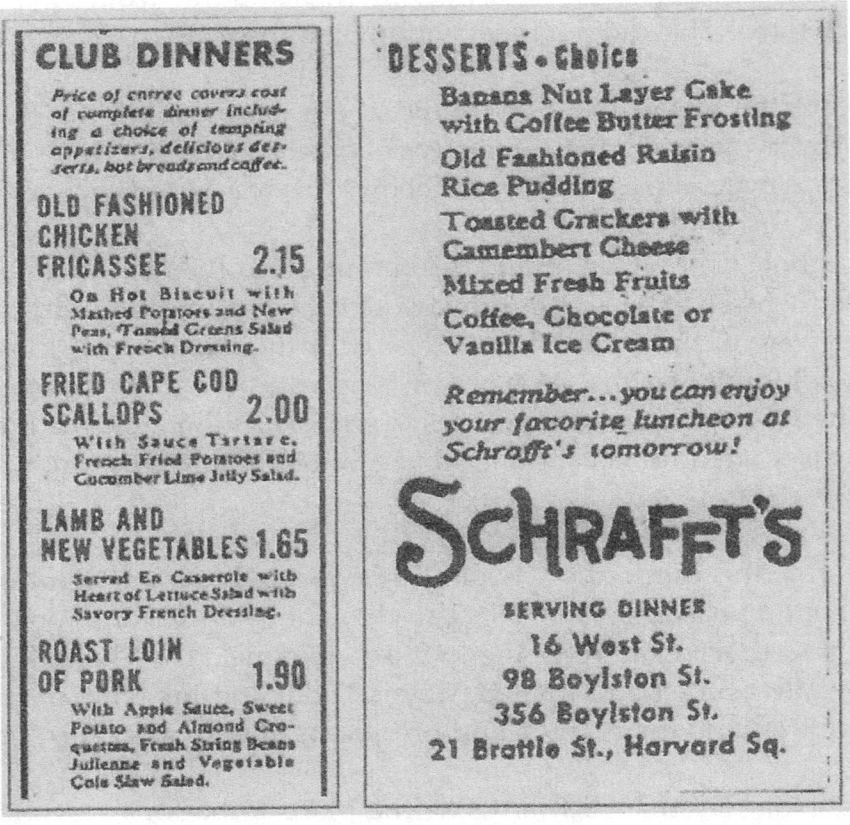

CLUB DINNERS

Price of entree covers cost of complete dinner including a choice of tempting appetizers, delicious desserts, hot breads and coffee.

OLD FASHIONED
CHICKEN
FRICASSEE   2.15
On Hot Biscuit with Mashed Potatoes and New Peas, Tossed Greens Salad with French Dressing.

FRIED CAPE COD
SCALLOPS   2.00
With Sauce Tartare, French Fried Potatoes and Cucumber Lime Jelly Salad.

LAMB AND
NEW VEGETABLES 1.65
Served En Casserole with Heart of Lettuce Salad with Savory French Dressing.

ROAST LOIN
OF PORK   1.90
With Apple Sauce, Sweet Potato and Almond Croquettes, Fresh String Beans Julienne and Vegetable Cole Slaw Salad.

DESSERTS - Choice

Banana Nut Layer Cake with Coffee Butter Frosting
Old Fashioned Raisin Rice Pudding
Toasted Crackers with Camembert Cheese
Mixed Fresh Fruits
Coffee, Chocolate or Vanilla Ice Cream

Remember... you can enjoy your favorite luncheon at Schrafft's tomorrow!

SCHRAFFT'S

SERVING DINNER
16 West St.
98 Boylston St.
356 Boylston St.
21 Brattle St., Harvard Sq.

The key point of this is a comparison can be made between the school nurses and Schrafft's. Would the school nurses, unlike Schrafft's, be able to change and cultivate continued growth and evolution over the years? Looking ahead, we will see them traverse the space, and observe another perfect symbol for school nurses: resiliency.

The Superintendent and the Boston School Committee's Messages

As Superintendent Arthur L. Gould discussed the Department of School Hygiene in his 1937

---

281 Boston, C. (2011, September 4). *Shopping Days in Retro Boston* [Web log post]. Retrieved from http://shoppingdaysinretroboston.blogspot.com/2011/09/retro-lunch-at-schraffts-in-bostonvery.html

report, he allowed us to observe the activities of the school nurses, which otherwise would not be available. He emphasized their duties were clearly defined, as were the duties and responsibilities of the School Committee concerning safeguarding the health of pupils and employees.

In Superintendent Arthur L. Gould's opinion, the principal function of the Department of School Hygiene was to "minimize the spread of communicable disease."[282] Mark these words. The question of course is what would be their function with the arrival of disease-preventable vaccines?

He noted the size of the Department of School Hygiene, which in later years would become a controversy. It consisted of the director, six supervising school physicians, 61 school physicians, one supervisor of nutrition classes, one sanitary engineer, one supervisor of health education and safety education, and one supervising nurse. Also, it included four assistant supervising nurses, 61 nurses, 23 school matrons, 21 nutrition class attendants, 19 assistant nutrition class attendants, 43 lunch attendants, and 13 cafeteria cooks. They maintained the ratio of one school physician to one school nurse.

Enrollment in all schools totaled 157,695 students.[283]

Regular day schools	140,398
Evening schools	15,000
Continuation School	1,006
Day School for Immigrants 751	751

Superintendent Gould summarized the successful school immunization campaign against diphtheria in 1936, during which the school physicians and school nurses immunized 7,000 children. The Superintendent praised them for their work calling it a "splendid tribute to the diligence, skill, and tact of the school nurse, who must enlighten and convince the parents (often against strong objection) of the

---

282   *Annual School Report of the Superintendent 1937*. (169) Retrieved from
      https://archive.org/stream/report1937bost#page/102/mode/2up/search/nurses

283   *Annual Statistics of the Boston Public Schools 1937-1938*: 5

necessity of such protection."[284]

The Department of School Hygiene implemented another new program in the fight against scarlet fever, an acute contagious disease of childhood caused by Group A hemolytic Streptococcus bacteria. It is characterized by sore throat, fever, enlarged lymph nodes in the neck, weakness, and a diffuse, bright red rash. Scarlet fever was difficult to control, according to the Superintendent, because of the mildness of the disease in some children, thus making it not easily recognized. This innovative program required the school, whenever they received notice of a new case of scarlet fever, to notify the school physician and school nurse immediately. With that notice, the school nurse inspected the child's classroom for similar signs of the disease. They excluded from school all children who had similar symptoms of the disease.

Since the implementation of this program, scarlet fever decreased from 1,485 cases in 1931-32 to 720 cases in 1935-1936.[285] This resulted in the school system's 51 percent decline in scarlet fever cases. The school nurses extensive class inspection program paid off in saving lives.

School Nurses Deal with Scarlet Fever and other Contagious Diseases

Superintendent Gould did not go into the details of scarlet fever, also called scarlatina, but it is characterized by a generalized erythematous (redness) skin eruption, or skin wound infections. Many different conditions produce similar rashes, and a single illness can result in assorted rashes with varied appearances. The differential diagnosis could be Kawasaki's syndrome or a viral rash or staphylococcal scarlet fever. The incidence of the disease is at its height in the five-to-eight-year age group, after which it decreases. The incubation period varies from one to seven days, most frequently it is from two to four days, with the causative streptococcus found most abundantly in the throat. The period of greatest communicability is during the febrile (fever) period, the first three-five days. It is spread through contact with droplets from an infected person's cough or sneeze. By the sixth day, the rash usually fades, but the affected skin may begin to peel, called desquamation. In mild cases, the rash and pharyngitis may pass unnoticed, and parents may seek medical care only when they notice the peeling skin.

284 *Annual Report of Superintendent 1937*: 171

285 *Annual Report of Superintendent 1937*: 171

The most common complications of scarlet fever are otitis media (inflammation of the middle ear), cervical adenitis (inflammation of the lymph nodes of the neck), and nephritis (inflammation of the kidney). The isolation period is based on the persistence of streptococci in the throat or the continuation of suppurative discharges, as pus coming from the skin rash or the ear infection.[286] Before the use of antibiotics, scarlet fever had a mortality rate of 15 percent to 20 percent. Now the infection can be cured with a ten-day course of antibiotics.[287]

Chapter 2 relayed the story of Boston's first school nurse, Annie McKay returning to Canada in 1919 to nurse several members of her brother's family with scarlet fever. Unfortunately, two of the children succumbed to the disease.

Do you remember Aloysius Ahearn in Chapter 10? He didn't have scarlet fever, but he recalls when he, his mother, and sister visited his father, and brothers' Ray and Jim, at Boston City Hospital, all with scarlet fever in the 1930s.[288] They could not visit them directly, but he remembers seeing them from the sidewalk. Father and children waved from their seventh-floor window down to the family below. That diagnosis would have precipitated a round of classroom inspections by the school nurses in the various schools the eight children attended.

Now, I picture the nurse going into a second-grade class of some 50 children, with her medical record cards, explaining her mission. The teacher would be happy to see her of course, because he/she wanted the least exposure possible. Therefore, the nurse would prevail upon the teacher to discreetly tell her what children had a runny nose, an ear discharge, or were sneezing and coughing. With this information, she would probably find a chair in the back of the room where there was a window to give her sufficient light, and call the children up to form a line, row by row. Hopefully, each child would be looked at individually, but if the nurse did not have the time, she would line about five students in front of her. Then she would instruct them to open their mouths so she could look down their throats and at their tongues, looking for a reddened sore throat and tongue, known as "strawberry

---

286 Blake, F.G., Wright, F.H., & Waechter, E.H. (1970) *Nursing Care of Children* (8th ed.). Philadelphia, PA. J.B. Lippincott Company. P. 353.

287 Benenson, A. (Ed.). (1995). P. 438. *Control of Communicable Diseases Manual* (16th ed). Washington, D.C. American Public Health Association.

288 A. Ahearn, personal communications, June 24, 2016

tongue," or ones covered with a whitish coating, early in the infection.

Some questions she might have asked:

"Does your tummy hurt?"
"Do you feel hot?"
"Does it hurt to swallow?"
at the same time demonstrating what she means by swallowing.

She would turn their faces to the window for the maximum light, making observations about the condition of their skin, looking for the telltale rash.
"Let me see your hands," as they stretched out their hands in front of her.

The question emerges as to whether she took the temperatures of all the students lined up in front of her. Using the glass thermometer of the time required five minutes to record a temperature, therefore, it is debatable whether a group of seven and eight-year-olds could control their behavior for that length of time. However, if one of them said, "I am hot," she would have taken his or her temperature to determine if they had a fever. Of course, if someone was sneezing, coughing, and had a runny nose, the child's name made her list for exclusions, along with all of the others who had the symptoms of scarlet fever.

The school nurses did not make home visits to communicable disease cases, but kept track of their exclusions, and would follow up on all cases. Just as Annie McKay, Boston's first school nurse, helped establish the system a quarter of a century earlier, they practiced health assessment, intervention, evaluation, and follow-up care for all their students.

The next step included notifying the parents. She gave all of the students who had suspicious symptoms a referral to see their doctor. Since the vast majority of the students did not have a phone, she doubtless kept them isolated in her office until dismissal. Hoping that a parent would then be home, she would escort them to their house.

The Superintendent continued his report covering other contagious diseases that occurred in the schools that year. I emphasize that school nurses had to be aware of, and know the signs, symptoms, and treatment of all these contagious diseases. He argued he did not consider the 3,055 cases of measles to be of epidemic proportions. Quarantine of the children in their homes who had measles reduced the spread of the disease. The MMR (measles, mumps, and rubella) vaccine, now available since 1971, is safe and prevents measles.

Stephen King, an author of more than 50 worldwide bestseller books, recalls in his book, *On Writing*, his bout at age six in 1953 with otitis media, a complication resulting from measles. He has never forgotten the repeated, painful trips to see the otologist for eardrum lancings. In one instance, as he was lying on the examining table, he humorously recalls this exchange, "'There,' the ear doctor's nurse said when it was over, and I lay there crying in a puddle of watery pus. 'It only hurts a little, and you don't want to be deaf, do you? Besides, it's all over.'"[289]

The first case of meningitis for the school year 1936 appeared at the Andrews School in the Quincy district, one of Annie McKay's former schools. The Superintendent referred to the surrounding residential area as "congested." A total of 14 cases were found, affecting both adults and preschool children. Despite the work of the Department of School Hygiene performing nasal cultures on possible carriers, no carriers were found. At the present time, 2020, there are two meningococcal vaccines available in the U.S. to protect against meningococcal disease, a serious bacterial infection that can lead to bacterial meningitis.

Boston faced a continuing problem with tuberculosis (TB). Public health officials revealed there were 20,000 known contacts of tuberculosis in 1936. The Superintendent expanded on his own case finding plan to x-ray all 9th graders at a cost of $5,000. "School nurses supervise all tuberculosis contacts as to their health and do an untold amount of good in delaying the onset of tuberculosis in these children, thus saving large sums of money that otherwise would be required for hospitalization, etc."[290]

Presently, treatment for TB includes a four-drug regimen, consisting of isoniazid, rifampin, pyrazinamide, and either ethambutol or streptomycin. Unfortunately, resistant strains of TB have developed, and further research is being conducted

---

289   King, S. *On Writing, A Memoir of the Craft*. (2010). P. 22-25. New York: Scribner.

290   *Annual School Report of the Superintendent 1937*. (173) Retrieved from https://archive.org/stream/report1937bost#page/102/mode/2up/search/nurses

to discover new cures.[291]

Due to reports in the January 1937 newspapers about the prevalence of influenza, colds, and grippe among school children, Superintendent Gould asked school nurses to conduct a survey of the causes of absenteeism during two weeks in January. Historically, school nurses routinely have been asked to do special surveys, despite barely having time to accomplish their normal workload. During the week ending January 16, the study showed absences of 22,584 students, and during the week ending January 23, the survey showed absences of 23,206. However, the Superintendent continued, the total number of absences during both of these weeks due to colds and grippe was 25,466. During the week ending January 30, the total number of absences rose to 53,876. These results, in his opinion, showed probably a contagious disease situation did take place. Although, it was "of short duration, of a respiratory nature, not accompanied by any serious complications and not to be considered as an outbreak of true influenza."[292] He denied that this event bore any resemblance to the influenza epidemic of 1918, which he did not want to see repeated.

At the end of his report about the Department of School Hygiene, he described the school nurse as a trained professional nurse, who must have other corresponding attributes requiring "tact, patience and untiring zeal" as she carried out her many functions. Examples of these functions ranged from escorting children to hospital clinics, arranging for admissions to summer health camps, coordinating the school with the home and social agencies, "finding means of relieving various pressing needs of children and families, and performing multifarious other services which cannot be fully appreciated from the statistics."[293]

To summarize, the Superintendent's Report demonstrated how the school nurses were making a positive contribution in keeping children healthy and in school while grappling with a cornucopia of issues. He recognized their presence, commitment, and dedication in promoting student health. How long that appreciation would last is yet to be seen.

---

291 *Medscape*. Retrieved from http://emedicine.medscape.com/article/230802-treatment#d11

292 *Annual School Report of the Superintendent 1937*. (173) Retrieved from https://archive.org/stream/report1937bost#page/102/mode/2up/search/nurses

293 Ibid. P. 175.

The Boston Public School Nurses Club

The Minutes of *the BPSNC* gave no mention of performing any particular survey regarding absenteeism. At this point, instead, their notes seem more focused on members retiring to be married, their gifts to be forwarded according to their number of years in service, and the total not to exceed $10.00.[294] The Elementary Teachers Club encouraged them to attend a play given for the benefit of undernourished children.[295] Notice how involved the school nurses were with malnourished children. They pointed out Patrick J. Foley, DDS was so helpful in obtaining their five-day work week. If he considered running for Boston School Committee, they would all vote for him. Now we can see some progress: they were learning to network.

The 1940s

An unknown author wrote a memoir about children of the 1930s and 1940s saying they were the last ones to grow up without television, instead imagining what they heard on the radio. They played outside until the streetlights came on, and they played on their own. It was safe to do so. There was no Little League, no soccer practice. Movies with newsreels, cartoon, and westerns occupied their Saturday afternoons. People walked a great deal, not jogging for their health, the way people do nowadays. They walked to get from one place to another.

World events took center stage for the second time in the twentieth century with the outbreak of World War II in Europe in 1939. The United States had to build a military strong enough to defeat the Axis powers, Germany, Italy, and Japan, as it became clear that it was only a matter of time before we would be drawn into the war. For the first time in our history, the United States instituted a peacetime draft on September

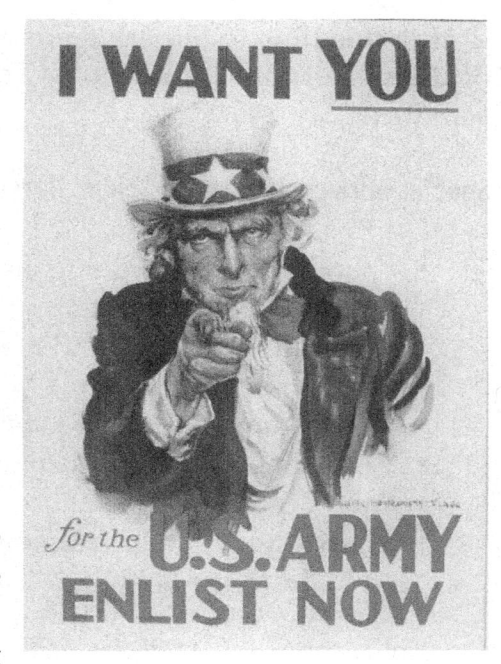

---

294 *BPSNC Minutes*: 2/9/1939

295 *BPSNC Minutes*: 3/7/1940

16, 1940. It required all men between the ages of 21 and 45 to register for the draft. The Selective Service only ended the draft on January 27, 1973, as the Vietnam War was winding down.

The Boston School Committee, with the Superintendent's approval, called upon Miss Helen F. McCaffrey, Supervising Nurse, to step in temporarily as the Director of the Department of School Hygiene during his absence on account of military service from January 1941 to September 1941. Apparently, they regarded her work as extremely competent. She received additional compensation of $45 per month for this endeavor.[296] See the image on the next page.

The school year proceeded on as usual with the school nurses going about their customary routines, trying like the rest of us to make sense of the world and their place in it. There were fewer incidences of contagious diseases being reported during this time to Superintendent Gould.[297] The following reports describe some of the school nurses' activities. Today, school nurses perform many of the same activities.

Special work performed by School Nurses included:

- Semi-annual weighing and measuring all children in elementary and intermediate districts
- Monthly weighing and measuring all malnutrition cases and the members of the nutrition group.
- Re-testing all defective vision and hearing cases.
- Assisting school physicians with physical examinations, daily inspections, and diphtheria preventive work.
- Assisting school physicians in examinations and re-examination of cardiac and other special cases.
- Making special reports on tuberculosis contacts.
- Addressing parents' meetings.

---

296 *Proceedings of the School Committee 1941*: 211

297 *Annual School Report of the Superintendent 1941*. P. 88. Retrieved from https://archive.org/stream/report1941bost#page/130/mode/2up/search/nurses

Social Work performed by School Nurses included:

- Securing social histories on all cases referred to welfare organizations.
- Referring pupils for vacations to various organizations
- Obtaining vacations for pupils at summer camps.
- Distributing food, including Christmas and Thanksgiving baskets, to needy children and their families.
- Collecting and distributing clothing to needy families.
- Selecting groups of needy children eligible for free milk.

Summary of School Nurse Daily Reports[298]

Visits to homes	26,618
Classroom talks on hygiene	9,625
Consultation with teachers	98,262
Consultation with pupils	173,553
Inspections of hair	434,185
Inspections of teeth	360,362
Treatments	57,964

Report on Correction of Defective Vision

(Intermediate and Elementary Schools)

Cases reported by teachers, after testing	6,732
School Nurse Re-Examined	5,833
Corrected: Glasses advised	4,503
Glasses obtained	4,367

---

[298] *Annual School Report of the Superintendent 1941.* P. 89-93. Retrieved from https://archive.org/stream/report1941bost#page/130/mode/2up/search/nurses

Strabismus cases	1,196
Under treatment	1,079
Not under treatment	117
Dental Work Summary	360,362
Number of pupils escorted for dental treatments	9,207
Classroom toothbrush drills	4,600
Number of pupils having dental work completed	29,737

Pupils Escorted to Clinics by Nurses

Clinic	Number	Revisits
Eye	483	245
Ear	57	16
Nose and throat	156	21
Medical	164	40
Surgical	99	14
Skin	44	10
Totals	**985**	**346**

Notice that school nurses escorted 985 pupils to various clinics and accompanied 346 pupils for revisits. Was this the best use of their professional skills?

Hearing Testing[299]

This report demonstrates the hearing testing program and the positive consequences that followed.

---

[299] *Annual School Report of the Superintendent 1942*. P. 87. Retrieved from https://archive.org/details/report1942bost/page/10

Audiometer Test	Number of Pupils
Tested by audiometer	10,038
Found defective by audiometer	1,310
Referred to otologist	578
Examined by otologist	578
Found defective by otologist:	
Advised treatment	362
Advised no treatment	176
Total	**538**
Advised to attend Lip Reading Class	100
Admitted to Lip Reading Class	65
Advised to continue in Lip Reading Class	24
Received treatment	
By family physician	9
By hospital	25
Total	**134**
Operations for the removal of tonsils and adenoids	20

    School nurses, of course, retested every child who failed the hearing test performed by the schoolteachers. If needed, they referred the student to an appropriate agency for follow-up care. Reliable resources state that in 1930, there were about 3,000,000 partially deaf children in the United States. Doctors recognized that tonsils, adenoid, and sinus diseases caused a great many ear conditions, resulting in varying degrees of deafness. A child with the beginning of a serious ear condition might not complain or give evidence of such a defect in hearing.

    Even despite close daily contact with their family and schoolteacher, suspicion frequently would not arise of a hearing loss. Hence, the importance of hearing testing was paramount. Students not hearing all the information in the classroom become inattentive. These children lose interest in school, and since they are unable to keep up with their schoolwork, they would become repeaters and could be held back several grades in school. Students would lose their full potential.[300] It falls to the school nurse to persuade the parent to take the children to the clinics and the specialists who work hearing miracles.

A high school student with a hearing loss of 15 percent in the right ear and 45 percent in the left ear sent the following letter to express her gratitude for the specialized education that she received:

> Boston, Massachusetts
> May 16, 1944
>
> Dear Miss_____ and Miss _____:
>
> *I would like to express my appreciation for the years of training you have given me in lip reading. I find it difficult to put into words just how helpful my knowledge of reading lips has been to me this past year. No one where I work has even suspected the slightest handicap. I probably would sound like an advertisement, but I really mean this.*
>
> *Well, thanks a lot, both of you, for your splendid work. And just in case you might be interested in how I made out, I passed a Civil Service examination, which rated me a position at a local Draft Board.*

Another yet unreported role of the school nurse involved supplementing the work of the attendance officer. The school nurse investigated the reasons for absence from school. Seventy-five percent of excuses given were for reasons of illness. State law protected this excuse. However, Boston School Superintendent Gould quoted former President Herbert Hoover concerning truancy as saying that a good nurse is better than 10 policemen. Of all the members of social agencies, courts, and school staff visiting the homes of truant boys stated the Superintendent, "there is no one more welcome and as generally sought for as is the school nurse."[301]

---

[300] Peery, V. Some Aspects of Deafness, Economic and Otherwise. (1930, August 2). *Daily Boston Globe (1928-1960)* pp. 18. Retrieved from http://search.proquest.com/docview/747682937.

[301] *Annual School Report of the Superintendent 1941*. P. 169. Retrieved from https://archive.org/stream/report1941bost#page/130/mode/2up/search/nurses

In November 1941, the Boston School Nurses Club mailed letters of congratulations to Dr. Foley and others on their election to the Boston School Committee. They discussed obtaining a lawyer regarding an increase in salary, but nothing was decided. After a while, though they were neophytes at this game, they sent letters about a salary increase to Dr. Keenan, the Director of School Hygiene, Miss McCaffrey, Supervising Nurse, Mr. A. Sullivan, Business Manager of the BSC, and members of the BSC.[302]

World War II

Little did the school nurses know when they held their meeting on December 5, 1941, of the events that would change their lives and those of the entire nation within the following days. The nation recoiled as this report blasted from the airways: *"We interrupt this program to bring you a special news bulletin. The Japanese have attacked Pearl Harbor…"* The Japanese surprise attack left 2,235 servicemen killed, 1,109 wounded and 68 civilians, dead. President Franklin D. Roosevelt declared the strike as, "A day that will live in infamy."[303]

Superintendent Gould responded in a clearly patriotic manner "that it subordinates everything else to the winning of the war." He referred to reports from military officials of the staggering percentage of draft-age youth who were declared ineligible for the armed services because of physical defects that were remediable in nature. These types of problems were the business of the schools, he argued, to teach the promotion of health and well-being.[304]

As a result of the declaration of war, the draft board called two school physicians to active duty. To protect staff and students in case of an anticipated enemy attack, Superintendent Gould and the Director of School Hygiene requested the Metropolitan Chapter of the American Red Cross to furnish instructors to give medical and nursing staff a first-aid refresher course. As a consequence, 60 school nurses and 40 school physicians attended a "Forty-Hour Course" furnished by the American Red Cross. These attendees then became qualified as instructors in

302   *BPSNC Minutes*: 12/5/41

303   John Daly, CBS Radio, December 7, 1941

304   *Annual School Report of the Superintendent 1942*. P. 10-11. Retrieved from https://archive.org/details/report1942bost/page/10

"Standard First Aid" and "Advanced First Aid" courses. They then, in turn, taught these courses at their schools where 3,200 staff members completed the course in Standard First Aid. The school department presented additional workshops in air raid precautions, blackouts, incendiary bombs, and supplies for disaster relief.[305]

The Committee on Defense Material allocated supplies for disaster relief to schools such as fracture pillows, wood traction splints, and Thomas arm and leg traction splints used by Boston City Hospital, now called Boston Medical Center. Nearly 50 years later, I found similar supplies buried deep in a closet in my nurse's office at the Thomas Edison Middle School in Brighton, where I had often speculated about their origins.

The *Boston Public School Nurses Club Minutes* resumed again on January 9, 1942. There was no mention of the war, but they were still obsessed with an increase in salary. And, so it continued through 1942. No meetings occurred in February and March due to extensive first aid classes for school nurses.

Boston faced more loss of life as a consequence of the Cocoanut Grove Night Club fire on November 28th, 1942, when 492 people perished, and hundreds were injured in that tragedy. Located on Piedmont Street in the Bay Village area, it was the scene of the deadliest nightclub fire in history. Under these circumstances, practicing their humanity to mankind, the Boston school nurses responded to the city's need for more nurses.

On the night of the fire, the club was entertaining about 1,000 people, all Thanksgiving revelers, wartime servicemen and their sweethearts in an area rated to hold a maximum of 460 people. Victims suffered from carbon monoxide poisoning and extensive burn injuries from the inferno. As a result of the fire, Boston instituted major improvements in the fire codes.

As has been pointed out earlier, the school nurses frequently volunteered their services to those in need, and they repeated this in the wake of the Cocoanut Grove Fire disaster. Nothing was noted in the school nurse minutes, but the Superintendent's Report included a summary of their activities. Thirty-four school

---

[305] *Annual School Report of the Superintendent 1942*. P. 18-19. Retrieved from https://archive.org/details/report1942bost/page/10

nurses gave 43 days of service in various hospitals, caring for the victims. Nine school nurses contracted to take a refresher course at MGH (Massachusetts General Hospital) to serve part-time during the summer months when they were off. Many other school nurses agreed to serve one month at various hospitals in Boston.[306]

But as the world knows all too well now, and is so often the case, the tragedy led to new advances in caring for burn and smoke inhalation victims. Survivors were among the first human beings treated with a new and unknown antibiotic called penicillin for staphylococcus bacteria. Doctors found this miracle drug to be crucial in combating skin graft infections. The U.S. government subsequently decided to support the production and distribution of penicillin for use in the Armed Forces.[307]

Life on the Home Front for School Nurses during the War Years

Numerous challenges confronted the American people at the onset of World War II. The country wanted to win this war and mobilized to support that effort. Immediately, the Federal government stepped in and was active at both the regional level and in local communities.

The government, through the use of ads, radio shows, movies, posters, and pamphlets, as no social media existed, insisted that Americans contribute to the war effort in every possible way. Four areas required immediate attention: 1) rationing and controlling prices, 2) defending the home front, 3) wartime research and development, and 4) war work and the employment of women.[308] The Federal government established agencies such as the War Manpower Commission and the Office of Price Administration to help address these concerns. These areas also had a direct impact on life in New England.

Now there was rationing. Do my readers know what that was? Some of us can remember what it was about. The American troops needed supplies. Therefore, at

---

306 *Annual Report of the Superintendent 1943.* P. 61. Retrieved from https://archive.org/stream/report1943bost#page/60/mode/2up

307 *Celebrate Boston: Cocoanut Grove Fire.* Retrieved from http://www.celebrateboston.com/disasters/cocoanut-grove-fire.htm

308 *America on the Homefront: Selected WWII Records of Federal Agencies in New England.* Retrieved from http://www.archives.gov/boston/exhibits/homefront/

home, fewer manufactured goods were available. The war caused shortages in gas, rubber, metal, clothing, and food. This, especially food, directly affected every American on a daily basis. The government asked Americans to conserve on everything. During World War I, the U.S. experienced problems with the shortage of manufactured goods, creating a black market and inflated prices where only the affluent could afford to purchase these items. Surprisingly, the government learned from this experience and developed a system of rationing and price controls during WWII.

Again, the Superintendent asked the school nurses to assist in such matters as the draft, sugar, and gas rationing registration process, generally through their work in the schools.[309] Since the school nurse knew so many families and their circumstances, she was able to add her expertise to the registration process. Officials asked each family to send only one member to register for the family and describe the members in order to obtain the "War Ration Book." Each of the stamps in the "War Ration Book" authorized a family's ability to purchase rationed goods in the amount and time within designated expiration dates.

Foods that required the "Red Stamp" were all meats, butter, fat, and oils, and with some exemptions, cheese. The "Blue Stamp" rationing book covered canned, bottled, frozen fruits, and vegetables, plus juices and dry beans, and such processed foods like soups, baby food, and ketchup. Sugar rationing started in 1943. As a result of rationing, sugarless cookies, eggless cakes, and meatless meals became the norm for homemakers.[310]

I recall accompanying my mother to an A&P supermarket to deliver the fat that we saved in cans for the war effort. This endeavor was part of the scrap drives for materials crucial to the war. My uncle's car stood on blocks in a garage because rubber tires were not available. Fashion complied by designing clothing that used smaller amounts of cloth. Women's dolman sleeves, patch pockets, and petticoats became out of style. Men's suits transformed from a four-piece double-breasted suit to a two-piece suit without pant cuffs. Virtually every household made adjustments to provide resources needed for the war.

---

309   *Annual School Report of the Superintendent 1942*. P. 80. Retrieved from https://archive.org/details/report1942bost/page/10

310   *Life in the 40s*. Retrieved from https://www.690kcee.com/nostalgia-lounge/life-in-the

Frequent sightings of German submarines along the New England coast fell under the auspices of defending the home front, their second prime concern. To protect the northern shipping lanes, a coalition of military and civilian groups trained to detect, defend, and attack the enemy if necessary.

Wartime research and development, the U.S. government's third concern involved the Massachusetts Institute of Technology (MIT), which furtively pursued an undisclosed program to develop new radar equipment for the war arsenal.

War work and the employment of women emerged as the fourth area of concern. Miss McCaffrey said some of the nurses had difficulty spending last year's allowance received from their annual, fundraising bridge party. This was due to the high wages paid to families working in defense plants. On the other hand, many households not employed in defense work had large families and inadequate income. These families would benefit from supplementary aid to obtain items like eyeglasses etc.[311]

The shortage of civilian labor due to the vast number of men joining the military and the need for peak production forced the federal government and the war industries to employ women to fill the gap. See the image on the next page. The increasing demand of the U.S. Armed Forces caused a shortage of civilian nurses. We know at least five of the Boston school nurses received a leave of absence without pay for the remainder of the war, to enlist and serve in the Armed Forces. The Nursing Council of National Defense worked with the American Red Cross to recruit nurses for the military. Besides, they partnered with Congressman Frances Payne Bolton of Ohio to pass the first bill that provided government funding to educate nurses for national defense. The Bolton Act in 1942 created the U.S. Cadet Nurse Corps, a program subsidized by the Federal government which prepared nurses as quickly as possible to meet the needs of not only the armed forces, but civilian and government hospitals, and war industries.[312]

---

311 *Boston Public School Nurses Club Minutes*: 6/10/1942

312 Egenes, K. History of Nursing. (17) Retrieved from jblearning.com/samples/0763752258/52258-CH01roux.pdf. 2/6/2014

BOSTON SUNDAY POST, NOVEMBER 8, 1942

Boston Girl Swings 10-Ton Crane

Close-Up View of Grace Currier Found at Red Cross Blood Donor Centre

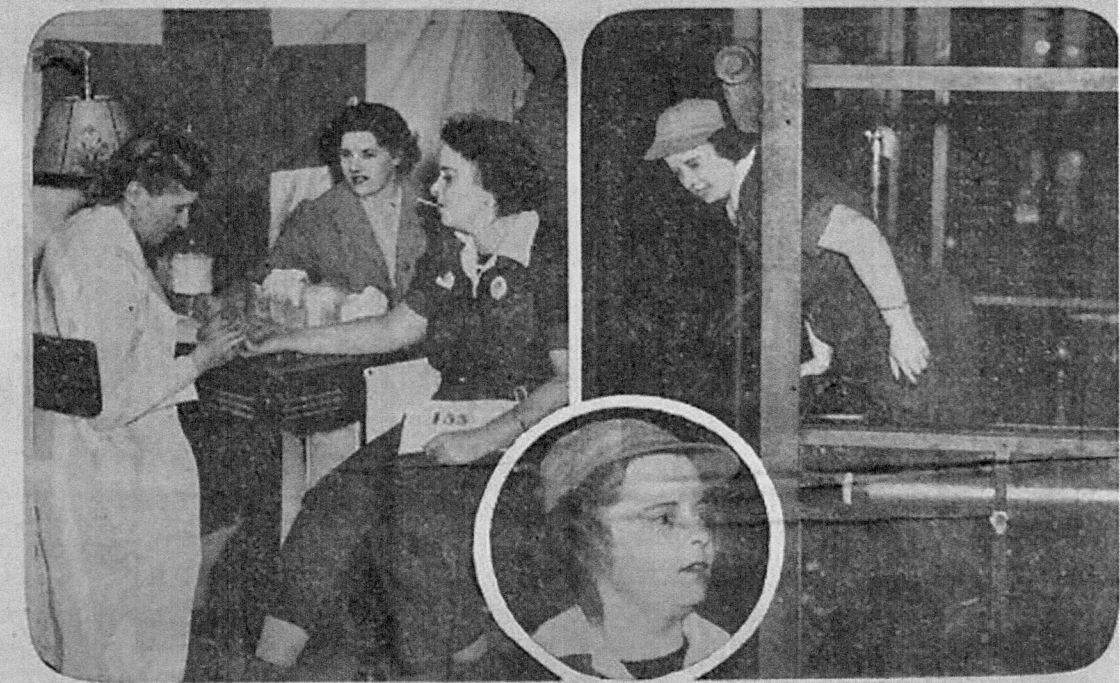

After working eight hours as a crane operator at the Watertown Arsenal, Miss Grace Currier goes to the Red Cross blood centre, still dressed in her oil-smeared overalls, to offer her blood as another contribution on her part in the war effort. Insert—Closeup of Miss Currier, who has pledged to give her blood to the Red Cross every eight weeks.

High above the factory floor, Miss Currier operates one of th 10-ton cranes at the Arsenal. She gave up her job as a masseus to work in the government defense plant.

As ordinary men and women continued to risk their lives to protect our fundamental freedoms, the Boston school nurses went about their duties and daily lives during the war. However, in November 1942, the nurses' salary committee continually pursued its demand for a salary increase by initiating a new proposal. It stated: 1) their nurses' duties, responsibilities had increased problems due to the war, and 2) the increase in the cost of living. When the draft caught up with young men, families experienced the sense of separation and loss, stress and confusion, grief, and fear when their loved ones journeyed to distant lands, maybe to never return. The school nurses, therefore, dealt with these issues involving children and staff, and maybe themselves.

The nurses thought that a lawyer who understood their situation could compile the material in a forceful, business-like manner, and write petitions for them. Of course, they would have to pay him. One of the school nurses said she knew of a lawyer whom she thought could handle the matter. Mr. Parker's name did not surface again. He was the lawyer who handled their case several years before.

Therefore, before the end of 1942, they contacted their supervisor Miss McCaffrey to make her aware of their position on salary. She responded by saying she wished they would have contacted her sooner. They, in turn, responded they had. She advised them to have a small committee of school nurses approach the Boston School Committee with their petition. They met with the President of the Boston School Committee, Mr. Ward, who confirmed the nurses were entitled to a salary increase. Additionally, he insisted several members of the Boston School Committee should receive the salary petition. The school nurses' salary committee decided to have their President of the BSNC, Miss Cronin, follow through with the request, and to include the number of nurses on maximum salary and the expected salary increase.

No meeting minutes were recorded from 1943, whether it means that no meetings were held, or so few attended we don't know. However, we are thankful for the notes that we have. They reactivated again in 1944 with salaries being discussed, and a petition to be presented to the Board of Apportionment. In contrast to past meeting minutes, they were reduced to only two-three sentences long, as opposed to a detailed one to two pages.[313] The question of course is what was happening? Perhaps the increased demands of their jobs and the general complexity surrounding the war superseded the need for detailed minutes.

By 1944, they had a lawyer, a Mr. Carney, who pushed that their salaries be recognized by the BSC for an increase. They presented a petition to their Supervisor, Miss Helen McCaffrey, and Miss Katherine McDonnell, an Assistant Superintendent, that school nurses' salaries should be comparable to that of elementary schoolteachers.[314] Thus, they found a new approach and staked out a position.

---

313 *Boston Public School Nurses Club Minutes 10/1942-12/1942*

314 *Boston Public School Nurses Club Minutes: 5/1944-11/1944.*

Simultaneously, other forces were at work in the form of organized labor union activity, forcing industries into concessions to maintain peak production. At that time, no labor unions existed for public employees, just the AFL, CIO, United Auto Workers, and United Mine Workers to deal with private companies. Tom Di Lorenzo, an uncompromising United Auto Workers leader, told *The Washington Post* in 1943, "Our policy is not to win the war at any cost."[315] The government hoped that organized labor would pitch in like the rest of the country to win the war by not going on production-slowing strikes. Unfortunately, that did not happen. Despite a no-strike pledge signed after Pearl Harbor, strikes and work stoppages continued throughout the war. In one case, at a North American aircraft plant, the workers defied the union and stayed on the job.

Barely one month after Pearl Harbor, the number of strikes leaped from 22 in January 1942 to 220 by July. In 1943, when the outlook for the war was at its lowest point, organized labor's actions still continued in the same manner, with 4.1 million labor days lost leaping to 13.5 million. President Roosevelt fumed when the United Mine Workers walked off the job for three days. He retaliated by ordering the Army to seize the mines and threatened to jeopardize the miners draft deferments. Congress immediately responded by passing the Smith Connally Bill, which instituted a questionable effect of requiring a 60-day notice before going on strike. This, however, did not defer work stoppages, because even in 1944, the last full year of the war, 4,950 work stoppages were costing 8.7 million labor days, enough time to build 2,000 B-17 planes.[316] What happened to their patriotism? Did they have no duty to their country?

By contrast, recall Superintendent of Schools, Gould saying, "It subordinates everything else to the winning of the war." Selective Service data revealed that a large number of enrollees, about 25 percent, were rejected because of disabilities. At the time, they considered this situation serious enough to influence national security. As a result, this fostered a renewed interest in preventive aspects of public health. To better prepare more young men to pass muster and be accepted into the military, the Boston schools approved a more thorough physical exam. Boys in their senior year received complete physical exams, without clothing. School

---

315 Herman, A. (2011, March 3). *Missing in Action: Unions in World War II*. Retrieved from http://www.writersreps.com/feature.aspx?FeatureID=214

316 Ibid.

physicians and school nurses then focused their attention on the application of remedial measures enabling students later on to pass the military physical.

The Department of School Hygiene extended their tuberculosis program, bringing x-ray machines to the schools, and eliminating the tuberculin skin test. They focused their attention on the senior high school boys and later included some intermediate schools. Out of the 15 high schools surveyed, 2,387 boys received X-rays. They found only one case of pulmonary tuberculosis. On the other hand, they discovered 41 cases of childhood tuberculosis. Students with this history, though, were accepted into the military.[317] At that time, school nurses were not assigned to high schools. As a result, school nurses appointed to this particular program did the follow-up work required, invariably realizing that many of these boys would never return. Undoubtedly, they kept a smile on their faces and wished the boys well.

Amidst all of the developments, the school nurses sent out a notice of an important meeting at the Hotel Lenox to elect officers. Besides Miss Cronin on the ballot for president, was a contender for the position, Margaret J. Ryan. The challenger won. The BPSNC extended a vote of thanks to Miss Cronin and the other officers for their splendid service. Miss Cronin would still be on the Salary Committee and the Executive Board.[318]

Though there is no mention in their minutes, I wonder what effect all the work stoppages and strikes had on the morale of the school nurses. It must have created some type of conversation among them, but, of course, we will never know. However, we can permit ourselves some thoughtful reflection here. I believe it just was not stitched into the fabric of their DNA to be involved with a work stoppage or strike for higher wages during wartime.

In 1945, the BPSNC went on record as opposing HB 894, which would have given the Mayor the authority to appoint members of the Boston School Committee. This was defeated despite the release of the Strayer Report in October 1944, which advocated a complete overhaul of the school administration, including obtaining

---

317 *Annual Report of the Superintendent 1943*. P. 56-57. Retrieved from https://archive.org/stream/report1943bost#page/60/mode/2up

318 *Boston Public School Nurses Club Minutes: 11/29/1944, 12/14/1944*

school committee members by a different method. The Report noted that Boston School Committee positions had become a "springboard to politics."[319] The BPSNC offered the supervisory staff nurses an invitation to join as honorary members of their club, which they promptly accepted. Though the war seemed to be drawing to a close, their president, vice president, plus another school nurse enlisted with the Army Nurse Corps.[320]

A petition, drawn up by the Salary Committee, outlined their request for an increase in the maximum salary of nurses to $2,208 per year in three annual increments of $96 each. The BSC had frozen their salary since 1936. Though they received an increase in their maximum pay, their maximum salary still remained lower than that of an elementary school teacher by $288 annually. As the headlines in *The Boston Daily Record* on August 11, 1945, shouted out, "B-29's Halt Jap Raids for Surrender Offer," the Boston School Committee issued new salary guidelines:

NURSES	*Starting Salary*	*Increment*	*Maximum*
Sup Nurse	$2,040	$120	$3,600
Assistant Supervisory Nurse	$1,824	$96	$2,304
School Nurses	$1,248	$96	$2,016
TEACHERS			
Teachers, (Intermediate Men)	$1,584	$144	$3,024
Teachers, (Intermediate Women)	$1,344	$144	$2,400
Teachers, Elementary	$1,248	$144	$2,304

---

319 Dudley, U. (1944, Nov 24). The Strayer Survey. *Daily Boston Globe (1928-1960)*, p. 10. Retrieved from http://search.proquest.com/docview/840048619?accountid=9675

320 *Boston Public School Nurses Club Minutes: 1/23/1945, 2/27/1945, 3/27/1945*

This is obvious gender bias. You will doubtlessly have noted that the male teachers received a higher salary than the women for performing the same job. The Massachusetts Historical Society's 2016 exhibition of Turning Points in American History displayed a letter that Abigail Adams wrote to her husband John Adams while he was at the Continental Congress working on the Declaration of Independence in 1776. She famously advised him to "Remember the ladies," something which the Boston School Committee obviously lost sight of in the interim.

During the war, over 77,000 nurses served in the Armed Forces, which at that time was more than two-fifths of the active nurses. Despite this, a nursing shortage still remained in the military. As a result, President Franklin D. Roosevelt, in his 1945 Congressional address, proposed a national draft of nurses. Leading nursing organizations, despite supporting a national service act for both men and women, did not support this resolution. This proposal became a moot point when we celebrated VE Day (Victory in Europe Day) in 1945 and later VJ Day (Victory in Japan Day) that same year.

A change in Boston school nursing leadership resulted when Helen McCaffrey retired, and Marion C. Sullivan, a former assistant supervising nurse, became the acting supervising nurse.[321]

The war was over but at a price. According to the U.S. Department of Defense, out of the 16.1 million personnel who served in the U.S. Armed Forces, 405,399 were killed. Two hundred and one nurses died. "The Greatest Generation" started returning home in 1945, as Tom Brokaw, a noted television journalist and author of later years, used this term in his 1998 book describing the men and women who grew up during the deprivations of the Great Depression. After that, he stated, these men and women went on to fight in World War II, as well as those on the home front. I am including Boston's school nurses because they made decisive material contributions to the war effort. Tom Brokaw insisted, "These men and women fought not for fame and recognition, but because it was the 'right thing to do.'" He argued, "It is, I believe, the greatest generation any society has ever produced."

Join me now as we follow the Boston school nurses in post-World War II America with so many new variables at play.

---

321 *Proceedings of the School Committee, City of Boston, 1945: 125, 127, 147*

Twentieth Century Milestones
Affecting School Nursing (Continued)

1935 - Sulfonamides identified
Passage of Social Security Act
National Council for War Service founded to coordinate nursing services during wartime.

1940s - Advent of mass-produced antibiotics
World War II 1941-1945

1943 - Nurse Training Act passed, making available free training for nurses
Streptomycin introduced as the first remedy for tuberculosis.

1945 - Penicillin produced

1946 - Communicable Disease Center established became Centers for Disease Control and Prevention

1949 - Association of Colored Graduate Nurses becomes part of the American Nurses Association

1950 - Boston's Population: 801,444.

1950s - School nurse roles expand to include health education. Polio becomes a major health issue.

1950-1953 - Korean War.

1953 - Structure of DNA identified.

1954 - "Separate but equal" schools for black and white students declared unconstitutional.

1955 - Advent of Salk polio vaccine. School nurses join with public health efforts to eliminate polio.

1957 - Sabin polio vaccine introduced.

1957 - Massachusetts School Nurse Law amended, requiring that a school nurse be a Registered Nurse.

Chapter 12

Post-World War II School Nursing

Part I

By the 1940s, over 80 percent of American households would own a radio, making it easier to listen to American music. During this big band and swing music era, returning troops post war often sang the popular homecoming song, "Back Home for Keeps," written by Carmen Lombardo and Bob Russell. The soldiers described their years away during the war, and their yearning to have everything remain the same when they return.[322]

This longing for untroubled times touched so many in the nation, including New England's veterans. They gladly returned home from far-flung locations to the Northeast's historic villages and verdant landscapes untouched by war. One Bowdoin College alumnus, while serving overseas during the war, wrote home to the president of his alma mater, pleading that nothing change when the war was over, that everything would remain the same in the much-loved school of his youth. After careful thought, President Kenneth C.M. Sills, according to *The Encyclopedia of New England*, replied to him, understanding that the young man wanted all beliefs and traditions that make New England this unique and richly endowed corner of America to remain unchanged. He wrote that it was "wishful thinking to believe that we shall return to the situation that existed before the war.

---

322   *World War II in American Music*. Retrieved from http://www.authentichistory.com/1939-1945/3-music/13-Homecoming/index.html"

We must gird ourselves for new tasks, new problems, new responsibilities." The President's prophecy proved true.

President, Franklin Delano Roosevelt, the only president to serve four terms in office, passed away in 1945. A former haberdasher, his vice president, Harry S. Truman, then stepped within the hallowed walls of the Oval Office. When those who served in the Armed Forces returned, they faced a dreary economic climate in Boston, unlike the rest of the country. Manufacturing peaked in 1916, as discussed in Chapter 10. The textile, shoe, and leather industries were decimated. Boston's heyday as a manufacturing center was past.

The government rapidly canceled military contracts, leaving employees and management in an unfortunate situation. Pratt and Whitney, the aircraft company, which employed 40,000 wartime employees in Connecticut and Massachusetts's towns, lost $400 million in orders within just a few days of the war ending. Wartime price controls were lifted as well as wartime wage controls, causing the unions to instigate work stoppages to resist the vast layoffs. During the war, as there were no luxuries to buy, people saved their money. In the immediate post-war period, consumers were eager to purchase goods, but because the economy changed so fast, there was a shortage of merchandise in Boston and Massachusetts.

Real estate development was also latent, with the 1915 Custom House Tower still standing as the city's tallest building. Boston had constructed no new office buildings since 1930. They built the last major hotel in 1927. Between 1929 and 1950, personal income fell by 20 percent.[323] The city's population peaked in 1950 at 801,444 people and then suffered a tremendous loss in the populace. Boston lost 30 percent of its population in the following 30 years, as automobiles made moving to the suburbs possible for more people. However, Boston still had assets in the form of banks, educational institutions, and health care that sustained growth in the succeeding years.

Strayer Report

The Boston Finance Commission released the Strayer Report in October 1944, earlier referred to in Chapter 11. It fought to push the Boston Public Schools (BPS) forward even as other industries lagged behind. The report continued to raise awareness of problems

---

[323] From Basket Case to Innovation Hub. (Spring 2015). *MHS Miscellany* No. 108, 8.

within the Boston Public Schools and tackle many thorny and intractable issues.

The survey found a variety of problems, such as unequal pay for men and women, weak personnel policies, and an absence of vigorous leadership and administrative planning. Other troublesome findings were a school curriculum that needed to be revitalized and modernized and an improvement in physical facilities, including closing down eight schools that were underutilized and possible fire traps. The report cited a system of costly and inefficient school maintenance and repairs and suggested finding another way to recruit school committee members. For example, the study discovered no soap or towels available for general use in any of the school buildings visited. The Boston School Committee balked at spending $15,000 for soap and towels, and instead appropriated a paltry $5,000. This decision denied 100,000 Boston school children the right to develop proper hand-washing habits.[324]

The Strayer Report unearthed the BPS's bizarre, sexist, and unpredictable pay scale hierarchy, another big issue. To illustrate this point, the survey cited that salaries of school custodians ranged from $35 to $103 a week, besides the $200 a year emergency compensation of all city employees since March 1, 1943. At the lowest end, a custodian could make a basic $1,820 per year in contrast to $5,356 at the top of the scale. Entrance requirements for the job description of a custodian as to education, age, the training, aptitude, or experience didn't exist, and they did not develop any organized training. An applicant had to meet the only requirement, which was to be a citizen who had lived in the state for one year and in Boston for six months. The survey found it absurd that there were 178 different salary scales for 247 senior custodians.[325]

The key idea here is to demonstrate the custodians were doing very well financially as compared to teachers. On the other hand, school nurses wanted to be on the same salary level as the elementary teachers. The survey found that Boston male teachers averaged $900 to $1,000 more than women teachers. Furthermore, they entered the Boston school system at a rate of $300 more than women, doing

---

324 Lyons, L. (1944, Oct 26) a. $15,000 saved on soap, towels," $250,000 wasted on repairs. *Daily Boston Globe* (1928-1960), pp. 1. Retrieved from http://search.proquest.com/docview/840029992?accountid=9675

325 Lyons, L. (1944, Nov 21) b. Urges equal pay for men, women; more state support. *Daily Boston Globe* (1928-1960), pp. 5. Retrieved from http://search.proquest.com/docview/840046949?accountid=9675

the same job, and could reach the top of the scale at $800 faster than a female in the same position. The highest-paid custodian made more in salary than the principal of Boston's largest intermediate school.

Likewise, the survey revealed though Boston salaries for high schoolteachers were greater than in most cities, wages for elementary and middle school staff were lower. The Strayer Survey suggested paying elementary and intermediate teachers the same salary as the high school teachers for equal qualifications and preparation.

As the practice was, then, men taught boys in high school, and women taught girls. Therefore, as we can see from the salary scales, the city paid more to teach boys than it did to educate girls, making teaching boys a higher paying job. Whereas a growing trend in American society was equal pay for equal work, regardless of sex, Boston remained bogged down with endless titles, classifications, and petitions by various teacher groups.[326]

"Legislators Secretly Vote to Shelve Strayer Bill" read the headline in the *Daily Boston Globe* on March 20, 1945, as the state legislators met in a secret session at the Parker House. This action prevailed, despite the recommendations of the Finance Commission that sponsored the survey, to adopt the suggested proposals to pull the school system out of what they claimed was its degenerative spiral.

Post-War Nursing: National Trends

A drastic shortage of nurses occurred after the end of World War II. This was due to several reasons:

1. Only one in six returned to their previous position.
2. Many nurses returning from the war wanted to pursue marriage and a family, and until the 1960s nurses, as well as teachers, were expected to resign when they married.
3. Nurses returning from the military, where they had profoundly autonomous roles with significant responsibility were reluctant to come back to a hospital

---

[326] Lyons, L. (1944, Nov 21) b. Urges equal pay for men, women; more state support. *Daily Boston Globe* (1928-1960), pp. 5. Retrieved from http://search.proquest.com/docview/840046949?accountid=9675

where they would have a subservient role as a hospital staff nurse.
4. Returning military nurses needed a change due to the intense war experiences.
5. They believed a professional should receive better wages and working conditions.

The Focus of School Health Shifted

In addition, nationally, school health experienced a shift in focus. It was the beginning of a philosophy that students and their parents should be more responsible for the protection and maintenance of their own health. Whether Boston's Department of School Hygiene would follow the rest of the nation in this regard would remain to be seen. School nurses became more involved with the health curriculum, working closely with schoolteachers to develop health lessons. This trend resulted in 40 states requiring nurses by 1949 to have a teaching certificate and 16 state Departments of Education, also requiring certification of the nurse who taught classes. By 1948, Congress defeated a National School Health Bill that proposed giving federal grant-in-aid to school health. This loss was partly due to the objections of the medical profession that feared federal funds for medical treatment given during school time would be provided to those who could afford to pay.

"Nurses were paid far less than elementary school teachers, the professional group to whom nurses were most often compared," writes Karen J. Egenes, contrasting nurses and teachers in *Issues and Trends in Nursing*.[327] The California Nurses Association prepared a study in 1946 and found that the majority of staff nurses were paid only slightly more than hotel maids and seamstresses. The Executive Director of the California Nurses Association, Shirley Titus, in 1946, at the American Nurses Association, successfully lobbied for economic empowerment for nurses. This plan included collective bargaining, insurance plans, benefits packages, and the right to consult with the state nurses' associations. By 1949, the American Nurses Association approved the right of nurses to use state nurses' associations as bargaining agents.

Once again, there were other forces at work. A 1947 revision of the Taft Hartley Labor Act exempted non-profit institutions such as hospitals and public schools

---

[327] Egenes, K. (2018) History of Nursing. In Roux, G., & Halstead, J. (Ed) *Issues and Trends in Nursing*, p. 21. Retrieved from jblearning.com/samples/0763752258/52258-ch01-roux.pdf2/6/2014

from the requirement to enter into labor negotiations with their employees to address workplace grievances. This affected nurses because the American Nurses Association had adopted a "no-strike" rule. Therefore, since hospitals and schools were not required to enter into labor negotiations with their employees, this left nurses with no way to improve their work conditions other than resigning or collectively pressuring their employers for improved working conditions. However, as noted in Chapter 11, a strike was not in the fabric of their DNA, and relatively few nursing strikes occurred.

What a bonus it would have been if the nurses had some knowledge of workplace negotiations. Did the school nurses have any transferable skills? Not many. Did they have a teacher? Did they have someone to pick them up should they stumble and fall? Not really. Nevertheless, they made slow but steady progress in collective bargaining. More about this in Chapter 15. Over time, through professional development and advanced education, school nurses would learn how to quantify the market value of their education, skills, and experience, and how to create a strategic pitch to the BSC to help them successfully negotiate for a new salary, ask for a raise, and build their self-confidence.

Boston Public School Nurses in the Post WW II Period

In the meantime, the BPSN made plans for a supper gathering but abruptly changed their plans at their February 28, 1946, meeting after discussing a bill pending at the State House. This bill recommended that, the appointment of school physicians and nurses be under the supervision of the Board of Health. It also urged that the Board of Health regulate the physical examinations of children. The bill did not pass. This debate over who is in charge of school health services continues to this day with the educators insisting that they are efficient administrators, and health departments responding in a counter argument that health personnel should operate health services.

Always forward-thinking, in 1946, BPSNC discussed a three-day sick leave that the other school "clubs" enjoyed, pursued a second and third increment, and possibly joining the Grievance Committee. They contemplated joining the "Teachers Alliance Club" with the potentiality of becoming Associate Members. Their salary discussions signaled a fresh round of debate asking for an increase of $800 and talk of changes in the pension plan. The school nurses received ongoing assistance in the form of letters supporting their request for a salary increase from their Supervisor, Miss Sullivan, the Supervising Physician, Dr. James Keenan, and Mr. Clement Norton, Chairman of the BSC.[328]

By 1947, the BPSNC received a letter from Superintendent Arthur L. Gould announcing the formation of a Grievance Committee to which they were to send a representative. Miss Miller, their vice president, became their representative. One of the issues they wanted to raise at the Grievance Committee concerned permission to attend lectures to gain information for the betterment of the club.[329]

Later in 1947, President Chapdelaine of the BPSNC received a surprising letter from the Department of Labor and Industries, State House, Boston, stating that the club acted like a "labor union." The Department of Labor and Industries asserted that the organization fell under the following definition that the Department used as a guide: *"Any organization of any kind, or an agency or employee representation committee or plan, in which employees participate and which exists for the purpose, in whole or in part, of dealing with employers concerning grievances, labor disputes, wages, rates of pay, hours of employment, or conditions of work."* Hence, the Department directed the BPSNC to file a statement required under the provisions of Chapter 618, Acts of 1946. The activities of the Club on behalf of the school nurses seemed to qualify. However, whether the Club undertook any actions is unclear, since there is no further reference of filing a statement.[330]

As was their custom, the BPSNC contacted the Chairman of the Boston School Committee (BSC), Clement Norton, extending their grateful appreciation for his efforts on their behalf in obtaining their salary increase. In response, Chairman Clement Norton urged them to attend the BSC meetings and make themselves known to the BSC members. Other groups did it, he continued, and "the creaking gate gets oil." He explained further that he wants to make, "our nurses the best-paid group in Boston."[331]

---

328 *Boston Public School Nurses Club Minutes*: 4/15/1946, 10/16/1946, 11/12/1946

329 *Boston Public School Nurses Club Minutes*: 2/24/1947, 3/11/1947

330 *Boston Public School Nurses Club Minutes*: 5/15/1947

331 *Boston Public School Nurses Club Minutes*: 5/20/1947

The BPSNC apparently followed his advice. A newspaper article reported that Mary C. Clifford, representing the assistant supervising nurses, submitted a request at a BSC public hearing where there were 17 teacher organizations presenting grievances, that they should raise the assistant supervising nurses' salary from $3,624 to $4,488. Charges filled this meeting of the BSC using political favoritism to fill positions.[332]

According to their *BPSNC Minutes* at this time, in their opinion a school nurse having a Bachelor of Science in Nursing called a BSN should receive any additional raises that other school departments were offered. Also recorded was a conversation with Miss McDonnell, an Assistant Superintendent, assuring President Chapdelaine of the BPSNC, that school nurses would receive a raise to $3,100 annually, at least retroactive to January 1, 1948. They discussed specialized fields of nursing versus generalized nursing and found that Miss McDonnell favored school nursing as a specialty.[333] These issues fell around two critical matters at hand, which were: a) their salaries linked to their level of education, and b) recognition of school nursing as a distinct specialty. As the school nurses stepped forward, trying to make changes, they recognized they had to focus on these themes of education and professional respect. We will see how they confronted these problems over time. I wonder what thoughts followed them in their lives during these days of uncertainty, bringing this poem of Emily Dickinson to mind:

Hope is the thing with feathers
That perches in the soul,
And sings the tune without the words,
And never stops at all.

And sweetest in the gale is heard;
And sore must be the storm
That could abash the little bird
That kept so many warm.

I've heard it in the chilliest land

---

332   Charges of Job Bootlegging Heard at Teachers' Session. (1949, Jun 25*). Daily Boston Globe* (1928-1960). pp. 3. Retrieved from http://search.proquest.com/docview/822232138?accountid=9675

333   *Boston Public School Nurses Club Minutes*: 5/25/1948).

And on the strangest sea;
Yet, never, in extremity,
It asked a crumb of me.

Salary[334]

Throughout this time, the BPSNC continued to advocate for an increase in their pay. See the image on the next page, for a comparison of school nurse versus teacher salaries from 1945 to 1955.

COMPARISON OF SALARIES 1945-1955

CATEGORY	SALARIES 1945			1947			1948			1949		
	MIN	INCRE	MAX	MIN	INCRE	MAX	MIN	INCRE	MAX	MIN	INCRE	MAX
Supervising Nurse	$2,040	$120	$3,600	$2,640	$144	$4,200	$3,480	$144	$4,920	$3,780	$144	$5,220
Ass't Sup Nurse Nurse	$1,824	96	2,304	2,616	144	3,100	2,616	144	3,624	2,916	144	4,212
Nurse	$1,248	96	2,016	2,040	144	2,616	2,184	144	3,336	2,484	144	3,636
School Medical Aid							$33.68 per week			$45.18 per week		
Nurse Certificating										$192 Additional		
Intermediate Teacher										2,484	144	3,924
Male	$1,584	144	3,024	2,184	144	3,624	2,184	144	3,624			
Female	$1,344	144	2,400	2,040	144	3,100	2,184	144	3,624			
Elementary Teacher	$1,248	144	2,304	2,040	144	3,100	2,184	144	3,624	2,484	144	3,924

CATEGORY	SALARIES 1951			1953			1954			1955		
	MIN	INCRE	MAX	MIN	INCRE	MAX	MIN	INCRE	MAX	MIN	INCRE	MAX
Supervising Nurse	$4,248	$144	$5,688	$4,368	$144	$5,808	SAME			$4,368	$144	$5,928
Ass't Sup Nurse	3,384	144	4,680	3,504	144	4,800	3,504	144	4,980	3,504	144	5,160
Nurse	2,952	144	4,104	3,132	144	4,284	3,312	144	4,464	3,492	144	4,644
School Medical Aid	$50.18 per week			$53.63 per week			$58.63 per week			SAME		
Nurse Certificating Office	$192 Additional			SAME			$230 additional			$288 additional		
Intermediate Teacher				3,312	144	4,752 4,752	3,492	144	4,932			
Male												
Female												
Elementary Teacher	$2,952	144	4,392	3,312	144	4,752 4,752	3,492	144	4,932	3,504	144	5,112

334 (*Proceedings of the School Committee, City of Boston, 1945*: 125,127)
(*Proceedings of the School Committee, City of Boston, 1947*: 163,165)
(*Proceedings of the School Committee, City of Boston, 1948*: 113,117)
(*Proceedings of the School Committee, City of Boston, 1949*: 202,205)
(*Proceedings of the School Committee, City of Boston, 1951*: 226,228)
(*Proceedings of the School Committee, City of Boston, 1953*: 449,501)
(*Proceedings of the School Committee, City of Boston, 1954*: 311,312)

No doubt, you can see that in 1945 through 1951, the elementary school teacher and the school nurse received the same starting salary. The breakthrough for teachers came in 1948 when, for the first time, elementary teachers received the same wage as middle school teachers, and male and female intermediate teachers received the same salary. In 1954, the Boston School Committee broke that tradition and rated the intermediate and elementary school teachers with a higher starting salary and higher maximum salary than school nurses. It seems that school nurses were good, but never good enough. The Boston school nurses needed time to sort this out.

New Massachusetts Vision Test

At one of their meetings, Miss Chapdelaine praised the Massachusetts Vision Test. She observed how it worked on a two-day visit to the Arlington Schools. Dr. James J. Regan, the department's ophthalmologist, started using the Massachusetts Eye Test in 1946. He implemented a pilot project in Mrs. Miller's Henry L. Higginson district.[335] Tests sought to bring vision screening procedures more up to date and utilize a method approved by leading eye specialists.[336] The school nurse would still retest all children with defective hearing. Note that this was the first time they referred to a nurse as Mrs.

Greater Boston Community Survey

Yet again, another study, the 1949 Greater Boston Community Survey, conveyed recommendations for a healthier Boston, including a review of the Boston school nurses. The Survey recommended the requirements for future school nurses be similar to those of public health nurses. The National Organization for Public Health Nursing and the American Public Health Association also supported these prerequisites. These recommendations, they noted, should be included in the qualifications for newly hired personnel, such as a staff nurse, assistant supervisor, and supervisor.

Another proposal advised they extend school nursing services to all the Boston Public Schools, including special schools and high schools. The Survey's suggestion for school nurse assignments using this model cited one nurse per 1,500 pupils, which they considered doable with the current staff.

---

335   *Annual Report of the Superintendent 1946.* P. 63. City of Boston Printing Department 1947.

336   *Boston Public School Nurses Club Minutes*: 1/7/1952

The third recommendation advised examining the school nurses' functions to concentrate on the most effective use of their time. Activities they considered superfluous and needing elimination included classroom talks, compiling of reports, taking children to clinics, and routine classroom inspections. What the Survey found to be the most crucial involved time for planned nurse-teacher conferences and nurses working with families.

Also, the Survey advised combining all three nursing services, which are the Department of Public Health, the Visiting Nurse Association, which was a private organization, and the Boston school nurses under the Department of Health. This entity would provide nursing services for the school health program as part of the generalized public health nursing plan of the Department of Health.[337]

The Greater Boston Community Survey highlighted several issues. Regarding public health experience and education, the Boston supervising nurse sent a letter in 1953 stating that 34 of the school nurses had less than one year of public health nursing education, and 23 had one or more years of public health nursing education. Just one year later, the *Annual Superintendent's Report 1950* asserted that they started to appoint registered nurses to high schools to strengthen their school program.

They voiced another concern related to the functions and activities of the school nurse, which seems to impart the definition-ambiguity of the school nurses' role and recognition by the school community and families. Definitely, they should eliminate nurses taking children to clinics for routine examinations. However, in the instance of an emergency situation at school, until a parent was located, school nurses should be prepared to accompany the pupil to the emergency room. As noted earlier in Chapter 5, Annie McKay, Boston's first school nurse, found it necessary, after a while, to ask for an assistant when a student needed a routine medical checkup, and the parent could not for a variety of reasons, accomplish this.

Compiling of reports or what we refer to as paperwork, on the other hand, continues to be crucial. Who would know what the school nurse did and if her activities had any effect on keeping the child in school, safe, healthy, and ready to learn? It is what we call today evidence-based strategies and interventions.

---

[337] Recommendations for A Healthier Boston. (1949, Feb 18). *Daily Boston Globe (1928-1960)*, pp.2. Retrieved from http://search.proquest.com/docview/839546908?accountid=9675

The Survey considered routine classroom inspections as another function to be on the chopping block. Nationally, health counseling replaced that term. The objectives and outcomes of the inspections became more critical, rather than the number of classroom inspections screened annually. It covered both the examination and the follow-up. Prevention and control of communicable diseases have always been one of the functions of the school nurse. These inspections discover signs and symptoms of contagious diseases, so, once again, I disagree with the Survey's recommendations.

Changing Times for Women

This was a time of change. A Federal Reserve bulletin in 1950 declared that there were more married women holding jobs outside the home than single women. Since the early part of the 20th century and beyond, women's place had been in the home. Until she married, she remained at home under the protection and support of her father or another male relative. Of course, there were exceptions. If a young woman did not find a husband and had to support herself, she could seek a job working for another woman, or in an office, or manufacturing and selling clothes. The point is that a working woman was predictably either a single woman or a widow. A few years down the road, many of these women did get married. Then, the next question was, should she continue to work, or stay home, look after a few rooms and her husband until children came. Economics enters the picture, and the young bride may decide that it was easier to run a household with two salaries than one.

On the other hand, the new groom may come from a traditional background, and oppose the idea of a working wife. Both sets of in-laws may not be trailblazers but embrace traditions. Life doesn't stand still. Customs change frightfully slow, but they made steady progress. More and more women were looking after both jobs, homes, and children.[338]

The Massachusetts League of Women Voters, many of them former teachers, asserted that women should be allowed to teach after marriage. "The behavior of male teachers and male elected officials at keeping women in a lower place today seems reactionary and reprehensible," writes Cronin.[339] This statewide teacher tenure law finally pasted in

---

338   Dudley, U. (1950, May 23). Working Wives. *Daily Boston Globe* (1928-1960), pp. 16. Retrieved from http://search.proquest.com/docview/821306662?accountid=9675

339   Cronin, J. M. (2008). *Reforming Boston School, 1930-2006. P. 45. Overcoming Corruption and Racial Segregation. New York*: Palgrave MacMillan.

1953, but not before some rancorous arguments at the Boston School Committee (BSC).

It took some time before the BSC addressed the new law. They passed an amendment to regulations Section 283 on July 1, 1954 that stated, "If a female teacher or a female member of the supervising staff shall marry, it shall be her duty to report such marriage forthwith to the superintendent and the business manager."[340] Anticipating this new regulation, on January 11, 1954, school nurse Marie Marotto reported that she married on October 3, 1953. Her new name was Marie Rubico.

About a week later, the regulation was brought up again for a vote, and BSC member Mr. Ward voted no, in opposition to married teachers within the schools.

> *"If this is simply a question that they report to the Superintendent after something is done, it's a technical subject. I again reiterate my firm stand and belief that we are going to stop juvenile delinquency; we are going to stop mothers teaching in schools and not taking care of the family at home. As I have stated before, if they want to visit their children in a reformatory in an automobile, which they own because there are two salaries coming in, they have a child in the reformatory. They should give the car up and keep the child at home."*

Despite his viewpoint, the order passed on a vote of four to one. This mandate was followed by another directive that stated the status of marriage should not affect a woman from taking the qualification exam for appointment as a teacher. As we can see, all of these new rules applied equally to school nurses.

A Boston School Committee Conversation

A thought-provoking and at times heated conversation and exchange of ideas occurred at a Boston School Committee meeting in 1952 between a new member of the BSC, Mrs. Alice Lyons, Assistant Superintendent Frederick J. Gillis, Chairman Isadore H.Y. Muchnick, and the BSC secretary Agnes E. Reynold. The subject concerned the disparity between the working hours and pay of the temporary school physicians and the nurse at the Certificating Office. The Chairman wanted to know why the nurses received $12 per day, and the school physicians received $10 during the periods July 21

---

340 *Proceedings of the School Committee of the City of Boston 1954.* P. 256. Retrieved from https://archive.org/stream/proceedingsofsch1954bost#page/38/mode/2up/search/married+teachers

through August 8, 1952, and September 2 through September 10, 1952.[341]

The secretary replied, "Doctors are only part-time. Nurses work all day."

Chairman: "And nurses stay the full day?"

Secretary: "I believe that is the difference."

Mrs. Lyons: "Mr. Superintendent, why do they need a nurse down there all day if the schools are not in session?"

Superintendent: "Mr. Gillis, would you answer that question on the school nurses in the Certificating Office?"

Mrs. Lyons: "Why do they need them down there all day if the schools are not in session?"

Dr. Gillis: "The day begins very early in the morning frequently about 7:30, and they work until after noontime, both the nurse and the doctor. They practically put in a full day, although they begin very early."

Mrs. Lyons: "Then that is not what Miss Reynolds just said when we asked why the doctor got $10 a day and the nurse $12 a day. The nurse gets more than the doctor; and if he works as long as she does, then can you explain why one gets more than the other?"

Dr. Gillis: "Well, the doctor does the examining, and the nurse keeps the records and fills out the records after the doctor has gone. I didn't know she got so much money. Her day will be longer than the doctor's. She doesn't leave when he leaves."

Mrs. Lyons: "Is she there all day?"

Dr. Gillis: "She is there for a full day's work."

---

[341] *Proceedings of the School Committee of the City of Boston 1952.* P. 156. Retrieved from https://archive.org/details/proceedingsofsch1952bost

Mrs. Lyons: "That doesn't quite answer my question. I said: Why do they have that office open when the schools are closed?"

Dr. Gillis: "Because every child who seeks employment during the summer must pass the doctor's examination, and that record must be kept in order to satisfy the requirements for Labor and Industries in the State House and the report sent to Washington as well. It is a state law. We have to examine them."

Mrs. Lyons: "I just wondered why they were open when the schools were closed."

The BSC, not pleased with the arrangement at the Certification Office during the summer months, voted the following year that school nurses assigned for temporary service in the Certification Office during the periods July 6 to 24, 1953, and August 10 to 28, 1953 would be compensated at the rate established for temporary school nurses. That is, they should receive $6 per session, not $12, and only one nurse was to serve at a time.[342] This course of action was justified as the nurse's salary was out of line with the physicians. It also demonstrated that the BSC was well informed when it wanted to be.

Part II - The 1950s: School Nursing National Trends

Across the U.S. in the 1950s, school health continued as it had in the 1940s, with the consensus that schools should not be adding medical treatment. The concept of educating the whole child was the priority, including his social and emotional skills alongside optimum physical health without disabilities. School nurses involved themselves more in teaching health.

Simultaneously, other forces intervened in the form of the Korean War, 1951-1953, prompting the beginning of the Cold War. Studies done during the 1950s found that when they drafted young men, they continued to fail the physical examination, and the U.S. medical services classified them as 4F. This same problem occurred during World War II when U.S. medical services rejected approximately one-

---

342 *Proceedings of the School Committee of the City of Boston 1953.* P. 422. Retrieved from https://archive.org/stream/proceedingsofsch1953bost#page/422/mode/2up/search/nurse.

fourth of the selectees because of physical defects.[343] They continued to show that draftees had physical and mental conditions that could have been corrected during childhood. They rejected American boys for short stature, being underweight, weak physique, venereal disease, heart abnormalities, defective hearing and vision, poor dentition, alcoholism, drug addiction, and foot deformities such as flat foot. Of course, some of these ailments would not have shown up during a boy's school career, but surely, they could have addressed maladies as defective teeth, being underweight, and defective hearing and vision.[344] This problem questioned the value of school physical examinations, which directly affected school physicians. Were these ailments noted, was there no follow-up, or were they both noted and followed-up, but the parents did not care to monitor it any further?

Heart Disease and School Work Study

School nurses participated in research regarding Cardiac Testing in 1939, 1945, and 1955, and engaged in a study of the public health aspects of heart disease, especially rheumatic heart disease in children. One of the goals of the study was to determine the number of children receiving home instruction because of heart disease and how their treatment plan affected their schoolwork.[345] Nurses reviewed the records and presented what cases would be included in the study.

The Boston Public School Nurses Club

In the early 1950s, the BPSNC experienced growing pains. The beginning of the 1952 school year for the BPSNC brought a lack of a quorum at their meetings, forcing them to send a letter out to their members. The letter highlighted the financial expenses of the club as compared to their income, the lack of members at their meetings, and what suggestions could be made to improve the unity of the club.[346] In response, over 30 nurses packed their meeting room on December 2, 1952, to voice support and unanimously voted Sally Givner as their new President. They

---

343 Wold, S. *School Nursing A Framework for Practice*. (1981). P. 9. North Branch, MN: Sunrise River Press.

344 Hoffman, F. Army anthropometry and medical rejection statistics. Retrieved from https://archive.org/stream/armyanthropometr00hoffuoft/armyanthropometr00hoffuoft_djvu.txt

345 *Department of School Hygiene Cardiac Testing 1939,1945,1955*. File. Boston Archive Collection.

346 *Boston Public School Nurses Club Minutes*: 10/7/1952

met at the American Congregational House at 14 Beacon Street, built in 1898, and near all transportation lines. It was a convenient site to hold their meetings.

Over the next few years, the school nurses' discussions included the possible passage of a state bill introduced by the Massachusetts Department of Education School Nurses Group concerning putting school nurses in a teaching category and forming a Salary Committee. They also discussed comparison salaries in other communities, and their lack of representation at School Department meetings. For example, they had no representation on the Planning Board. As noted earlier in this chapter, putting nurses in a teaching category was following a national trend.

Sometimes out of conflict flows new life; sometimes, those rocky periods in our lives turn out to be surprising sources of growth. Consequently, the BPSNC made some decisions: two members, preferably officers, should attend all future dinners of the School Department, at the expense of the club. They would join nursing organizations so that school nurses have representation and sponsor an in-service program for college credit during the summer. School Committeeman, Mr. Lee, suggested that they compile a report showing the duties of the school nurse, the scope of their program, and send it to the Assistant Superintendent, Philip J. Bond.[347]

Their Supervising Nurse forwarded a summary of the school nurses' education to the Boston School Committee.

General College Education
Some college but no degree	44 nurses
One or more collegiate degrees	13 nurses

Public Health Nursing Education
Less than one academic year	34 nurses
One or more academic years	23 nurses

At this time, 1954, there were 61 nurses, four assistant supervising nurses, and one supervising nurse.[348]

Miss Crowe, a Malden Supervising School Nurse, and speaker at one of the

---

347   *Boston Public School Nurses Club Minutes*: 4/7/1953, 9/11/1953, 1/7/1954, 3/9/1954

348   *Boston Public School Nurses Club Minutes* 2/12/1954

BPSNC meetings, encouraged the school nurses to organize, and become associated with national and local education associations. She also suggested applying for a conference cluster within the Public Health Group of the Massachusetts State Nurses' Association.

Elections at the BPSNC in November 1954 produced a new President, Marguerite McLaughlin. She commented, as did her predecessors, on the difficulty and lack of knowledge of how to develop the recommended report since the persons sending the document had no previous expertise in producing a technical report. At this time, they discussed having a single salary for all nurses, regardless of whether they had acquired a college degree. The BPSNC believed, however, that such a plan would discourage others from obtaining a college degree. Miss McLaughlin urged the members to join the Massachusetts State Nurses Association, the Boston Teachers Club, and as well as the School Nurses Association of Massachusetts (SNAM).

During the next few months throughout several meetings, the nurses again discussed the yearly report. Some nurses stated the annual reports did not present an accurate picture of their duties and responsibilities. Their job included many intangibles and matters outside of routine work and daily activities. The question was how to capture the expanse of their role so the Superintendent, Boston School Committee, parents, and the public could understand the extent of their assignments.

Once again, a member of the Boston School Committee advised the nurses to draw up a petition which stated the requirements for school nursing, their number who hold college degrees or degree credits, the purpose of the school nursing program, etc. and include a request that the nurse's salary be on par with that of the teachers. The school nurses decided to add the term "social work," and that they worked with juvenile adjustment counselors. They talked about obtaining a list of salaries of different school nurse groups from Miss Crowe as mentioned above. Another change occurred when Dr. James A. Keenan retired, and Dr. Martin H. Spellman became the new Director of School Hygiene in December 1955.[349]

The disparity in pay in Boston between teachers and school nurses finally came to a head in February 1956 when they submitted their formal petition to the Boston School Committee. In their appeal, the Boston School Nurses Club, as it was then called, urged

---

349   *Boston Public School Nurses Club Minutes 4/5/1955, 5/3/1955*

the BSC to equalize the pay for nurses to that of teachers based upon their educational training and services being performed not only to the students under their care but also extending to the community at large. Already, the petition pointed out that across Massachusetts, 28 school nurse groups received equal wages to that of teachers.

Indeed, by comparison to teachers, nursing qualifications were as rigorous if not equal. In terms of educational requirements, the petition listed that Boston nurses had to have achieved the bare minimum of a three-year diploma from a program of nursing, plus at least eight college credits. Furthermore, nurses had to not only be registered by the MA State Board of Examiners but also pass an exam given by the Boston School Department of Examiners.

As an indication of their pursuit of education, the petition mentioned that an additional 17 Boston school nurses already possessed a BS degree in Nursing or Education while three held master's degrees. Many others were taking courses to obtain their college degrees.

Moving on to their responsibilities towards school children and the communities, the petition itemized 11 different functions, and 24 subcategories that school nurses performed on a daily and weekly basis. Other activities involved their tasks performed after regular work hours, and away from the school, such as in notifying parents, escorting children to hospitals, and home visits.

Within the school environment, school nurses coordinated a range of functions with the school physician, involving various physical exams and preventive immunizations. In addition, the nurse treated minor injuries and performed periodic classroom inspections for dental defects, pediculosis, symptoms of infectious diseases, and cleanliness. The nurse kept detailed records of each child. Other responsibilities included following up on all physical defects, such as defective vision and hearing, physical handicaps, and absences due to illness. The school nurse carried an average workload of 1,200-1,500 students. In a recent school year, they don't say which one, school nurses made 21,261 home visits for 29,261 reasons.

In conclusion, the petition respectfully requested that maximum salaries for Boston school nurses be equalized to that of teachers in recognition not only of the requirements for the position, but also of the myriad of services they performed that benefitted the City as a whole.[350]

At a meeting in April 1957, school nurse Miss Madeline Dolan reported a conversation she had with BSC member, Mr. Herlihy. Frank J. Herlihy informed her that the BSC received their petition, and the salary adjustment committee acted on it favorably. The BSC rated school nurses in Class A with the teachers and those who held an A.B. degree. Were they referring to an Associate degree? This progression to the single salary schedule occurred over a few years. See the following image.

SALARIES	COMPARISON 1955			NURSES AND 1956			TEACHERS 1957		
	MIN	INCRE	MAX	MIN	INCRE	MAX	MIN	INCRE	MAX
Supervising Nurse	$4,368	$144	$5,928	$5,172	$144	$6,048	$5,772	$240	$6,648
Ass't Supervising Nurse	3,504	144	5,160	3,504	144	5,280	4,004	240	5,780
Nurse	3,492	144	4,644	3,504	144	4,824	3,768	240	5,088
School Medical Aid	SAME			$58.63 per week			SAME		
Nurse Certificating Office	$288 additional			SAME			SAME		
Intermediate Teacher				3,504	144	5,292	3,863	240	5,652
Male									
Female									
Elementary Teacher	3,504	144	5,112	3,504	144	5,292	3,768	240	5,556

In 1955, the starting salary for a school nurse was $3,492 as compared to that of an elementary school teacher $3,504.[351] An increase occurred in 1956, raising the school nurse to the same $3,504 starting income as that of an elementary school teacher, intermediate teacher, and assistant supervising nurse, though the maximum for the school nurse tumbled lower than for other staff members.[352] The precedent broke in 1957 when the school nurse, the elementary school teacher, the intermediate schoolteacher and the assistant supervising nurse all received salary hikes, however, only the school nurse and the elementary school teacher obtained an equal starting salary. Yet, the elementary school teacher still picked up

350   *Boston Public School Nurses Club Minutes* February 3, 1956

351   *Proceedings of the School Committee of the City of Boston 1955.* P. 265. Retrieved from https://archive.org/stream/proceedingsofsch1955bost#page/148/mode/2up/search/nurse

352   *Proceedings of the School Committee of the City of Boston 1956.* P. 168. Retrieved from https://archive.org/stream/proceedingsofsch1956bost#page/n3/mode/2up

a higher maximum pay than the school nurse. The intermediate schoolteacher and the assistant supervising nurse received higher minimum and maximum wages than the school nurse and the elementary school teacher.[353] At the time, the Boston Teachers' Alliance cited the shortage of middle and high school teachers as their need to offer them a higher salary.[354]

They were fed up with being predictable, reliable, and perennially underestimated. Therefore, was the time-consuming letter worth it? In the long run, the results stand on their own. See the image on the next page for a comparison of salaries. The school nurses had to speak up for themselves. If they didn't, no one else would. See the chart on the next page comparing salaries in 1961.

COMPARISON OF BOSTON SCHOOL NURSE SALARIES AND TEACHERS 1961

GROUP I

School Nurses and Teachers			Master's Degree		
MIN	AN INCRE	MAXIMUM	MIN	AN INCRE	MAX
$4,740	$240	$6,900	$5,220	$240	$7,380
Step		Salary	Step		Salary
1		$4,740	1		$5,220
2		4,980	2		5,460
3		5,220	3		5,700
4		5,460	4		5,940
5		5,700	5		6,180
6		5,940	6		6,420
7		6,180	7		6,660
8		6,420	8		6,900
9		6,660	9		7,140
10		6,900	10		7,380

GROUP 2 RANKS			GROUP 3 PART A RANKS		
Ass't Sup.Nurse, other Supervisors			Super. Nurse + Guidance Councelors		
MIN	AN INCRE	MAXIMUM	MIN	AN INCRE	MAX
$7,380	$240	$7,860	$7,540	$240	$8,260
Step		Salary	Step		Salary
1		$7,380	1		$7,540
2		7,620	2		7,780
3		7,860	3		8,020
			4		8,260

353   *Proceedings of the School Committee of the City of Boston 1957*: 209

354   Teachers Ask Salary Boost, Single Schedule. (1957, Jan 06*). Daily Boston Globe (1928- 1960).* Retrieved from http://search.proquest.com/docview/845304981?accountid=9675

The American Nurses Association (ANA)

At the dawn of 1958, two school nurses reported on their attendance at a meeting of the ANA where they represented the BPSNC. The American Nurses Association, during a "roll call," a nationwide membership campaign during which thousands of nurses would seek out colleagues, urged them to join the ANA. The campaign's objectives proposed to strengthen the nursing profession, the professional organization, and each individual nurse.

The nurses distributed a vital survey at this meeting. See the following image.

Seattle 9, Washington
NURSES SALARY SURVEY
Thirty Cities Over 300,000 (7 did not report)

CITY	SALARIES 1956-57				COMPARISONS				CONDITIONS OF EMPLOYMENT					
	NURSE		TEACHER		Same Schedules Same in Same Ways	Different	Paid by Altogether	Other Agency Other Duties Than School		Same Hrs. as Teachers		Same Mos. as Teachers		Travel Allowance
	Min. With BAO	Highest Attainable	Min. With BAO	Highest Attainable					Yes No		Yes No			
New York	$4000	$6080	$4000	$8000		X		X	X		X		X	X
Chicago	4000	7500	4000	7500	X				X		X			X
Philadelphia	3600	5900	3600	6200		X			X		X			X
Los Angeles	4250	7800	4250	7800	X				X		X			X
Baltimore	2508	3036	3600	6600			X		X		X			X
St. Louis	3150	3800	3600	6200		X			X		X			X
Washington, D.C.	3630	4480	3900	6500		X	X	X	X		X			
Boston	3504	4624	3504	5292	X				X		X			X
San Francisco	4920	5640	4250	7700			X	X	X		X		X	X
*Pittsburgh	3900	6400	3900	6400	X			X	X		X			X
Milwaukee	4822	5225	4000	6800		X	X	X			X		X	X
Houston	3600	5900	3400	5900	X				X		X			X
New Orleans	3372	4524	3600	6700		X					X		X	X
Minneapolis	3650	5200	4000	6750		X	X		X		X			X
SEATTLE	3600	5800	3600	5800	X				X		X			X
Kansas City	3600	6000	3600	6500	X						X			X
Newark	3520	5520	4000	7300		X			X		X		X	X
Dallas	3500	5900	3500	5900	X				X		X			X
**Indianapolis	3800	6250	3800	6250	X		X		X		X			
Denver	3900	6975	3900	6975	X						X			X
San Antonio	3005	3903	3450	5525		X			X		X			X
Oakland	4002	7107	4002	7107	X				X		X		X	X
Columbus	3700	6350	3700	6350	X				X		X			X
Portland	3756	4416	3700	6600		X	X	X	X		X		X	X
San Diego	4000	7350	4000	7350	X				X		X			X
*Atlanta	3264	6264	3264	6264	X		X		X		X			X
Birmingham	3000	5000	3000	5000	X				X		X			X
St. Paul	3620	4330	3800	6600		X	X		X		X		X	X
Toledo	3400	6000	3400	6000	X				X		X			
Jersey City	3000	5400	3600	7000		X			X		X		X	X
MEDIANS	3610	5720	3700	6550										
TOTALS					13	4	13	10	6	12	18	19	11	27

*Only 5 nurses are employed by schools, all others by county
**All nurses in elementary schools employed by Board of Health

The Executive Committee of the ANA appointed a select committee of the ANA Research and Statistics Unit of the School Nurse Branch. This committee, as part of the School Nurse Branch of the American Nurses Association Public Health Nurses Section, conducted the survey. The subsequent report, called "Salaries and Employment Conditions of School Nurses Employed by Boards of Education," covered 30 United States cities with populations over 300,000, including Boston.[355] It was a long time coming, but at last, an organization stepped forward, offering school nurses some support. The nurses distributed the document during their meeting, but unfortunately, it was not part of the *Minutes*. I located the Survey at the Boston Archives, folder School Health, Nurses.

Data paints a more complete picture for several notable reasons. The survey demonstrated to the BPSNC where they stood regarding salary and working conditions among comparable size cities. The ANA summarized the study this way:

- 43 percent or 13 of the 30 cities reporting pay the same salary schedule. Of these 13, nine have same time schedules, days and months, for both teachers and nurses.
- 43 percent or 13 of the 30 cities have salaries different in all respects. Of these 13, 11 report time of service required in days or months is greater for nurses than teachers.
- All 13 report higher maximums for teachers.
- An agency other than schools pays eight.
- Schools pay five.

This chart revealed how Boston's nurse salaries were similar in some respects to other cities in the survey. As you may undoubtedly see, Boston had both the lowest minimum and maximum salary for school nurses. Though their starting salaries were the same, the maximum for Boston teachers was $468 higher than the school nurses. New York school nurses and teachers had the same starting salary, but the peak for teachers was $2,920 higher, a considerable difference. Boston school nurses worked longer hours than teachers.

Unfortunately, there is no discussion in the *Minutes* about the Survey. Nevertheless, there must have been some conversation and exchanges between

---

355 *Boston Public School Nurses Club Minutes*: 12/4/1957

those concerned about these facts and how they affected their future plans.

Comparison of Massachusetts School Nurse Salaries

The 1955 Minutes contained a conversation about obtaining a list of wages from different school nurse groups in various Massachusetts towns, which would be helpful. They would ask Miss Crowe, who later became the president of SNAM, for some guidance on how to proceed. Still, the Minutes did not mention it again.

I found a chart called Salaries of School Nurses-1960 at the Boston Archives in Folder Nurses 1957-1974. See the image below.

SALARIES OF SCHOOL NURSES - 1960 — Massachusetts

	Population	Salary Minimum	Maximum
Quincy	87,000	5,300	6,700
Malden	57,000	4,200	6,600
Waltham	55,000	4,400	6,400
Melrose	29,000	4,200	6,600
Norton	4,401	5,440	6,700
Saugus	17,162	5,225	6,525
Concord	8,623	---	6,200
Needham	16,313	---	6,100
Northbridge	10,476	4,150	6,100
Winthrop	19,496	4,500	6,100
Greenfield	17,349	---	6,050

Boston's population at that time was 697,197. To compare the compensation of Massachusetts school nurses in 1960, Boston school nurses received a minimum of $4,020 and a maximum of $6,420.[356] Certainly, the reader can see that their salary ranked lower than the eleven towns listed and placed sixth in maximum salary

---

356 *Proceedings of the School Committee of the City of Boston 1959. P. 171.* Retrieved from https://archive.org/stream/proceedingsofsch1959bost#page/n3/mode/2up

attainment. In particular, Quincy sported the highest maximum salary, causing repercussions that we will hear more about later. As a consequence, it was not surprising Boston school nurses continued to seek higher remuneration and to be brought up to the comparable status of other professional school personnel. One question is, why did it take five years to compile this chart's data? Did people move at a slower pace?

Collective Bargaining Agents Emerge

Several early organizations competed to represent teachers and other school personnel in seeking to improve their salaries and working conditions. The Boston Teachers Union, Local 66, organized in 1945, emerged as a branch of the American Federation of Teachers. At the same time, the Boston Teachers Alliance in 1946 developed out of three separate groups, the Elementary Teachers Association, the Schoolmen's Economic Association, and the principals. It became an umbrella group linking these nonunion teachers and administrators together.

Both organizations gained new inroads for teachers, though the Boston Teachers Union was critical of the Boston Teachers Alliance. The Alliance advocated for a single-salary scale for all teacher levels in 1948, and opposed salary increases for high school teachers until they achieved wage parity. Because of this position, about 1,000 members, mostly high school teachers, left the Alliance. They advocated for a three-day paid sick leave, and fought for raises from $600 to $1,200, especially for the lower-paid elementary teachers.[357]

Led by an English teacher, Mary Cadigan, since 1945, the Boston Teachers Union fought with the Boston School Committee. In retaliation, in 1948, the BSC reassigned her from her high school teaching position to a health education class. She refused the assignment on the grounds that she did not have the proper qualifications and preparation. In turn, the BSC accused her of insubordination and started dismissal proceedings. Throughout Massachusetts, a groundswell of Union support arose for Cadigan, forcing the BSC to cancel her reassignment. But by 1953, members replaced Cadigan as President and voted in a male teacher who opposed her support of a single salary scale for both men and women.

---

357 Cronin, J. M. (2008). *Reforming Boston School, 1930-2006. P. 42. Overcoming Corruption and Racial Segregation. New York*: Palgrave MacMillan.

The Boston Teachers Union, in the 1950s, guided only 400 teachers, just 10 percent of the teacher force. However, they successfully campaigned with the BSC to obtain "sick leave," which doubled their membership. Since 1960, Massachusetts permitted public employees the right to bargain with their employers, including teachers, though not required to do so. Teachers requested an election in 1964 to determine who would represent them, but the BSC voted and denied the request. Again, in 1965, they made the same request, but this time it was approved, when it became evident that the state would require public employee bargaining. At that time, in 1965, the teachers elected the Boston Teachers Union as their exclusive bargaining agent.

Discontent Among Nurse Groups

The BPSNC Minutes included an editorial from the *Quincy Patriot Ledger*, February 8, 1958. It accurately compared the salary of Quincy school nurses and nurses working for Quincy City Hospital. In the opinion of the Quincy Patriot Ledger, there should be no difference in the wages of a Quincy school nurse and a Quincy City Hospital nurse. Though they were both employed by the City of Quincy, the Quincy School Committee granted raises to the school nurses, and the City Council governed hospital nurses' wages. Historically, as described in this editorial, the School Committees were independent of the City Council. They suggested there should be more cooperation and responsibility between the City Council and the Quincy School Committee when they were considering raises for non-educational personnel such as school nurses and custodians.

However, Mayor Amelio Della Chiesa revealed the nurses in the hospital and Health Department were disturbed and suffered lower morale since the school nurses received raises by the School Board. Because of this dispute, the mayor called for a meeting of school nurses, public health, and hospital nurses to discuss their wages, hour, and working conditions.

Nevertheless, the unhappy Quincy nurses were not alone. *The Boston Globe* ran a series of articles about the desperate shortage of nurses in Massachusetts. Hospitals resorted to closing down beds and postponing elective surgeries. They attributed the shortage to the expansion of hospital beds to accommodate the advances in medicine that have brought many more people to the hospital, a greater variety of jobs open to women, and high academic standards in schools of nursing. Other prevailing forces given were: living in a high-cost state on low wages, working on weekends and nights with little time for gratifying bedside care, and nurses, as well as other young girls, were marrying at a younger age and having larger families than they did in the 1930s. Earlier in 1957, Massachusetts nurses' salaries ranked in the lowest third of nurses' wages in the nation. Their new starting pay was $70 per week, which would place them at the middle third of national nurse salaries. In 1957, a new Boston school nurse earned $3,768 annually. Divide that by 52 weeks to receive a weekly salary of about $72, which made Massachusetts nurses and school nurses about equal.

Though compensation proved to be an essential issue, education also persisted in being of great consequence. At the Boston School Nurses Club meeting in February 1959, then President Louise Holthaus reported on a session of the School Nurses Association of Massachusetts (SNAM) held at Boston City Hospital that discussed a bill before the legislature on school nurses under Boards of Education. The subject brought up at the SNAM meeting revolved around the minimum educational requirement for school nurses. As the legislature has argued, since schoolteachers were required to have a degree, then for school nurses to receive the same salary and status as teachers, they should also be required to have a degree. Hearing this, the Boston School Nurses Club immediately made plans to raise its standards and entrance requirements.[358]

The advances in medical science required more skilled and better-educated nurses. One answer to this dilemma suggested increased and new funding for nursing education and nursing students, and the expansion of schools of nursing.[359] However, someone on the horizon was thinking outside of the box. Mildred Montag wrote her college dissertation on how to produce more registered nurses in a shorter time than the traditional three-year hospital diploma programs and the four to five-year college programs. She envisioned the two-year associate degree in nursing program, the ADN. In 1951, they began pilot programs. The new ADN was a success. Evaluators found that the new programs produced nurses who were proficient in technical skills and could successfully function as registered nurses. These programs opened up the nursing profession to men, married women,

---

[358] *Boston Public School Nurses Club Minutes*: 2/4/1959

[359] Menzies, I. (1957, Sep 02). Governor's Commission Reports Why Shortage of Nurses is Desperate. *Boston Daily Globe* (1928-1960) pp. 1. Retrieved from http://search.proquest.com/docview/845589388?accountid=9675

mature students, and other groups that were traditionally locked out of nursing programs.[360] The question of the Bachelor of Science in Nursing, BSN, as the entry-level into nursing remains up for debate. It takes time and financial resources to produce a nurse with the education and skills necessary to take care of more and more patients and deliver quality health care.

Next, follow the Boston school nurses as they join the public health effort to eliminate polio.

---

[360] Egenes, K. (2018) History of Nursing. In Roux, G., & Halstead, J. (Ed) *Issues and Trends in Nursing*, p. 21. Retrieved from jblearning.com/samples/0763752258/52258-ch01-roux.pdf2/6/2014

Chapter 13

School Nursing During the Polio Epidemics

School Nursing During the Polio Epidemics – The City

The Boston Globe ran a story in 1950 that wrapped up how their editors felt about Boston: "Boston was a dead city, living in the past," and urged young people to "seek their fortunes elsewhere."[361] "Charlie and the MTA (Massachusetts Transportation Authority) … riding forever 'neath the streets of Boston," hit the top of the song charts in 1959, protesting Boston transit fare hikes. Boston harbor was foul from overuse and neglect. *Fortune* magazine in June 1964 contained an article titled "Boston: What Can a Sick City Do?" Nightlife in the city was lackluster, with the number of nightclubs declining from 26 to 4. Completed in 1958, Route 128 drained Boston of people and jobs thanks to high-tech industries in the suburbs.

As a result of America's successful wartime experience overseas, and proud of it they should be, city fathers convinced the townspeople they could solve their problems at home just as they had abroad. Their promises evolved into a new program to modernize urban housing and bring middle-class families back to the city under the guidance of the Boston Redevelopment Authority (BRA). As mentioned in Chapter 5, the BRA called it urban renewal, but it became part of the federal slum clearance program. "Federal funding was used to demolish an entire neighborhood and displace its residents with total disregard to the hardship

---

361 Cronin, J. (2008) *Reforming Boston Schools, 1930- 2006: 4. Overcoming Corruption and Racial Segregation.* New York, NY: Palgrave Macmillan

it would cause them," said West End Museum Curator Duane Lucia. Residents also lost a close-knit, ethnically differentiated, and working-class community in the West End, after relocation, 48 percent of the residents experienced a shift to a middle-class way of life, another 32 percent of the residents showed no change in their quality of housing, while a further 23 percent lived in more inferior housing than before.[362] Working with relocated families developed another role for the school nurse, providing comfort, reassurance, and compassion for the students and their families.

Boston's Early Polio Epidemics

People knew in the 1950s that polio was a serious, contagious disease. Parents remembered seeing pictures of President Franklin Delano Roosevelt in his wheelchair, making great efforts to learn to walk, to diminish and hide his disability. They responded to the polio outbreaks by not allowing their children to swim or even play with other children. An epidemic is said to occur when one case occurs per every 1,000 in the population. At that rate, Boston experienced polio epidemics in 1916, 1927, 1931, 1935, 1949, and 1955. Then it was gone.

Polio or poliomyelitis derives from the Greek; *polios* means "grey," *muelos* means "marrow" and *itis* means "inflammation." According to The Centers for Disease Control and Prevention, polio is a crippling, deadly infectious disease caused by the poliovirus. The virus spreads from person to person and can invade an infected person's brain and spinal cord, causing paralysis. The virus lives in the infected person's throat and intestines. Mild flu-like symptoms such as sore throat, fever, tiredness, nausea, headache, and stomach pain occur in about one out of four affected people. There are no symptoms in up to 70 percent of infections. But in about 0.5 percent of cases, there is muscle weakness resulting in paralysis. This muscle weakness generally involves the legs but can affect the muscles of the diaphragm. In those with muscle weakness, about 2 percent to 5 percent of children and 15 percent to 30 percent of adults die. An infected person may spread the virus to others immediately before and about one to two weeks after symptoms appear. The virus can live in an infected person's feces for many weeks and thus contaminate food and water in unsanitary conditions.

---

362 Fisher, S., & Hughes, C. (Eds.). (1992). P. 84. *The Last Tenement Confronting Community and Urban Renewal in Boston's West End*. Boston, MA. The Bostonian Society.

Scientists now believe that improved sanitation in the 20th century was the cause of polio hitting older children and adults, and excessively the middle class. Previously, water supplies were always contaminated, and children would be exposed to the poliovirus from infancy, causing them diarrhea, but on the other hand, bestowing upon them lifelong immunity. With strict sanitation policies in place, people had clean drinking water, and, therefore, probably would not stumble upon the virus until later in childhood. At this time, the virus would more likely spread to the brain and spinal cord, causing paralysis. As we review the polio epidemics that follow, note the important role the school nurse's knowledge, critical skills, and skilled decision-making played.

1916

Children under school age comprised the majority of cases during the outbreak of acute anterior poliomyelitis (Infantile Paralysis) in 1916. The period covered during this outbreak incorporated nine weeks during late summer and early fall. Superintendent Franklin Dyer conferred with medical authorities. Considering the facts that contagious diseases in general always increased among children with the opening of the schools, and the nervousness and suspicion of parents regarding the possible spread of the disease, this inclined the medical establishment toward the opinion that a school opening delay of two weeks was desirable. [363]

Dr. Devine, Director of Medical Inspection, with the approval of Superintendent Dyer, forwarded a circular to all principal and headmasters, to be shared with teachers, regarding their plan to combat the spread of polio in the Boston schools. However, they admitted not everything was known about the disease, referring to it as a specific bacillus, not yet isolated, rather than the poliovirus. A cadre of 40 school physicians and 38 school nurses would visit and be available for school inspections so that either a doctor or nurse would call upon a school every day. The schoolteacher, an essential part of the team, would refer suspicious cases and any child exposed to the disease to the school physician.

The school physician would promptly examine the child and exclude any child exposed to the disease. Doctors knew that the germ existed in the discharges from

---

363   *Annual Report of the Superintendent 1916*. P. 81. Retrieved from https://archive.org/stream/report1916bost#page/22/mode/2up/search/nurses

the nose, throat, and intestines. Additionally, medical authorities warned children and families should be advised about the dangers of personal contact, such as the sharing of candy, gum, pencils, using the same drinking utensils, etc., and the avoidance of public assembly places as "moving picture shows."

When the schools finally opened in October 1916, hospitals reported to the Boston Health Department lists of 173 cases from July 15 to September 25, 1916. Schoolteachers received the names, addresses, and wards of these victims so they would know the exact extent to which the disease had prevailed in the sections of the city where their students resided.[364] Apparently, privacy was not their primary concern.

Age Distribution of Massachusetts Polio Cases and Deaths in 1916

Age Groups (Years)	Cases	Percent	Deaths	Percent
0-4	1,289	69.7	297	65.7
5-9	366	19.8	91	20.1
10-14	62	3.4	8	1.8
15 and over	133	7.1	56	12.4
Totals	1,850	100.0	430	100.0

This chart demonstrates that children in the 0-4 group show the largest number of cases. The 5-9 group climbs to second place in the number of cases. The highest death rates were distributed in almost the same proportions; 297 or 65 percent were under five years of age, and 388 or 85 percent were under ten years of age.[365]

364　Ibid. P. 84.

365　The 1916 Infantile Paralysis Epidemic in Massachusetts

The Iron Lung

Pulitzer Prize-winning novelist Jeffrey Eugenides said, "Biology gives you a brain. Life turns it into a mind." At this time, a man with creative intelligence developed a device for desperate patients paralyzed by polio. In 1928, Philip Drinker, a medical engineer at Harvard, invented the iron lung. Designed as an airtight tank, the iron lung regulated airflow in and out of the lungs. It enclosed the whole body except the head and proved to be a lifesaver to polio victims who could not breathe on their own. See the image on the next page - Children in the iron lung.[366] A typical polio patient with a paralyzed diaphragm would spend about two weeks inside an iron lung while recovering.

1931, 1935

The polio outbreak in 1931 started in early August, lasting for approximately nine weeks, as did the occurrences in 1916, 1927, and 1935. From the study of past epidemics, medical authorities believed that all indications pointed to a course of the disease running out in a period of nine weeks' time. Polio seemed to strike every four years, as can be seen in the sharp increase in the number of cases. Doctors explained the four-year incidence in this way: 75,000 children were born in Boston over that time, thus making a new population susceptible to attack by the virus.

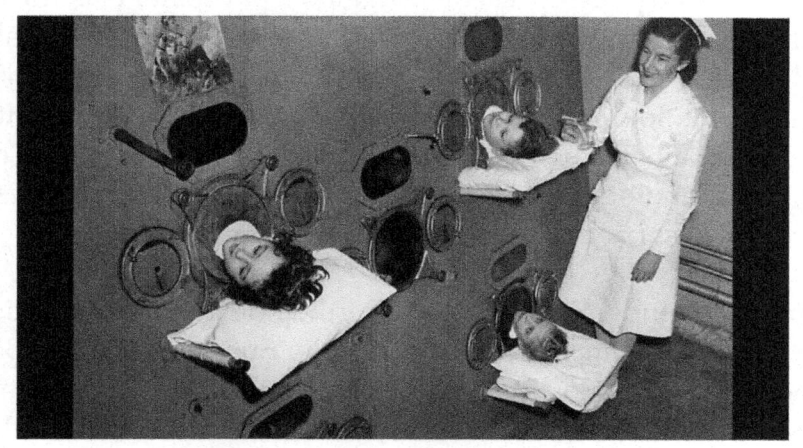

During the peak of the polio epidemic in the U.S., some hospital wards even had large, room-like iron lungs where multiple children lived.
Courtesy of Boston Children's Hospital Archive

366 Courtesy of https://www.npr.org/sections/healthshots/2012/10/16/162670836/wiping-out-polio-how-the-u-s-snuffed-out-a-killer

See Figure 2 below. Polio cases across the U.S.[367]

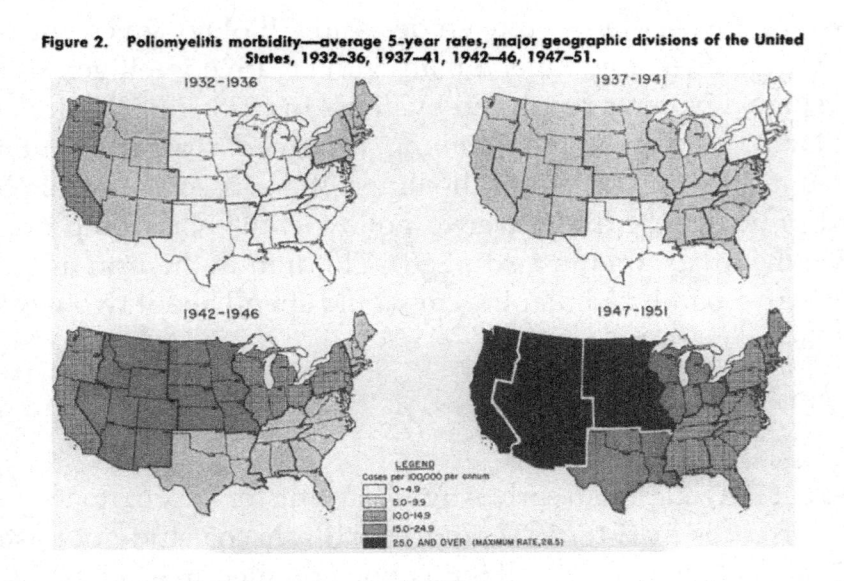

Figure 2. Poliomyelitis morbidity—average 5-year rates, major geographic divisions of the United States, 1932–36, 1937–41, 1942–46, 1947–51.

LEGEND
Cases per 100,000 per annum
0-4.9
5.0-9.9
10.0-14.9
15.0-24.9
25.0 AND OVER (MAXIMUM RATE, 28.5)

Doctors traced the start of the 1935 semi-epidemic to a boy who recently moved to Boston's Roxbury neighborhood from Fitchburg and enrolled in the public schools in late May 1935. He had a slight limp from paralysis of his foot. Let's call him Michael. One of the school physicians who was interested in how Boston became entangled in the polio crises, investigated a particular class that claimed the distinction of having the first known polio case in Boston. The date was June the 6th. A six-year-old child, we will call him Joe, had symptoms of paralysis of the muscles involving swallowing. Joe was in the same class as the boy who recently moved to Roxbury. A school physician discovered Michael's limp during an examination. Subsequently, epidemiological experts and public health authorities considered Michael to be the first carrier of the 1935 disease in Boston.[368]

During the 1935 epidemic, school authorities delayed the opening of school for several weeks to contain the spread of polio. Specially trained Boston school physicians and school nurses interviewed hospitalized polio patients collecting their case histories. They would follow-up on the information derived from

367 Polio cases across the U.S. Courtesy of https://europepmc.org/backend/ptpmcrender.fcgi?accid=PMC2024019&blobtype=pdf

368 *Anterior Poliomyelitis*. Polio General File 1936, 1946-1961. Boston Archive Collection.

these interviews, specifically about their contacts, first symptoms, places visited, etc. Superintendent of Schools, Dr. Patrick T. Campbell, thanked them for their remarkable self-sacrifice and cooperation.

1955: Why Was It Worse Than Ever Before?

Public health officials in Washington knew another polio epidemic loomed on the horizon for Massachusetts in 1955. Actually, officials expected it the year before. Their reasoning for this was the same as explained earlier in this chapter. These factors can produce a new epidemic: a non-immune population resulting from six years with comparatively little polio in that community, and a neighborhood that has a high birth rate where people live and play close to each other. As a consequence, these issues produced Boston's worst polio epidemic. The 1955 statistics show the number of children under five years of age diagnosed with polio amounted to 327 cases of the 834 total cases of polio in Boston. The five to nine-year-old's totaled 225 cases.

Children's Hospital and the Haynes Memorial Hospital, an isolation hospital in Brighton, overflowed with polio patients. As a result, Mayor John B. Hynes called an emergency meeting on August 3, 1955, of city and health officials, hospital authorities, and representatives from the medical, nursing, and physical therapy community, to mobilize and make plans to control the outbreak. People were terrified. Vacationers who had planned to visit Boston flooded state officials with phone calls. To allay fears, officials issued reassuring statements saying they had reached the peak of the outbreak. In reality, it had not. August witnessed 1,727 new cases of poliomyelitis in Massachusetts compared to 421 on July 1, 1,008 in September, and 476 in October.[369] Those adults and children stricken by polio had no idea what fate had in store for them. For many, it was a time of isolation wards, spinal taps, braces, several orthopedic operations, social reproach, and confinement inside an iron lung, sometimes for years, just to breathe.

The Salk Vaccine

Obviously, a preventative vaccine was desperately needed. Finally, Dr. Jonas Salk, on April 12, 1955, introduced the Inactivated Poliovirus Vaccine (IPV) called the

---

[369] Burns, F. (1955, Dec 05). The Polio Year We Won't Forget--II. *Daily Boston Globe (1928-1960)*, pp. 14. Retrieved from http://search.proquest.com/docview/840600842?accountid=9675

"killed-virus," announcing the vaccine was effective and safe. Two years prior, Salk injected himself, his wife, and his three sons, with the vaccine in his kitchen after boiling the needles and syringes on his stove.[370] What a courageous man.

Clinical trials of the vaccine began all over the United States, and by the end of June 1954, 1.8 million people had become "polio pioneers." Researchers used the double-blind method where neither the patient nor the one administering the injection knew if they were giving the vaccine or a placebo. Regardless, there was no shortage of volunteers. People just queued up to receive whatever doctors offered.

Renowned newsman, Edward R. Murrow, interviewed Dr. Salk on April 13, 1955, the day after he made his announcement about the vaccine. During that interview, Salk praised the financial assistance he received through the March of Dimes that funded the vaccine's research and clinical trials. When asked who owned the vaccine's patent, he replied, "Well, the people, I would say," in light of the poster child campaign that brought in millions of dollars in small contributions.[371] In other words, the vaccine did not have a patent. Unfortunately, this led to problems when manufacturers replicated the vaccine.

As Dr. Alexander Langmuir, chief of the Communicable Disease Center of the United States Public Health Service, in Atlanta, Georgia commented, by the middle of May 1955, "All hell broke loose" (Burns: 12/11). Shortly after authorities declared the Salk vaccine safe, more than 200 cases of polio cropped up in California and Idaho. Contacts of children who received the vaccine developed paralytic polio. As a result of an investigation, epidemiologists discovered that the children had received a bad batch of the Salk vaccine manufactured by Cutter Laboratories in Berkeley, California. Eleven people died. In retrospect, the federal government rushed to make the vaccine. They had not provided proper supervision of the major drug companies who had contracts with the March of Dimes to produce 9,000,000 doses for 1955. The U.S. Surgeon General halted any more inoculations. Regardless, people continued to receive polio injections. See

---

370   Klein, C. (2014, October). 8 Things You May Not Know About Jonas Salk and the Polio Vaccine. *History in the Headlines*. Retrieved from http://www.history.com/news/8-things-you-may-not-know-about-jonas-salk-and-the-polio-vaccine

371   Ibid.

the following image – A girl with a nurse and doctor, receiving a polio injection in a Boston school. Photo courtesy of the Boston Archives Collection

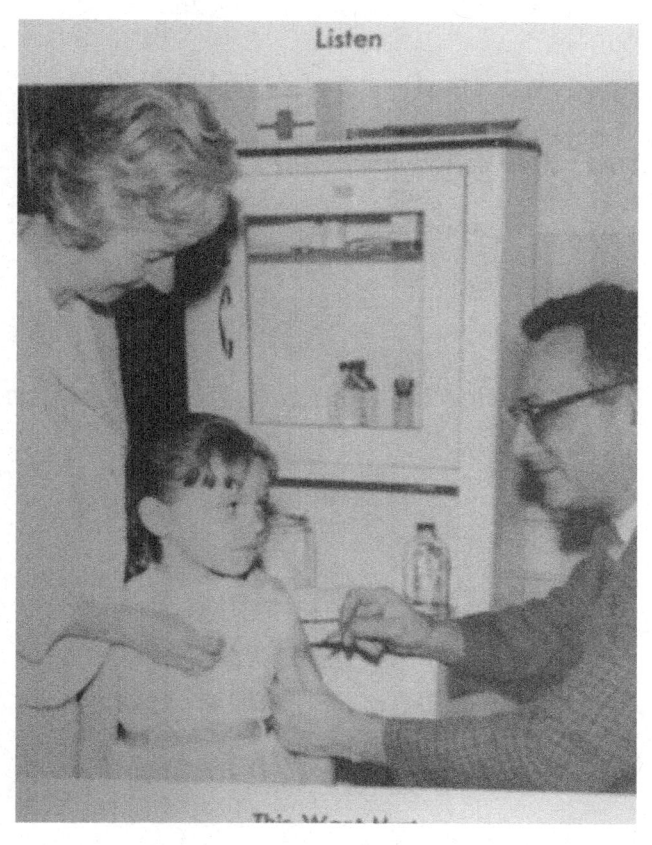

Massachusetts had its own concerns. Did the vaccine produce the 1955 Boston polio epidemic? Uncertainty prevailed. In April, although the state Advisory Board halted the Massachusetts Public Health Polio Program, Boston persisted and proceeded with their Salk program in June 1955.

The Boston Public Schools jumped on the bandwagon and gave one injection during May and June of 1955 to children in Grades 1 and 2. The result of the anti-poliomyelitis vaccination program was as follows:[372]

---

372 *Department of School Hygiene, Poliomyelitis Vaccine Program Report, December 9, 1955*

Total number enrolled 15,409

    Total number vaccinated   11,286

    Total number not vaccinated   4,123

Twenty people contracted poliomyelitis among the 11,286 vaccinated

    Paralytic   12

    Nonparalytic   8

Seventeen people contracted poliomyelitis among the 4,123 not vaccinated.

    Paralytic   12

    Nonparalytic   5

Rates for total cases:

Vaccinated	20/11,286	= .0018	= 1.8 per 1,000
Non-vaccinated	17/4,123	= .0041	= 4.1 per 1,000

Rates for paralytic cases:

Vaccinated	12/11,286	= .0011	= 1.1 per 1,000
Nonvaccinated	12/4,123	= .0029	= 2.9 per 1,000

    This report, though discomforting to read, showed the promise and effectiveness of the Salk vaccine. To complete the Salk vaccination program required a series of three injections. If a person just received one shot, but they already harbored the polio virus, the one inoculation was not enough for immunity.

    The summer of 1955 arrived in Boston along with record-breaking heat. At a Boston School Committee (BSC) meeting on August 8, 1955, they asked Miss Marion C. Sullivan, Supervising Nurse, as a public service, to canvass the school nurses to find out who would work as a relief force for nurses in the hospitals. This relief force would release staff nurses to care for polio patients on infectious disease units. On an entirely voluntary basis, 13 school nurses were willing to roll up their sleeves and work on hospital floors. But, Dr. Spellman, Medical Director of the Department of School Hygiene, did not want them working with polio cases.[373]

On September 6, 1955, the BSC discussed whether to delay the opening of schools to September 22, due to the hysteria and concern of parents. Mr. Lee, a Boston School Committeeman whom we have heard from many times, regarding the fate of school nurses, commented on the current state of events concerning the polio crises and the schools. Additionally, Mr. Lee said he received two letters urging that schools open later:

> *"What impresses me is that, like almost everything else, there seem to be two sides to this thing. On the one side are the medical men, who, according to all the newspapers, think the children are as well or better off in the unrushed, clean atmosphere of the classroom, with nurses in attendance, as we have in every school district, and with a physician making daily visits, and an alerted force of teachers.*
>
> *So that the men who have dedicated their lives to protecting the health of children seem to be on one side, saying that we might as well open. And on the other side are those whom these same medical men describe as giving way to psychological worries against the weight of evidence.*
>
> *I may perhaps be influenced by the situation in the West End where I live, and where there have only been two cases of polio. I happen to know the father of one of the girls who came down with the disease. He is a close friend of mine, and I happened to walk in on him at his place of work on Sunday and heard him saying that if schools had been opened during the summer, his daughter would not have had polio, and he hoped for the sake of his other daughters that schools would open promptly.*

---

[373] *Proceedings of the School Committee of the City of Boston 1955.* P. 221. Retrieved from https://archive.org/stream/proceedingsofsch1955bost#page/148/mode/2up/search/nurse
https://archive.org/stream/proceedingsofsch1955bost#page/284/mode/2up/search/Mr.+Lee

As I said, outside of the personal appeal of another person, a woman in the West End who is very well acquainted with people there and is very active-this was the only call I received. This woman, for her part, said it had been a hard summer with a great deal of heat in the big buildings of the West End and the crowded streets, and she hopes that schools would open on time and the kids could go back to an atmosphere where their conduct was more controlled and more serene, and where there were nurses and medical men around."[374]

The schools delayed the opening to September 22, to alleviate the anxieties and worries of the parents.

Dr. Spellman, Medical Director of the Department of School Hygiene (DSH), wrote to the School Committee in December 1955. He said he was disturbed and distressed the Massachusetts Health Department was not allowing school doctors to inoculate school children. Still, they were not prohibiting private physicians from immunizing children against poliomyelitis. By February 1956, a bill passed in the Massachusetts legislature to buy vaccine. The DSH restarted inoculations in the summer of 1956. See the image on the following page showing children being inoculated. Photo courtesy of the Boston Archives Collection, Superintendent's Report.

During the school year of 1956-1957, the DSH inoculated all students and school personnel who wished to receive the vaccine. Doctors estimated they could immunize 125 children in two and one-half hours in the same school. School doctors gave an amazing 101,512 inoculations. Medical personnel gave the Salk vaccine intramuscularly or IM, as they would refer to it. They gave the second inoculation one week after the first, and the third inoculation four weeks after the second.[375]

The Department of School Hygiene received a letter from school nurse Miss S. in a Boston elementary school, alerting them to a situation occurring in her school. The mother of a little girl who died from paralyzing bulbar polio sent the letter. The story unfolds that the mother signed consent slips last May 1955 to have both of her children inoculated. Because of problems with the fifth-grade pupil, at the last minute, the mother signed a refusal form and telephoned the assistant principal to verify this request. In 1956, the following school year, she insisted that her remaining child be given a second inoculation as she received her first last year in school. This situation could not have happened, the nurse responded, as

[374] *Proceedings of the School Committee of the City of Boston 1955*: 284-285
[375] *Polio General File 1936, 1946-1961*. Boston Archive Collection.

she had the mother's consent slip in the drawer with the other withdrawals. The classroom teacher confirmed the child did not leave the room to receive the inoculation. Miss S. repeated they would never let a child in line without a consent form. Offering support and encouragement, Miss S. added the school would be only too glad to inoculate her surviving child this year. The mother said she would take it up with her family physician.[376]

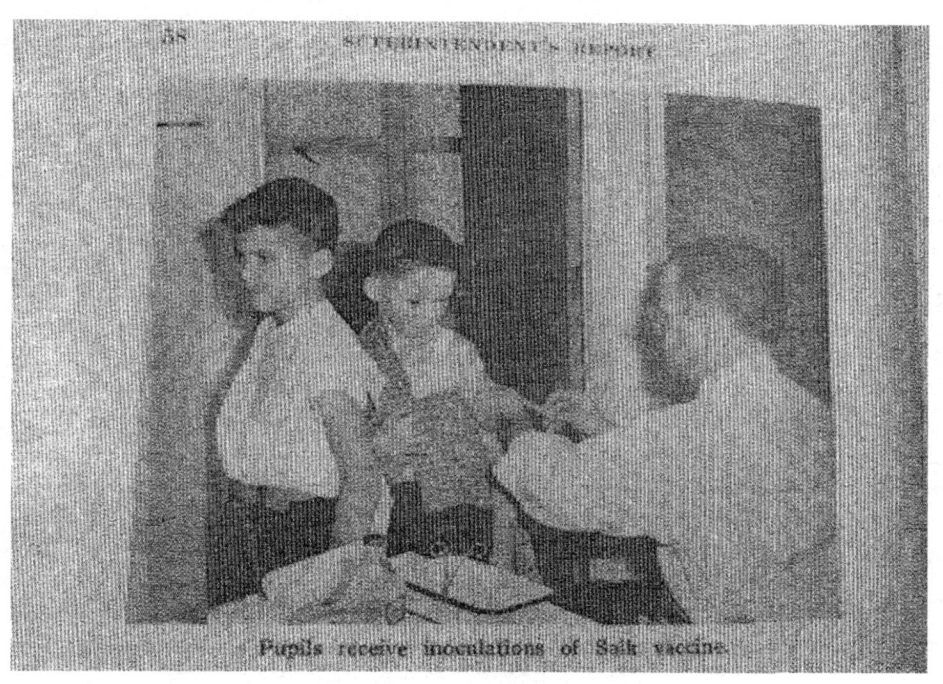

Pupils receive inoculations of Salk vaccine.

It is understandable how confused parents were considering the complexity of the times. On the one hand, they heard reports of people dying after receiving the vaccine in other parts of the U.S. Then, on the other hand, school doctors were administering the Salk vaccine. Who to believe and what to do? If the little girl in the Boston elementary school had received only one injection, would that have saved her life? It goes without saying, these grief-stricken parents, after losing one child to polio, would ponder their decision to withdraw the permission slip for the rest of their lives. School nurses had a daunting job arranging these immunization sessions, obtaining permission slips and supplies, running the program, and in all likelihood, making home visits to follow-up with families. Helping a parent to understand the risks they faced, while at the same time, assisting them in preventing or managing problems effectively, may have relieved the parent's anxiety.

376   *Letter from School Nurse*. Boston Archive Collection, Polio General File (2) January-May 1956

By January 1956, the schools distributed 90,000 flyers produced by the National Foundation for Infantile Paralysis, founded by Franklin D. Roosevelt. The pamphlet stated some children received their first shot in 1955, at a time when polio was on the rise in their communities and their systems already contained the virus. Thus, sadly, the vaccine was given too late to stop the disease.

Dr. Martin H. Spellman, Director of School Health Services, sent out an Emergency Poliomyelitis Prevention Program Letter from the Department of Public Health on April 28, 1960, to school physicians and school nurses. The letter requested schools to do their part in a community-wide mass inoculation program against poliomyelitis. The Department of Public Health provided the schools with free vaccine to immunize staff under the age of forty.[377] See the image on the next page - a report of the Salk polio vaccines given by the Department of School Hygiene, a total of 308,203 injections.

DEPARTMENT OF SCHOOL HYGIENE
BOSTON PUBLIC SCHOOLS

Number of Poliomyelitis Vaccine Inoculations
Given by School Physicians

	School Year	Number of Injections Given	Injections	Given to:	Vaccine Provided by:
I	1954-1955	13,251	1st	Grade I, II	State
II	1955-1956	60,013	1st, 2nd	Pupils up to 15 years	State
	Summer 1956	18,185	1st, 2nd	Pupils up to 15 years	State
	Summer 1956	1,337	1st, 2nd	Pupils+Parochial and Preschool	State
III	1956-1957	101,512	1st, 2nd, 3rd	Pupils up to 19 years and Personnel	State
IV	1957-1958	8,927	1st, 2nd, 3rd	" " "	State through Nov. 1957
	Spring 1958	3,584	1st, 2nd, 3rd	" " "	Purchased by School Committee
V	1958-1959	46,340	1st, 2nd, 3rd	Grades Kdg. Gr. I	Purchased by School Committee
VI	1959-1960	15,587	1st,2nd,3rd,4th	" " "	State
	May and June 1960	39,467	1st,2nd,3rd,4th	Grades II through XII and Personnel	State
	Total	308,203			

377 *Polio Program (6).* Boston Archive Collection

The Sabin Vaccine

The rival oral poliovirus vaccine (OPV), called the "live-virus" vaccine, developed by Dr. Albert Sabin in 1962, began replacing Salk's Inactivated Poliovirus Vaccine (IPV). OPV was cheaper to produce and easier to administer. The Boston Public Schools carried on a continuous Poliomyelitis Prevention Program. In 1965, SHS dispensed 1,214 vials of Sabin Oral Polio Vaccine to school nurses at their monthly meeting to begin the program. School nurses distributed the vaccine on a cube of sugar, no injections. Do readers remember receiving this in school? The Department of School Health Services (DSHS) anticipated having all school children completely immunized against poliomyelitis. Therefore, the DSHS offered the trivalent oral vaccine (Types I, II, III combined) to any kindergarten or Grade 1 pupil to complete their polio immunizations. Only children with a consent slip signed by parent or guardian requesting this immunization received this service.[378]

Unfortunately, vaccine-associated paralytic poliomyelitis (VAPP) still occurred, forcing medical authorities to change their recommendations from an all OPV vaccination schedule back to an all-IPV schedule. The overall risk for VAPP was roughly one case in 2.4 million doses of OPV. However, since 1997, the immunization schedule has included a combined IPV-OPV vaccine. Later, an enhanced-potency IPV vaccine developed in 1997 improved the immune response of IPV.[379] "Outside of the Cutter Incident, not a single case of polio attributed to the Salk vaccine was ever contracted in the United States."[380]

The school nurses worked tirelessly during the polio epidemics rounding up students and staff to receive the polio vaccine. Since that time, another issue has come into play, that of parents not wanting to immunize their children. Given the seriousness of paralytic polio, and its aftermath in the subsequent years, why would a parent ever consider submitting their child to that suffering?

Now we will follow the school nurses through the turbulent 1960s.

---

378 *Polio Program (7)*. Boston Archive Collection.

379 *Poliomyelitis Prevention in the United States*. Centers for Disease Control and Prevention. Retrieved From https://www.cdc.gov/mmwr/preview/mmwrhtml/rr4905a1.html

380 Klein, C. (2014, October). 8 Things You May Not Know About Jonas Salk and the Polio Vaccine. *History in the Headlines*. Retrieved from http://www.history.com/news/8-things-you-may-not-know-about-jonas-salk-and-the-polio-vaccine

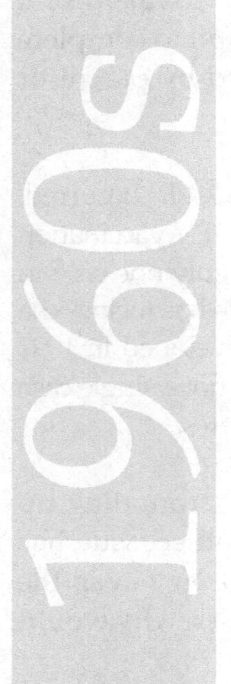

Twentieth Century Milestones Affecting School Nursing (Continued)

1960 Some states require nurses to have teaching degrees. Boston's Population: 697,000.

1960-1980 Specialization of nursing; Debate over entry level of practice (BSN vs. ADN).

1964 American Nurses Association adopts motion supporting baccalaureate education as educational foundation for the registered nurse.

1964 Economic Opportunity Act passed to provide poverty assistance.

1969 Man walks on the moon.

Author note: I am choosing to refer to race in the vernacular of the times as it was related to me by the subject and does not in any way intend to promote racist language.

Chapter 14

Threatened Policy Changes and Voices from the Past

Evolving School Nurse Functions

The following events and stories are a window into the times in the 1960s and part of our American story. In sixty years, the United States graduated from the horse and buggy to putting a man on the moon, a gigantic leap of science and technology. Science fiction had become fact.

On the other hand, a visitor to Boston in the 1960s arrived in a city, that had not changed much in the past 50 years. Boston's Civil Rights Movement started along with protests against segregation in the Boston Public Schools, and basketball's Celtics had a winning team. Locals referred to the adult entertainment district in downtown Boston as the Combat Zone, and John F. Kennedy was in the White House. The Woodstock Music and Art Festival drew flower children enjoying music performances and visions of peace. By 1963, the nation endured the pain of Kennedy's assassination, followed by his brother Robert in 1968, as well as the Reverend Martin Luther King Jr.

The 1960s brought its own set of challenges with the U.S. escalation of the Vietnam War and then the capture of Saigon in 1975, marking the end of the war. The United States' involvement in South Vietnam, eventually turned public opinion against the war, and this developed into a strong peace movement. President Lyndon B. Johnson, who succeeded President Kennedy, announced a "War on Poverty" through his "Great Society" programs.

The positive outcome of the "Great Society" was a renewed interest in public health agendas and the development of new school health programs. In 1966, Title 1 of the Elementary and Secondary Education Act provided federal funds for expanded school health programs in areas where there were large disadvantaged populations, providing food for children and salaries for school nurses and doctors. Legislators added Early Periodic Screening, Detection, and Treatment (EPSDT) to Title 19 (Medicaid) of the Social Security Act via 1967 amendments to provide ongoing health care for children receiving welfare assistance. This agenda included a standard health test, immunization, well-child health supervision, and dental care services. In addition to dental education, school fluoride programs for the prevention of tooth decay increased dramatically during the 1970s. By 1974, the focus of Title 1 had changed to providing priority to educational purposes, and health purposes would be secondary. The federal government made all of these funds available to Boston, and we will follow how they utilized them.

In the 1960s, Boston school nurses still battled communicable diseases. Nurses in the high schools conducted a special tuberculosis (TB) case-finding program in 1960 after doctors diagnosed two high school pupils with tuberculosis.[381] Again, in the 1961-1962 school year, a pupil in English High School was diagnosed with an active case of TB. This particular case presented its own set of challenges, as the family were Christian Scientists. In all likelihood, the school nurse visited the family on several occasions, listened to frightened and anxious parents share their story, and gave the family anxiety-provoking information about tuberculosis. The family finally agreed to hospitalize their son.

Active cases of tuberculosis required all the contacts in English High School, both pupils, and teaching staff as well as others in the building, be tuberculin or tine tested. The tine test is a multiple-puncture tuberculin skin test. Protocols required all who tested positive receive a chest x-ray. As a result of the follow-up work, one positive case needed treatment.[382] During the school year 1965-1966, pupils in kindergarten and grade 1, and all newly admitted pupils from outside Boston in all classes 1 through 12 were tine tested. See the image on the next page - students line

---

381 *Annual Report of the Superintendent 1960*. Retrieved from
https://archive.org/stream/report1960bost#page/24/mode/2up/search/nurses

382 *Annual Report of the Superintendent 1961-62*. P. 117-119. Retrieved from
https://archive.org/stream/report196162bost#page/116/mode/2up

up to receive a tine test in a Boston elementary school - Photo courtesy of Boston Archives.

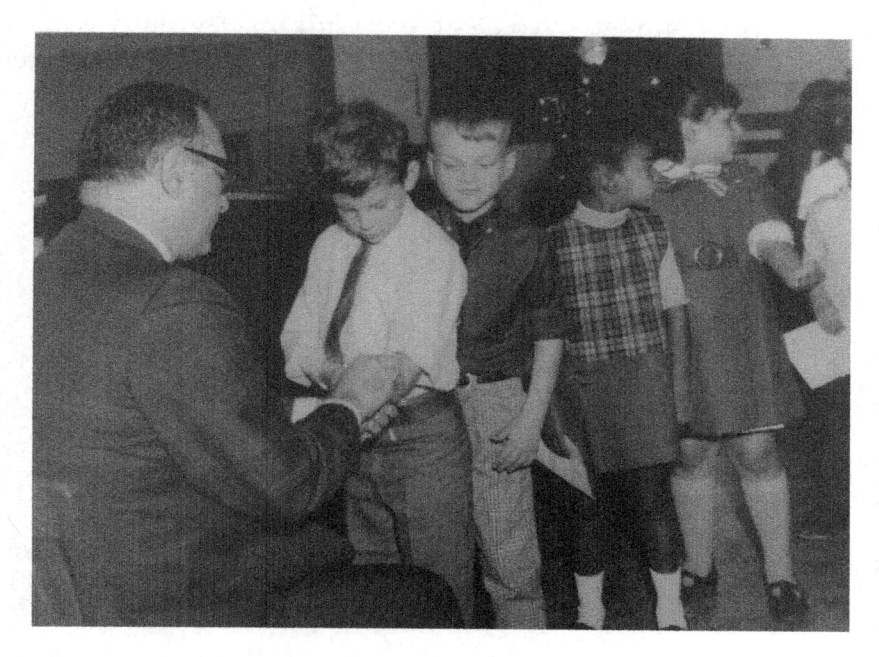

One of the nurses' roles pertained to reading the tine tests. Of the 17,689 students tested, 181 read positive. These tests revealed 11 pupils with active tuberculosis. Of these students, four required hospitalization, and seven received treatment at home under medical supervision. This screening program exposed eight cases of active tuberculosis within one family, a powerful benefit for the community.[383]

Another role of the school nurse involved follow-up on the students' contacts and referring them for a tine test. School staff understandably became very anxious about TB, and the school nurse would offer support and encouragement, and explain to staff the significant aspects of the follow-up work she was doing.

Nurses' Education

In 1964, Miss Sullivan, the Supervising Nurse, sent a memorandum to Dr. Gorman, the Medical Director, pertaining to the education of newly appointed school nurses.

---

[383] Tuberculosis Cases. Boston Archive Collection. Folder *School Health*

SCHOOL NURSES – DEGREES WHEN APPOINTED

School Year	No. of Nurses Appointed	No Degree	with BS Degree	with M. Ed Degree
1963-64	3	0	3	0
1962-63	9	4	5	0
1961-62	4	1	1	2
1960-61	5	4	1	0
1959-60	3	0	3	0
1958-59	2	0	2	0
1956-57	8	3	5	0
1955-56	5	4	1	0
1954-55	6	3	2	1
1953-54	4	1	3	0
Totals	**46**	**20**	**23**	**3**

This survey indicates at that time, in 1953-1964, 50 percent of school nurses had a BS Degree, but 43 percent had no college degree. These figures did not match teacher credentials, indicating the nurses needed to make some changes. A bachelor's degree with a major in nursing became a requirement for appointment as a Boston school nurse in January 1964, similar to requirements among many large cities.[384] Surprisingly, this, too, would undergo modification in the future.

Dr. Gorman returned a memo to Miss Sullivan, agreeing with the minimum requirements of a BS Degree for school nurses. He acknowledged this would be in keeping nationally with what the school nursing departments in the large cities were doing. These school systems used school nurses with degrees in public health and education to teach in the physical education departments. He hoped Boston

---

[384] Nurses *1957-1974* Boston Archive Collection, Folder *Nurses 1957-1974*, Boston Municipal Research Bureau, Boston, MA

school nurses armed with a degree might be utilized in this way in Boston.[385]

Unfortunately, that model did not last. The Boston School Committee voted to eliminate the degree requirement for school nurses in 1967. This decision would not affect those persons on the current eligible list for appointment as a school nurse.[386] Was there difficulty acquiring nurses? That is the only factor I can consider for this new ruling. For that reason, whether the school nurse had a BS Degree or not, she would still be on the first step of the salary scale. As has happened before, no mention of this action appeared in the school nurse minutes.

A Nursing Voice from the Past

I had the opportunity to meet Ann Donovan, a former Boston Public School Nurse, at a 2011 Nursing Archives Associates Annual Meeting at Boston University. At 95 years young, she was wonderfully upright, giving her a presence, and her eyes were both merry and intelligent. Her gray and wispy hair complemented her face.

We talked about stories from long ago and accounts from her past. Immediately after her graduation from Mount Auburn Hospital School of Nursing in 1943, she joined the Navy Nurse Corps, serving in the Navy for the next 20 years. While a naval nurse, Donovan served during WWII in the Pacific, directing operating rooms. During the Korean War, she served on four carriers and was assigned stateside to San Diego Naval Hospital during Vietnam. She said, being in the Navy, "I got to see a lot of the world. It was a widening and educational experience." In the 1950s, the Navy sent her to the University of Minnesota, where she obtained a BS in Nursing Education. As far as any particular stories from her Navy career, she confides, "I wouldn't like to put it in print." Donovan retired in 1963 as a Colonel in the Navy Nurse Corps.

Following retirement, Donovan was not sure in which direction she wanted to go in adjusting to civilian life. She explored various avenues of nursing and took many tests for certification in different fields, often ranking at the top of their list.

---

385   *Dr. Gorman Memo*, Boston Archive Collection, Folder School Nursing

386   *Proceedings of the School Committee of the City of Boston 1967*. P. 358. Retrieved from https://archive.org/stream/proceedingsofsch1967bost#page/n3/mode/2up

After some thought, she decided to give school nursing a try. School nursing offered more or less the same independence she experienced in the Navy. At that point in her life, working in a civilian hospital did not appeal to her.

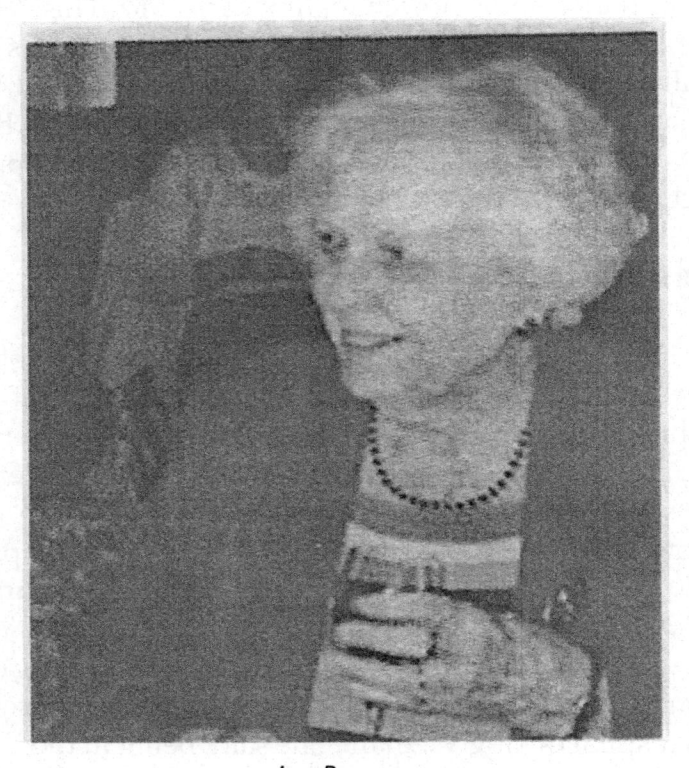

Ann Donavan

After applying to the Boston Public Schools in 1965, she received an assignment as a school nurse to three Dorchester Schools, the Mather, Edward Everett, and Edward Southworth, as she had the required BS degree in Nursing. Formerly located in the old Mather School on Meeting House Hill, the Southworth closed in 1974. The Mather School, represented today by its lineal descendant situated on 1 Parish Street in Dorchester, was the first free public school in America, established in 1639. From the beginning, a direct tax or assessment of the town's people supported the school. When Donovan was at the Mather, she remembers how proud the teachers were of the picture hanging in the auditorium that was painted by Winslow Homer, the artist, while he attended 4th grade at that school.

Despite the passage of years, she still laughingly remembered her interview for the position. One of the questions asked was if she would be able to handle the antics of the high school boys. She replied that surely if she could handle the behaviors of sailors returning from shore leave, she could manage schoolboys. Her reply settled the question.

This was the time in 1965 Boston before the occurrence and turmoil of school busing. Children often came to the school nurse's office with "headache" as their complaint, generally because they left home without breakfast. Donovan set aside peanut butter, crackers, and leftover milk in the school refrigerator to give them a quick snack and return them to their classroom. In her view, the children in Dorchester were neglected. Do these statements have a familiar ring? Annie McKay, Massachusetts' first school nurse, made the same comments in 1906. She commented children left home without a proper breakfast, drank too much coffee, and stayed up till 11 o'clock at night. No matter how the times change, some situations in school nursing remain the same.

Donovan considered the Mather's school doctor "very good." A dentist at the Forsythe Dental Clinic examined the children's teeth. As a school nurse, her duties included first aid, checking for head lice, vision and hearing screening, and following up on physical exams. In her opinion, the role of the school nurse then was not as well defined as today.

Donovan harbored concerns about exposed radiators in classrooms, which, when the heat was on, were hot enough to burn a child. She lobbied the school administration for radiator covers, but they ignored her request until a girl received a radiator burn in the classroom.

While at the Mather School, a male teacher approached Donovan asking if she would teach his female students in the 5th and 6th grade about their "monthly," and personal hygiene. In the ensuing weeks, she held classes for these girls but found the school principal had some objections. He objected to her teaching in the classroom because she did not have the credentials to teach, despite being certified as a health educator.

Donovan fondly remembered the nursing supervisors who she worked with, namely Louise Holthouse and Mrs. Baugh. She also worked with a social worker, Ms. Mahoney, who was active in starting Boston's METCO program in 1966. I admire Donovan's ability to recall their names after all these years. She respected the Boston Public School nurses she worked with and felt "they did a great job."

Unfortunately, she did not involve herself with the BPSNC.

Subsequently, on December 31, 1966, Donovan left school nursing. She moved on to other positions, such as the Massachusetts State Nurses Association Board of Directors, New England Sinai Hospital, and the Nursing Archives Associates at Boston University.

Donovan commented about school nursing and nursing today. She related, "It encompasses far more than it did in my day since now both parents work, and the kids are exposed to so much. It's a whole different world. So, few women were educated back then. They [meaning returning nurse military veterans] were the leaders in their day."

She recounted, "Nurses today are no longer the handmaids of doctors as they were before WWII. Before the war, nurses were dominated by what the doctor said. When WWII nurses returned, they were accustomed to practicing independently and were ready to do that in civilian life. The GI Bill of Rights [passed in 1944], gave returning veterans the ability to move on and get an education." Armed with that education, "It opened up more doors for women and really changed nursing."

Ann Donovan, an astute, smart nurse, experienced school nursing in the mid-1960s. In retrospect, I wonder, given her extensive military background, whether school administrators would not have grasped this unique opportunity to seek her out to assist them in modernizing school health services. Policy and procedure manuals that were not updated since 1935 would have benefited from her expertise. However, in no way did Donovan make this suggestion.

At the end of our discussions, Ann was 96 and thanked the Lord for her excellent health. I thanked Ann for her service to our country and our nursing profession. Sadly, Ann has since passed away.

New Challenges Arise Over Hiring of School Nurses

An explosive report compiled and published by the Boston Municipal Research Bureau in 1961 stated that Boston should unify school health services. Needless to say, it caused a furor. The Boston Municipal Research Bureau was initially founded in 1932 as a fiscal watchdog for the administration of James Michael Curley (Recall him from Chapter 10).

Two separate school health programs existed, the report argued, one for public schools and another for parochial. The cost of the public-school health program per pupil was two-and-one-half times that of the parochial school program, administered by the Boston Public Health Department (BPHD). School health services for the city cost a total of $900,000.

	Number of School Children	Cost	Total Cost
Public Schools	89,000	$10.00 per child	$800,000
Parochial Schools	35,000	Less than $4.00	$100,000
TOTAL COST			**$900,000**

A united program, the report pointed out, would eliminate duplications and make more productive use of health staff. The Boston Municipal Research Bureau demanded the programs unify under the BPHD. According to the assignment of nurses to public schools at the time, one nurse served about 1,300 pupils on the average in the junior high and elementary schools. In the high schools the staff consisted of one nurse (including medical aides) for 1,400 pupils. Physician's averaged one for every 1,700 pupils.

The Boston Globe ran an article on January 16, 1961, outlining the two programs. The public-school program included 140 permanent employees, 10 temporary employees, and 16 part-time employees. In addition to the Director of School Hygiene, the permanent staff included 53 school physicians, 2 medical specialists, a supervising nurse, 4 assistant supervising nurses, 67 school nurses, 8 medical aides, a supervisor of nutrition, a sanitation engineer, and 2 clerks. Salaries for the entire department exceeded $790,000 a year.

The parochial school program consisted of 15 physicians, 9 of them full-time doctors, dedicating one-third of their time to school health. The other 6, including 5 part-time doctors gave 80 percent of their time to school health, plus a part-time ophthalmologist. Eleven public health nurses and an audiometer tester completed the staff. The entire program cost $92,000 annually.

On January 26, 1961, Superintendent of Schools, Dr. Frederick Gillis, joined the BPSNC meeting as a guest speaker. He named Dr. Michael J. Donavan, MD, as the acting head of the School Hygiene Department, on the retirement of Dr. Gillis. Superintendent Gillis told them that their destiny was in the hands of the five school committee members and he opposed 100 percent the unification of public and parochial school programs. He pointed out they should ascertain if this question of unification required legislation, and if so, he advised the school nurses to obtain a lawyer. He also mentioned school doctors were not in favor of unification. However, he had no reassuring words for them as to their future. I might ask, why he wasn't asking the school's lawyers whether this proposal required legislation His lack of support indicated he really didn't care who performed the job as long as it got done.

After Superintendent Gillis departed from their meeting, the school nurses jumped into action. They formed three committees. Group I would visit the Chairwoman of the Boston School Committee (BSC). Group II would present a complete resume of the duties and program carried out by the school nurses in the Boston Public Schools to the BSC. Group III would obtain a copy of the program carried out by the public health nurses in the parochial schools. They also elicited letters of support from school principals to maintain the present status of the school nurses.

Again, on February 2, 1961, they met and reviewed their plans. The question arose, "Could a bill for unification be passed without legislation from the State or by the City of Boston, and is there a city law pertaining to Boston School Nurses?"[387] At the time, there were no definite answers to these questions, though these inquiries would be raised again in the future. The answer, however, remained the only agency that could hire and fire Boston school nurses was the Boston School Committee, which hired them in the first place. But never mind that, first, they would contact the lawyer for the BPS, Mr. E. Kief, to ask for some legal advice on how to proceed.

Health services offered to schoolchildren in the Boston Public Schools and the parochial schools differed in several ways. The newspapers followed up with articles attempting to sort it out. A commentary in the *Boston Herald* on March 8, 1961, "School Hygiene Challenge" referred to the costs of each plan. At a cost of less than $4 per pupil, the parochial school's program cost less than the $10 per student price tag in the Boston Public Schools. The Health Department argued they were the logical agency to perform children's health services since it had overall responsibility for community health. Shortly after that, Acting Director of the School

---

387 *Boston Public School Nurses Club Minutes*

Hygiene Department, Dr. Donovan, submitted his resignation. This opened the door for the BSC to initiate the merger, particularly since they planned to eradicate Dr. Donovan's position. If the School Committee wanted the position filled during the process of the consolidation, according to the *Boston Herald*, it should appoint Health Commissioner F. Robert Freckleton.

Differences: Health Services in Public Schools/Parochial Schools

Massachusetts State Law, Section 57 Chapter 71 of the General Laws requires the physical examination of school children in public schools, whereas, parochial schools were considered private schools and were not subject to state laws. Parochial schools, however, observed these regulations in part. Parochial schools performed physical exams in grades 1, 5, and 8, and to all newly admitted children. Grades 1, 3, 5, and 7, and any referrals from other grades received a routine vision test.

On the other hand, the state laws were compulsory for public schools. They required physical exams every three years, preschool or kindergarten, or grades 1, 4, 6, 9, 11, and successful vaccination against smallpox for admission to school. Public school physicians needed to visit every school every day. Public school nurses were full time, generally working 8:45 AM to 2:30 PM. After school closed, they visited homes from 2:30 PM to 4:00 PM.

The City Health Department administered The Parochial Schools and conducted their program for children in kindergarten through grade 8. The 15 physicians mentioned earlier provided this service. In conjunction with the Bureau of Public Health Nursing, the City Health Department appointed the parochial school nurses. Part-time schedules at the parochial elementary schools limited nurses' time allotment for those schools to only part of the day. The full-time equivalent of 11 public health nurses and an audiometer tester provided the nursing service. Health Department assignments supplied the full-time equivalent of one physician for every 2,300 pupils and one nurse for every 2,300 pupils. One hundred thousand public and parochial school children in kindergarten through grade 8 received dental service via the Health Department.

The Boston Municipal Research Bureau offered an intriguing interpretation of the controversy, insisting that the merger would eliminate duplicating administration, supervision, and overhead, while providing needed oversight where it apparently did not exist at that time. All schools in an area would be served by the same medical and nursing personnel, as was the case with the Health Department Dental Service. The latest comparative data on health service expenditures for 1957-1958, published by the U.S. Office of Education, showed that Boston's $7.97 per pupil for health services was the highest of all large cities in the country. In many cases, Boston cost at least twice that of comparable cities.[388]

The public controversy continued with an interview on February 26, 1963, by Bob Hey of the *Christian Science Monitor* with Dr. Richard J. Gorman, the new Director of School Hygiene.

Mr. Hey, Question: "How does Dr. Gorman account for the discrepancy per capita cost between the public and parochial schools?"

Dr. Gorman, answered:

"Public schools are governed by state laws which have to be complied with to the letter; parochial schools are private schools and therefore not subject to state laws. We give excellent service in high schools with daily visits by school nurses and doctors. School physicians give all athletes a complete physical examination. In the parochial schools, there are no doctors or nurses in attendance in the high schools at all except in special programs."

"Elementary parochial schools are not covered full time every day as public schools are. Our nurses are in school all day. Since they have several schools to visit each day, they are on call all day by their other schools in case of (an) accident or illness of pupils. The nurses take the pupils home or to the hospital.'

"All parochial school children who are problem children are transferred to the public schools. Special services such as an ophthalmologist, otologist, working certificates, all classes of special instruction; vision classes, special classes, Horace Mann School for the Deaf, Speech Improvement, Conservation of Eyesight, Cerebral Palsy Class, and Lip Reading come from public school costs and are used by parochial school children. Minor boys over 16 years of age and minor girls over 18 years of age are licensed for certain trades and have to be examined

---

[388] Nurses *1957-1974* Boston Archive Collection, Folder *Nurses 1957-1974*, Boston Municipal Research Bureau, Boston, MA

in the Certificating Office by our doctor and nurse in attendance there. There are some pupils who are from 12-16 years of age."

"Our health services are all inclusive, tending to keep up with major cities in (which) health services are under boards of education. The following large cities have their health services under the board of education:

Chicago, Illinois	Houston, Texas
Philadelphia, Pennsylvania	New Orleans, Louisiana
Los Angeles, California	Cincinnati, Ohio
Baltimore, Maryland	Dallas, Texas
Cleveland, Ohio	Denver, Colorado
San Francisco, California	San Diego, California
Pittsburgh, Pennsylvania	Birmingham, Alabama
Richmond, Virginia	

"There are approximately 200 kindergartens in the public schools as against 11 in the parochial schools."

Mr. Hey, *"Dr. Gorman is definitely against the transfer."*[389]

During the next few months, the Boston school nurses consolidated their reports about their school nurse activities and public health nurse activities. They submitted a copy of their report to their supervisor Miss Marion Sullivan and Dr. Gillis, the former Medical Director. When approved, they planned to send a copy to all of the BSC members. For the first time, the name of the Boston Teachers Union came up, and they considered joining that group. As was noted in Chapter 12, they ultimately joined the Boston Teachers Union in 1965.

Health Commissioner F. Robert Freckleton, MD, MPH., sent a letter to Boston's Mayor John F. Collins, on March 28, 1961, which declared his view of the merger. In it, he stated Health Department programs already address infants and pre-school children, and the Health Department nurses render a complete family service. *"The consolidation of School Hygiene services in the Health Department will serve*

---

[389] Hey, B. (February 26, 1963). Boston Archive Collection, Folder School Nursing *Merger with Health Department, 1961.*

to avoid reduplication and splintering of service," and to utilize existing personnel and resources more effectively.

Unfortunately, there are no other BPSNC Minutes to consult after March 1961 until September 1965. Despite the furor raised, we can assume that the school nurses' efforts to remain under control of the Boston Public Schools emerged successful. In 1965, the Boston Public Schools still employed the school nurses.

How Should School Nurses Be Funded?

During this debate, Boston School Committeeman (BSC), Joseph Lee, in 1961, made a plea for a lower and fairer city tax rate that would benefit both the city and the schools. He declared that the BSC spent a smaller percentage of its tax dollars on education than any city or town in America. (It spent only half of the state average. Nationally, cities and towns disbursed 30 cents of the tax dollar, whereas Boston laid out 20 cents of the tax dollar.)

In his customary attack, Mr. Lee stated both he and Mayor Collins agreed the Boston School Committee overpaid certain personnel in the school system, but they didn't agree who these individuals were. He continued that the BSC paid school nurses twice as much as the Mayor paid nurses at City Hospital (now Boston Medical Center). On the contrary, Mr. Lee informed the Mayor by letter and suggested the BSC pay school nurses no higher than hospital nurses. The Mayor expressed disinterest and seemed not to agree, since he never answered his letter.[390]

On the salary scale, the BSC placed school nurses into Group 1 category along with elementary, junior high school teachers, and high school teachers. However, Mr. Lee persisted and requested again to give a lower amount of maximum wages to school nurses, and place high school teachers in Group 2, due to the shortage of these teachers. They did not follow his request. The details of those who fell under the Group 2 Master's degree were those who had a master's degree, and or a bachelor's degree, and had worked under specific certificate approved by the BSC. As noted, a nurse could not apply for a Group 2 Master's degree category even if she had worked for 15 years under a specific certificate.

---

390   *Proceedings of the School Committee of the City of Boston 1961*. P. 15-16. Retrieved from https://archive.org/details/proceedingsofsch1961bost

Simultaneously, the BSC worked just before the opening of the school year developing Group 2 Ranks to include four assistant supervising nurses, along with supervisors from the fine arts, music, physical education, handicraft, vocational education, and assistant in industrial arts. Group 3 Part A Ranks encompassed the supervising nurse, guidance counselors, division heads, vocational instructors, vocational assistants, research assistants, and school adjustment counselors. As may be seen, the BSC placed school nurses, assistant supervising nurses, and the supervising nurse in categories with teachers who had similar responsibilities.

See the following image - 1961 Salary Scale.[391]

COMPARISON OF BOSTON SCHOOL NURSE SALARIES AND TEACHERS 1961

GROUP 1

School Nurses and Teachers — Master's Degree

MIN	AN INCRE	MAXIMUM	MIN	AN INCRE	MAX
$4,740	$240	$6,900	$5,220	$240	$7,380
Step		Salary	Step		Salary
1		$4,740	1		$5,220
2		4,980	2		5,460
3		5,220	3		5,700
4		5,460	4		5,940
5		5,700	5		6,180
6		5,940	6		6,420
7		6,180	7		6,660
8		6,420	8		6,900
9		6,660	9		7,140
10		6,900	10		7,380

GROUP 2 RANKS — Ass't Sup. Nurse, other Supervisors

GROUP 3 PART A RANKS — Super. Nurse + Guidance Councelors

MIN	AN INCRE	MAXIMUM	MIN	AN INCRE	MAX
$7,380	$240	$7,860	$7,540	$240	$8,260
Step		Salary	Step		Salary
1		$7,380	1		$7,540
2		7,620	2		7,780
3		7,860	3		8,020
			4		8,260

[391] *Proceedings of the School Committee of the City of Boston 1961.* P. 244. Retrieved from https://archive.org/details/proceedingsofsch1961bost

Although the school nurse and teacher salaries were the same in 1961, once again, in 1964, the situation changed. The school nurse salary and increment remained the same, while the minimum teacher salary increased from $4,740 to $4,980, an increase of $240, including one significant increment of $480. Notice that they did not recognize a nurse having a doctorate.[392]

The following 9 images show salaries from 1964 through 1970.

1964

COMPARISON OF BOSTON SCHOOL NURSE SALARIES AND TEACHERS 1964

GROUP I TEACHERS 1964				TEACHERS WITH MASTER'S DEGREE				TEACHERS WITH DOCTOR'S DEGREE			
STEP	MIN	INCRE	MAX	STEP	MIN	INCRE	MAX	STEP	MIN	INCRE	MAX
	$5,400	10 at $240 / 1 at 480	$7,860		$5,400	10 at $240 / 1 at 480	$8,340		$5,940	10 at $240 / 1 at 480	$8,820
1			$4,980	1			$5,460	1			$5,940
2			5,220	2			5,700	2			6,180
3			5,460	3			5,940	3			6,420
4			5,700	4			6,180	4			6,660
5			5,940	5			6,420	5			6,900
6			6,180	6			6,660	6			7,140
7			6,420	7			6,900	7			7,380
8			6,660	8			7,140	8			7,620
9			6,900	9			7,380	9			7,860
10			7,140	10			7,620	10			8,100
11			7,380	11			7,860	11			8,340
12			7,860	12			8,340	12			8,820

GROUP 12-A SCHOOL NURSES				SCHOOL NURSES WITH MASTER'S DEGREE				GROUP 12-B ASSISTANT SUPERVISING NURSE			
STEP	MIN	INCRE	MAX	STEP	MIN	INCRE	MAX				
	$4,740	$240	$6,900		$5,220	$240	$7,380	Salary	$8,340		
			Salary				Salary				
1			4,740	1			5,220				
2			4,980	2			5,460				
3			5,220	3			5,700				
4			5,460	4			5,940				
5			5,700	5			6,180	GROUP 12-C SUPERVISING NURSE			
6			5,940	6			6,420				
7			6,180	7			6,660				
8			6,420	8			6,900	Salary	$8,740		
9			6,660	9			7,140				
10			6,900	10			7,380				

392 *Proceedings of the School Committee of the City of Boston 1964.* P. 103. Retrieved from https://archive.org/stream/proceedingsofsch1964bost#page/n3/mode/2up

1965

COMPARISON OF BOSTON SCHOOL NURSE SALARIES AND TEACHERS 1965

GROUP 15	BANK SCHOOL	NURSE		GROUP 1	BANK	TEACHERS	
SCHOOL NURSES SALARY				**SCHOOL TEACHERS SALARY**			
	Bachelor's /	Master's		Bachelor's /	Master's or	Doctorate	
Step	Other Cert.	Degree		Equivalent	Equivalent		
1	$5,260	$5,740		$5,400	$5,880	$6,360	
2	5,500	5,980		5,670	6,150	6,630	
3	5,740	6,220		5,940	6,420	6,900	
4	5,980	6,460		6,318	6,798	7,278	
5	6,220	6,700		6,696	7,176	7,656	
6	6,460	6,940		7,074	7,554	8,034	
7	6,700	7,180		7,452	7,932	8,412	
8	6,940	7,420		7,830	8,310	8,790	
9	7,180	7,660		8,208	8,688	9,168	
10	7,420	7,900		8,910	9,390	9,870	
GROUP 16 BANK							
Supervising Nurses		$8,860					
GROUP 17 BANK							
Chief Supervising Nurse		$9,260					
School Nurse Certificating Office Stipend $288							

Proceedings of the School Committee 1965, p 75,76

Figure 5

1966

COMPARISON OF BOSTON SCHOOL NURSE SALARIES AND TEACHERS 1966

GROUP 13	Rank					
	SCHOOL	NURSES	SALARY			
	Bachelor's or		Master's			
	Other Cert.		Degree			
Minimum	Annual Increment	Max Salary	Minimum	Annual Increment	Max Salary	
$4,980		$7,860	$5,460		$8,340	
Step						
1	8 @ $240	$4,980		8 @ $240	$5,460	
2	2 @ $480	5,220		2 @ $480	5,700	
3		5,460			5,940	
4		5,700			6,180	
5		5,940			6,420	
6		6,180			6,660	
7		6,420			6,900	
8		6,660			7,140	
9		6,900			7,380	
10		7,380			7,860	
11		7,860			8,340	
GROUP 14	RANK					
Supervising Nurses	No Change					
GROUP 15	RANK					
Chief Supervising Nurse	$9,340					
School Nurse Certificating Office Stipend $288						

Proceedings of the School Committee 1966, p 230,232

Figure 6

COMPARISON OF BOSTON SCHOOL NURSE SALARIES AND TEACHERS 1966

GROUPS — Rank SCHOOL TEACHERS SALARY

		Bachelor's or other Certificate		Master's Degree or 15 years special Certificate	
Minimum	Annual Increments	Max Salary	Minimum	Annual Increments	Max Salary
$5,550		$9,300	$6,000		$9,800
Step					
1	6 @ $300	$5,550		6 @ $300	$6,000
2	2 @ $400	5,580		2 @ $400	6,300
3	1 @ $500	6,100		1 @ $500	6,600
4	1 @ $700	6,400		1 @ $700	6,900
5		6,700			7,200
6		7,000			7,500
7		7,300			7,800
8		7,700			8,200
9		8,100			8,600
10		8,600			9,100
11		$9,300			9,800

Proceedings of the School Committee 1966, p 230, 232

Figure 7

1967

COMPARISON OF BOSTON SCHOOL NURSE SALARIES AND TEACHERS 1967

GROUP 12 Step	RANK SCHOOL Bachelor's or Other Cert.	NURSES SALARY Master's Degree		GROUP I Bachelor's or Equivalent	RANK Master's or Equivalent	TEACHERS Master's / 30 Credits	Doctorate
1	$6,000	$6,500		$6,000	$6,500	$7,000	$7,500
2	6,288	6,788		6,400	6,900	7,400	7,900
3	6,576	7,076		6,800	7,300	7,800	8,300
4	6,864	7,364		7,200	7,700	8,200	8,700
5	7,152	7,652		7,600	8,100	8,600	9,100
6	7,440	7,940		8,000	8,500	9,000	9,500
7	7,728	8,228		8,400	8,900	9,400	9,900
8	8,016	8,516		8,800	9,300	9,800	10,300
9	8,304	8,804		9,300	9,800	10,300	10,800
10	8,592	9,092		10,000	10,500	11,000	11,500
11	8,880	9,380					

GROUP 13 RANK		
Supervising Nurses		$10,440

GROUP 14 RANK		
Chief Supervising Nurse		$11,340

1968

COMPARISON OF BOSTON SCHOOL NURSE SALARIES AND TEACHERS 1968

GROUP 12 Step	RANK SCHOOL Bachelor's or Other Cert.	NURSES SALARY Master's Degree		GROUP I Bachelor's or Equivalent	RANK Master's or Equivalent	TEACHERS Master's / 30 Credits	Doctorate
1	$6,420	$6,970		$6,500	$7,050	$7,600	$8,150
2	6,728	7,278		6,900	7,450	8,000	8,550
3	7,036	7,586		7,300	7,850	8,400	8,950
4	7,344	7,894		7,700	8,250	8,800	9,350
5	7,652	8,262		8,100	8,650	9,200	9,750
6	7,960	8,510		8,500	9,050	9,600	10,150
7	8,268	8,818		8,900	9,450	10,000	10,550
8	8,577	9,127		9,400	9,950	10,500	11,050
9	8,885	9,435		10,000	10,550	11,100	11,650
10	9,193	9,743		10,700	11,250	11,800	12,350
11	9,660	10,160					

GROUP 13 RANK		
Supervising Nurses		$11,170

GROUP 14 RANK		
Chief Supervising Nurse		$12,134

1969

COMPARISON OF BOSTON SCHOOL NURSE SALARIES AND TEACHERS 1969

GROUP 12	RANK SCHOOL NURSES	NURSES SALARY		GROUP I	RANK SALARY	TEACHERS	
Step	Bachelor's or Other Cert.	Master's Degree		Bachelor's or Equivalent	Master's or Equivalent	Master's / 30 Credits	Doctorate
1	$7,000	$7,600		$7,000	$7,600	$8,200	$8,800
2	7,500	8,100		7,500	8,100	8,700	9,300
3	7,900	8,500		7,900	8,500	9,100	9,700
4	8,400	9,000		8,400	9,000	9,600	10,200
5	8,900	9,500		8,900	9,500	10,100	10,700
6	9,300	9,900		9,300	9,900	10,500	11,100
7	9,700	10,300		9,700	10,300	10,900	11,500
8	10,200	10,800		10,200	10,800	11,400	12,000
9	10,800	11,400		10,800	11,400	12,000	12,600
10	11,300	11,900		11,300	11,900	12,500	13,100

GROUP 13	RANK						
Supervising Nurses		$13,066					

GROUP 14	RANK						
Chief Supervising Nurse		$14,194					

1970

BOSTON SCHOOL NURSE SALARIES AND TEACHERS 1970

	GROUP I SALARY	RANK		
Step	Bachelor's or Equivalent	Master's or Equivalent	Master's / 30 Credits	Doctorate
1	$7,600	$8,200	$8,800	$9,400
2	8,200	8,800	9,400	10,000
3	8,900	9,500	10,100	10,700
4	9,600	10,300	11,000	11,700
5	10,200	10,900	11,600	12,300
6	10,800	11,500	12,200	12,900
7	11,400	12,200	13,000	13,800
8	12,100	12,900	13,700	14,500
9	12,900	13,700	14,500	15,300

GROUP II
Supervising Nurses
$15,480 $16,280 $17,080

Chief Supervising Nurse
Base $16,000

Salary Schedule for 1972

	SALARY SCHEDULE						
	Bachelor's	Bachelor's	Master's	Master's	Master's	Master's	Doctorate
Step		*l* 15 Credits		*l* 15 Credits	*l* 30 Credits	*l* 45 Credits	
1	$8,459	$8,809	$9,159	$9,509	$9,859	$10,209	$10,609
2	9,127	9,477	9,827	10,177	10,527	10,877	11,277
3	9,906	10,256	10,606	10,956	11,306	11,656	12,056
4	10,685	11,085	11,485	11,885	12,285	12,685	13,135
5	11,353	11,753	11,600	12,553	12,953	13,353	13,803
6	12,021	12,421	12,200	13,221	13,621	14,021	14,471
7	12,688	13,138	13,000	14,038	14,488	14,938	15,438
8	13,468	13,918	13,700	14,818	15,268	15,718	16,218
9	14,359	14,809	14,500	15,709	16,159	16,609	17,109
GROUP II							
BASE		$17,229		$17,679	$18,129	$18,579	$19,079

By 1965, both nurses and teachers received an increase, raising the nurses to $5,260 and the teachers to $5,400, respectively. See the 1965 Salary Scale.[393]

Likewise, 1966 produced more of the same, with the nurse starting salary of $4,980 and the teachers receiving $5,550. See the 1966 Salary Scale.[394] A break in this pattern developed in 1967, when the nurses and teachers received the same starting salaries and starting a master's degree, but a lower maximum for nurses. They recognized teachers only with a master's plus 30 credits. See the 1967 salary chart.[395]

Unfortunately, in 1968, the BSC returned to their former pattern when they granted nurse's a raise from $6,000 to $6,420, but increased the teacher's pay from $6,000 to $6,500. See the 1968 salary chart.[396] They scored in 1969 when both

---

[393] *Proceedings of the School Committee of the City of Boston 1965*. P. 76-77. Retrieved from https://archive.org/stream/proceedingsofsch1965bost#page/n5/mode/2up

[394] *Proceedings of the School Committee of the City of Boston 1966*: 230-232

[395] *Proceedings of the School Committee of the City of Boston 1967*: 247-248

[396] *Proceedings of the School Committee of the City of Boston 1968*: 167

nurses and teachers received the same starting salary, same maximum, and equal compensation for a master's degree. See the 1969 salary chart.[397] The following year, 1970, was similar. See the 1970 salary chart.[398] However, the 1972 schedule included additional categories, such as Bachelor's + 15, Master's + 15, and Master's + 45. These did not apply to school nurses. On the other hand, the Bachelor's, Master's, Master's + 30, and Doctorate did include school nurses. The nurses made slow but steady progress.[399]

Harvard - MIT Report

Amidst all of this, Harvard-MIT released a contradictory report in late 1969 and 1970 about the physicians and nurses in the Boston School Health Service. After reviewing their history of being the first in the nation in 1894 to bring physicians, then called medical inspectors, into the schools to improve the health care of school children, the report cited that the 54 medical doctors conducting physical examinations were not up to par. Each doctor visited three or four schools a day, mostly in the morning, announcing their presence in the school by ringing a bell, and left within five minutes. One teacher wittingly remarked, "But if you had a foot or leg injury, heaven help you, because you couldn't get to the office in time. In five minutes, the doctor would have gone on to the next school." Generally, they attended to their private practice in the afternoon. The physicians were in their senior years, the oldest being 78, and among the 54, only one was a pediatrician. They collected $5,500.00 annually for a ten-hour week.

The Harvard-MIT Report then attacked the next recipients, the school nurse. Seventy-five school nurses staffed the schools, one to each high school and the others assigned from two to five elementary and junior high buildings. Though by law, they could not administer medicines nor treat patients, because of malpractice laws, they tested vision and hearing and checked the height and weight of students every year. Maintaining health records required 50 percent of their time.

The report referred to this as "light lifting" as compared to employment in a

---

397 *Proceedings of the School Committee of the City of Boston 1969*: 261

398 *Proceedings of the School Committee of the City of Boston 1970*: 241, 243

399 *Proceedings of the School Committee of the City of Boston 1972*: 310

hospital setting. They worked the same hours as teachers and enjoyed the same vacations. Additionally, they paid school nurses $5,000 more than their nurse counterparts at Boston City Hospital. "The Harvard-MIT report noted 'turnover is low, and the waiting list is long'"[400] The team recommended discontinuing the daily medical inspector visits, and instead partnering with neighborhood health clinics.

Regarding the school nurses, the report delivered a harsh, incomplete, and limited analysis of the Boston school nurses' workload. Wouldn't it be jolly if their job description only included performing vision and hearing tests, and heights and weights? They did not mention a school nurse implemented a myriad of activities on any given day, such as a) complying with all the preventive immunization campaigns that the school required; b) daily pupil inspections; c) classroom instruction in health and safety habits, and personal hygiene; d) periodic classroom inspection for dental defects, pediculosis, symptoms of infectious diseases, and cleanliness; e) first aid care; f) escorting children to clinics; and g) home visits after the close of school, just to name a few.

Though a school nurse dealt primarily with well children, she also needed an understanding of normal growth and development, be able to recognize deviations from the normal, and to recognize signs and symptoms of disease. Had they not demonstrated to the public that their services were worth the cost? What outcomes did they expect? At the same time, the federal government sponsored new programs and grants to expand and provide funds for school health services in districts with large disadvantaged populations, thus making Boston eligible. We will continue to monitor the path and response of the school nurses to these new challenges.

More Controversies

The ensuing years bring to mind the Book of Job, with multiple travails experienced by the school nurses in the form of a teacher strike, the discontinuation of the school nurse exam, another Task Force proposal of transfer to Health and Hospitals, Boston's desegregation order, and the loss of the Chief Supervising Nurse and Supervisors. Again, sadly, the history lacks the input of continued Minutes from 1961-1965, and again 1974-1975 from the BPSNC. We can only contemplate their

---

400 Cronin, J. *Reforming Boston Schools, 1930-2006: Overcoming Corruption and Racial Segregation.* (2008). New York, NY. Palgrave McMillan.

multiple reasons for this loss of their history. Were they so busy? During one point, September 1974 to May 1975, the first year of desegregating the schools, their account read, "No meetings were held during this period, but we haven't been idle." Similarly, were they so caught up in the turmoil that they were reluctant to express themselves on paper? Was there no desire to be together for a sense of community? Did they experience such agonizing darkness and hopelessness that they didn't hold meetings or attend them? Their journals are silent.

Every journey, whether physical, emotional, or spiritual, begins with leaving something behind. Maybe the reason we feel like we never get anywhere new in life is because we are unwilling to leave anything, much less everything, behind. Yet, C. S. Lewis said, "There are far, far better things ahead than any we leave behind." Did they hear the suggestions of their adversaries? Just as they listened to their student's and staff's problems, in the same way, were they listening to their critics? The journey continues as we listen to their voices.

Listen to Their Voices

Let me introduce Shirley Ericson Garagna. I had the pleasure of visiting Shirley and her husband John at their home in Newton on a bright, sunny summer day in June 2015. Large blooming, enticing, blue hydrangea flowers in the front of their house greeted me as Shirley invited me in. Shirley's is a compelling story. Her account allows us to see a young, black woman* breaking down the color barriers in school nursing as the Boston Public Schools addressed segregation. See the image to the right - Shirley Ericson Garagna.

Nursing, Shirley revealed, was not her first career choice. Shirley wanted to be a social worker. However, her father intervened and said, *"You should not be among the starving millions. Be a nurse."* That is what she did. At the time, the 1950s, all occupations were not open to black women, or any women.

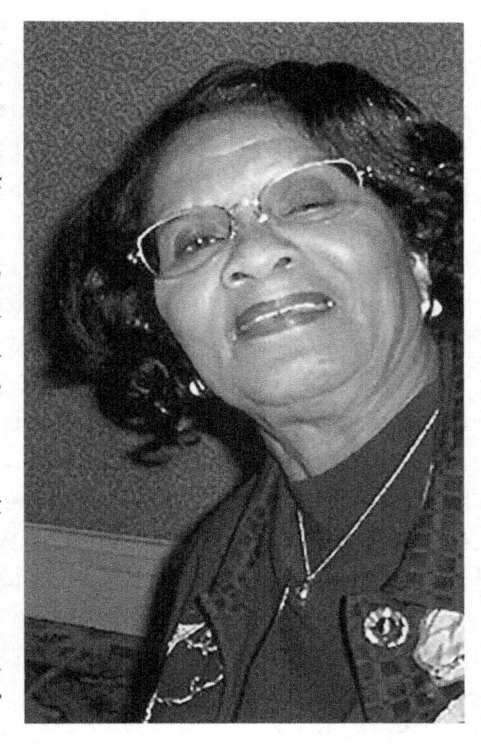

A product of the Boston Schools herself, Shirley attended the Higginson, Ellis, and Lewis Schools and graduated from Burke High School. After graduating from the four-and-a-half-year nursing program at Boston University (BU), Shirley went into public health nursing. Her career there included working in a well-baby clinic and a tuberculosis clinic. Subsequently, she took the school nurse exam and received a very high grade. She thinks it was because of the excellent preparation she received at BU. Later on, she returned to BU and received her master's degree in maternal and child health. This was a time before the busing crises in 1974.

Her first assignment to the BPS included three schools. Every day a nurse went to two schools, spending a morning in one, the afternoon in the other one, and fitting the third one in during the week. Her post incorporated the Dillaway School District in Roxbury, including the elementary schools, Dillaway, Nathan Hale, and Abbey May. All have since closed.

Shirley made home visits every day. Were the parents glad to see the nurse? *"Well, it depended on what you were there for,* she explained. *"You couldn't make a whole host of visits, because the schools ended later in the day. I think I walked between my schools,"* Shirley recalls. *"I did not have a car. If you were a nurse with a car, you had a different assignment."* Nurses with a car had assignments spread out over a larger area, possibly covering more than one district. *"Our meetings were at Beacon Street,"* she explained. *"In later years you would share things like a hearing machine. You would not know the nurses in the other districts."*

Shirley believes that children have changed, but then again, she stated, she was so much younger then. Besides, she also lived in Roxbury. She continues, *"The children were well disciplined. Most had two parents, not like now. They had more whole families. The children were mixed, white and black, girls, and boys."* Eventually, more families of color moved to Roxbury. She explained that the Abbey Mae was in a mixed community. Many of the white children attended parochial schools, such as St Joseph's. She did not dispense any medications. Some students had a treatment for asthma, but they carried it with them. As it happens, she doesn't recall ever giving diabetic insulin. The incidence of Type I diabetes was lower in that era as compared to today. The nurses would go to the classrooms to check the hair for lice, just as they still do.

School nurses did not receive an equal salary with teachers back then. She couldn't remember if having a degree made a difference in your pay, granted that she was just happy to receive a check. When she started in 1962, Shirley resumed, *"not all of the nurses had a bachelor's degree. Most of the nurses came from hospital schools of nursing. Very few had been to college."*

Referring to the school physicians, *"The doctor came to the district. He came on certain days. Three bells would ring, and the students would come to see him. He didn't go to every school every day. The day I was at school, the doctor would come."* The doctor would perform physicals but first had to have parental permission. Students did not undress for the exam. Nurses explained to the students the assessments the doctor would perform during the exam and stayed with the student during the examination.

There was a lot of respect for the nurses. The nurse was a special person, regarded as a professional in the school ... *"I worked primarily in Roxbury. A supervisor from downtown, from the main office, would come to your school to see how you were doing. There was no Faculty Senate back in 1962."*

During the Poliomyelitis Prevention Program, Shirley recalls that the doctor came to the school to give injections of the Salk vaccine, and the nurses helped prepare the setup. The nurse drew up the polio vaccine and had the needles ready, retrieved the signed consents, and sent out the notices. *"We paid for cards with the children's name on it. It was a lot of paperwork."*

"In the black community," Shirley recounts, *"most of the kids did not have private doctors. The families went to Boston City Hospital or another clinic. They did not have a private physician that came to the house."*

When recalling the time, she became a supervisor in 1976, Shirley laughed. *"I worked as a nurse for a number of years before I became a supervisor. I became a supervisor under Marguerite McLaughlin. She asked me to work downtown at the BPS headquarters on Court Street and become a supervisor."* Staff tension, Shirley related, existed at Court Street. Shirley worked at the Jeremiah Burke High School when the administration called her to become a supervisor. She would be the only person of color on the nursing supervisor's staff.

Shirley admits she liked being a supervisor. *"You would have to go out and see these nurses. The nurses were doing a good job. Some of them you had to pay more attention to. For the most part, they were professional, did a good job, and liked their work."*

When she became a supervisor, commuting to Court Street presented new challenges. She had to make after school pickup arrangements for her children. Regardless, more than money, the position offered her an advancement.

"If you had an opportunity to move yourself along, you did it. For a black woman, it was the way I was brought up. You had no right to refuse an opportunity. They knew I was qualified. I did not have the right to say no."

Her picture and story made headlines in the local black newspaper.

Asked about desegregating the schools and busing, Shirley and her teacher-husband John related that this time period presented challenges. School nurses accepted any student that came through the door. The demographics of schools changed.

John Garagna shared his comments:

"Prior to actual busing, there was a great deal of discussion, especially in the newspapers. In anticipation of busing, in the late 70s, the white students left the system. People were moving out, getting their own homes, wanting bigger houses. The student population changed. The city changed."

"During that time, students born in this country left the system. The Chinese (families) primarily moved to Quincy and Newton. Students who were not born in the U.S.A., and who never had their shots replaced them. They tended not to bring in the documentation. Unfortunately, they were not all legal. They did not want to be required to go someplace, where it would be discovered that they were illegal. This proved to be a difficult time for school nurses."

"Vietnamese and Hispanic students replaced the Chinese students." John said, *"When you are a teacher, the city walks into your school every morning."* The same applies to school nurses. For instance, the Superintendent instituted a class in Spanish for school nurses because of the massive influx of Puerto Rican students.[401]

---

401 *Annual Report of the Superintendent 1962-63. P. 37.* Retrieved from https://archive.org/details/report6263bost

In 1982, the school department took drastic measures when cutting their budget. I asked how that affected her. "*I left Court Street (school headquarters) to go to West Roxbury High School (WRHS). They took the nurse supervisor jobs away. I was there for about ten years.*"

Did you have any laughs, any memorable incidents that come to mind?

"*It was always keeping the sanctity, a balance between being kind and being firm. I did not make the nurses' office a student hangout. I maintained discipline, and tried to balance qualities of kindness, gentleness, and caring. I still see some of my former students at church. Some students would do anything to escape class. They try to be sick, not feeling well; wanted to lie down. Their purpose was to be in school. We had heard of some gun-toting, but there were never any shootings while I was there. Principal Pelligini was a wonderful human being, a great principal. The kids were very engaged in the school.*"

Shirley Ericson Garagna's account of her school nurse career has covered many years and many accomplishments, including being the first minority nursing supervisor. Her journey traversed budget cuts and school desegregation, but she persevered against continual adversity and endured. Additionally, she challenged the status quo.

Listen In

Let us now recount an interview in 2015 with another retired, Boston school nurse, taking place in a South Shore library. Our source prefers to remain anonymous, so we will use a fictitious set of initials, JK. Her account points out the changes that occurred in school nursing over the last 50 years and counting.

"*I graduated from St. Elizabeth's Hospital School of Nursing in Brighton, Massachusetts, a three-year program.*" JK started at St. Elizabeth's Hospital School of Nursing on October 4, 1944 and completed the program on October 4, 1947.

"*Before I even graduated from there, I started at Boston College for my BS degree. They had just started their five-year* [nursing] *program. Many of the nurses were veterans. I was in the first group that started for their bachelor's degree. Before I graduated from St. E's* [St. Elizabeth's Hospital], *I took morning classes at Boston College, then worked 3 to 11 at the hospital for two weeks. ... I eventually got my degree from Boston College in 1950. If you lost time, you had to make it up.*"

When did you start working for the Boston Public Schools?

"I worked at Tufts New England Medical Center (Tufts Medical Center) as a staff nurse and eventually went into the school department in October 1951 ... I knew there was an exam for it. I took the exam when it was given. Nurses didn't have to have a degree when I came in 1951, but I did have my degree. I was a permanent nurse. I was not a substitute nurse." JK took pride in that.

"After some time, they had vision and hearing nurses. When I first went in, the nurses did recheck the vision on some of the students. I can't remember when they [the vision and hearing nurses] *came in for that."*

Did most nurses have a BS Degree, or were most of them RNs?

"When I first started, I would say not too many. ... Probably the only ones having a degree were the supervisors in those days." JK remembers when she was taking the exam given by the city for school nurses, a few supervisors were checking the nurse's credentials. When the supervisors checked her documents, they said, *"wonderful."*

What was your day like? What schools did you serve?

"My schools were the Benjamin F. Tweed, grades kindergarten, 1, 2 and 3 combined; Bunker Hill School, grades kindergarten - 6; O. Holden School, grades kindergarten, 1, and 2.; and Clarence Edwards Junior High School, grades 6-8; a total of four schools. We had to get all of the immunization records and were busy. The doctor gave the inoculations. We set it up for him. Though the doctors came every day, the nurse might not be there." [The doctor and nurse worked together when the doctor was giving immunizations or doing physicals].

"I was at the Holden Monday afternoon and Thursday morning. The Tweed eventually closed. I did not have it for too long, and I can't remember when [it closed]. *Monday's was the Edwards Junior High School. I did it every day or some part of it. The Bunker Hill School I did Tuesday and Thursday morning and Wednesday afternoon. I would take a group on Wednesday at noon to the dental clinic. ... I took another group on Friday morning from the Edwards Junior High to the dental clinic. Eventually, that was phased out* [they phased out the dental clinic.] *You had to have parental permission. They did cleanings and dental work. There was no charge for that work. Up until I went to the high school that was done. They would give dental certificates if everything was ok. ... All of my schools were in Charlestown."*

"Eventually, I went to Charlestown High School in 1963. I might have been there a year or two before, but I was there when Kennedy was killed. I was there until I retired in 1988." People always remember where they were when President Kennedy was assassinated.

How did you travel between schools?

"I walked between the schools. Once in a while, I would take a bus from the Holden up to the Bunker Hill School. ... I did not have one [a car]. Some nurses had cars."

What did the doctor do?

"The doctor came every day even though you would not be there. He would ring the school bell. If anyone had to see the doctor, the teacher would send him or her down, and that was it. I don't know how many schools he had. The same physician went to all of my schools."

"The 1950s and 1960s were a different time." We talked about the students. *"I feel the blacks* were lenient with their children. I did not work with blacks. My schools had all neighborhood children, all community schools. Basically, it was fine until desegregation came. There were not many blacks* in Charlestown High School. They had all Charlestown people, except in the electrical program, which was a technical program. This specialized curriculum was open to the city. In the technical curriculum, the students had two weeks on the academic side, and two weeks on the technical side, out in the field. In the 9th and 10th grade, they were in the school shop and had their academics in the main building. Junior and seniors went out to work [for two weeks] like internships. Wonderful program."*

"In another part of the city, you might have plumbing. Good, it gave them a vocation and educated them. ... Teachers would weed them out in 9th and 10th grade, who would make it, who would not. ... They would graduate and become electricians. Excellent program, until desegregation came in, and then it went down the tubes. Judge Garrity said you had to move these people around."

At this point, we discussed retiring Superintendent Frederick Gillis' *Annual Report from 1962-1963*. He reported that over 60 girls received academic instruction in homes for unwed mothers. This program enabled them to return to their schools, continue with their classes, and graduate with their class. In his opinion, the schools had changed, and in his words, *"New concepts are in vogue."* As an example, he claimed that the community-centered school, *"has become suspect. Ability grouping, educationally sound, is frowned upon as socially undemocratic. District gerrymandering is the panacea for eliminating unit raced school."*[402]

The Superintendent rightly predicted the turmoil that would overcome Boston in the next ten years. Superintendent Gillis retired in 1963 after three years of service, followed by William Ohrenberger, who served from 1963-1973, retiring one year before the start of forced busing.

How were you affected by desegregation and busing, or did that affect school nurses?

"Desegregation started in 1974. I was at Charlestown High School at the time. It was kind of an unsettled situation because the kids were torn between what their parents were telling them to do and what the schools were telling them to do. You had a lot of sit-ins and walking out of school and the like. I had detectives sitting in the office, just trying to keep things down. Desegregation blew the whole system apart." She paused. *"People wanted to stay in their own communities. All they wanted was an equal education for their children."* See the image below.[403] The first day of school, Charlestown H.S. (1975, September 8).

First day of school, Charlestown

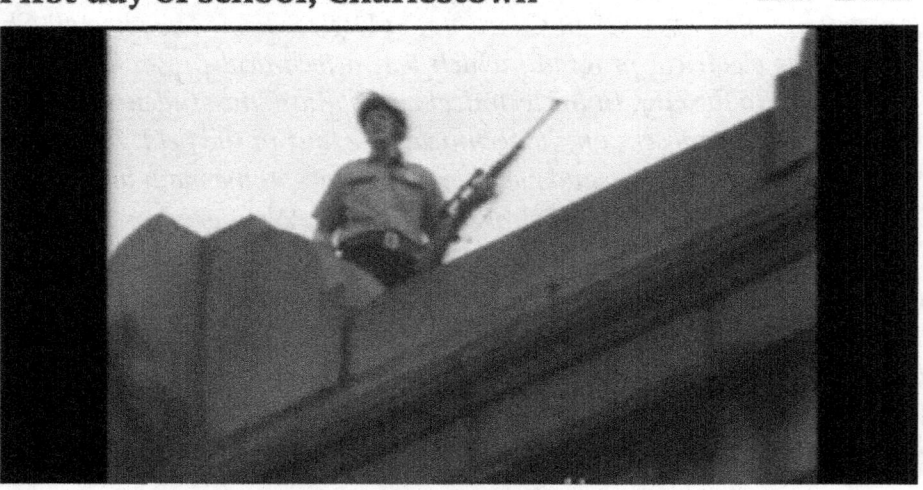

402 *Annual Report of the Superintendent 1962-63. P. 18, 70.* Retrieved from https://archive.org/details/report6263bost

403 The first day of school, Charlestown H.S. (1975, September 8). Retrieved from https://www.digitalcommonwealth.org/search/commonwealth-oai:vq280697z

The conversation turned to nurse and employment practices. One such issue was working after marriage. JK couldn't remember when that all came about. School nurses followed the regulations set for teachers. As discussed in Chapter 12, the legislature passed a law permitting teachers to work after marriage in 1954. Therefore, when JK first started in 1951, school nurses could not work after they married.

How were the substitutes obtained? Did you have to find your own?

"You had to call into Marion Sullivan, the chief supervising nurse. There were four assistant supervisors, or at least three. ... You had to call Miss Sullivan and tell her you would be out sick."

Did you have medications to give?

"No."

Were there any technology dependent children or diabetics?

"There were no technology dependent children. ... At least I did not have them. You did not have to worry about the diabetics."

If the students were on crutches, were they able to come to school?

"I do remember I had one little fellow. He was somewhat of a paraplegic. He couldn't get around that much. ... Eventually, he went across the street to the Warren School. He was very independent. He would go up and down the stairs on his backside. He was the only real problem that I recall. He was seven or eight."

Were most of the students from two parent families?

"Pretty much, in Charlestown, they were."

How did the school department regard the nurses? Did they respect them?

"We were on the same salary schedule as the teachers. We might not have had all of the benefits that the teachers had. From the time I went in, I was always on the teacher's salary schedule." Some Massachusetts school nurses just received that designation in 2015.

Did you make home visits?

"Yes, I did. After school, if you didn't have the authorization for the inoculations, [(student]) failed their vision or hearing [tests], and the parents had not done anything. We needed their permission. You would go and push them on a little bit for failed vision tests and consent for immunizations. Most mothers were home; in those days, they were. Sometimes they had a phone and sometimes not. Usually, you could get them. Sometimes you would have to walk the child home."

JK recalls this incident.

"A child came to school, and the child was sick. I tried to get the telephone number, but he had an unlisted phone number. I ended up getting the chief operator. It is unheard of having a sick child in school and not being able to contact someone. I didn't want the phone number, I told them, just to reach the parent. They did do the connection."

Were there any particular programs in which the school nurses were involved? Were there any epidemics?

"We did at least two programs, the Salk vaccine and Sabin oral (for Polio). We gave those in school. ... The Salk was a shot. The school doctor gave the Salk injection. The Sabin was easy. We did it without the school doctor. It was much easier. We would just go in the back of a classroom and bring cups. We did not have to take them [students]out of the classroom."

This plan must have pleased the teachers. They didn't lose classroom time.

"Kids generally went to their own doctor. ... We did physicals, not really involved, cursory thing, you know. The schools were required to do certain grades. The students could send it in from their own doctor."

Were there any other programs?

"Not unless something came up. You would receive notification from the Department of Public Health as I did when I was at the high school. They found that one of my students had tuberculosis. I had to do those screenings [tine tests]. The Department of Health would notify you."

Were you active in the Nurse Faculty Senate?

"No. I was not involved."

Was it called the Boston Public School Nurses Club?

"I don't recall that. We always had a meeting once a month when we were in school with the supervisors. Various groups would go out to eat afterwards."

Was the Boston Teachers Union active then?

"Eventually we did go into the teachers' union. The nurses were not in it for quite a while, and I don't remember exactly when. I don't remember when the Nurse Faculty Senate started."

"If you were out one day, you lost a half-day's pay. You got the school vacations and all the vacation periods, the same as the teachers. We were always contributing to pensions. We did get sick time. The teachers got sick time first, and eventually, the nurses got them."

Were you on a higher salary scale than the nurses without a degree?

"No, it was the same at that time. ...We had a salary scale, increments, a BS Degree plus so many credits, depending on what you had, and a master's degree. Eventually, we got everything."

Do you think nurses are a lot different now?

"They wanted to be on the same schedule as teachers. The nurses got along."

What do you think of school nursing then and now?

"Well, when we first started, it was put on a band-aid. Now they have to do so many other things. You have to do so many nursing procedures that should not be in the schools. They decided to take the children out of the institutions and mainstream them into classrooms. Now nurses do tube feedings, catheterizations, and glucose monitoring [just to name a few]."

If the girls became pregnant, were they in schools?

"I did not have any pregnant girls at Charlestown High School. ... Most of the pregnant girls were black people.* That was my impression. ... I was basically in Charlestown, and there weren't that many blacks*. I don't know about the inner city. ... There might have been more in Dorchester. Charlestown was mostly white until desegregation came in. I just knew of some who had been pregnant at another school. Some of them went to an unwed mother's school. They had a pregnancy previously, but not while I was there. There were not many occupations that were open to girls. Girls are doing things [now] that you would not think of."

JK pointed out the developments that ensued in the schools during and following desegregation in 1974, the immunization programs the school nurses participated in, the plans for pregnant girls, and the school nurses escalating salary schedule and benefits. Nurses faced further challenges resulting from the newly enacted Federal laws, Section 504 of the Rehabilitation Act of 1973, and the Individual with Disabilities Act, known as IDEA, passed in 1975. As Superintendent Gillis commented in his report, the schools had more than 1,000 physically handicapped or emotionally disturbed children in home or hospital instructions.[404] Under the new legislation, the schools mainstreamed these children into regular classrooms as much as possible. Another transition occurred, permitting pregnant students to continue their studies in their high school.

In reviewing the records, JK's presumption she was always on the teacher's salary scale proved to be incorrect. The nurses only received identical compensation, starting in 1969, as outlined earlier in this chapter.

In this day and age, it is difficult to recall there was a time before cell phones and smartphones when making a phone call might require contacting "information" and obtaining an operator's assistance. JK's dilemma with the phone company, and the emergency card in the main office without a phone number, left her in a position of not being able to contact a parent. The "information" operator notified JK the family indeed had a telephone, but the number was unlisted, which meant they could not give it out. However, common sense and good judgment saved the day when the chief operator made the connection without revealing the phone number.

---

[404] *Annual Report of the Superintendent 1962-63. P. 70.* Retrieved from https://archive.org/details/report6263bost

Would a phone company react that way today? I doubt it with all of our current privacy regulations. Do readers recall the dispute between Apple and the FBI? Whether right or wrong, Apple fought against unlocking an iPhone belonging to one of the San Bernardino terrorists.[405]

Surprisingly, JK's schools are still functioning, although three are under different sponsorship. The Bunker Hill School closed and is now on the National Register of Historic Places. The Holden is now a private, coed Christian high school called Holden School. The historic B.F. Tweed School closed, and the Edwards continues as a junior high school.

At this juncture, my readers deserve a further explanation of what happened during Boston's desegregation of the public schools.

Racial Imbalance Act

In 1965, the state legislature passed the Racial Imbalance Act. This law defined a racially imbalanced school as one with over 50 percent non-white students and stated that any imbalanced school system could lose state funds. Court-ordered desegregation in Boston forced the reassignment of 15,000 children in September 1974 to schools outside of their neighborhoods. Because of geographic barriers between black and white communities, a federal court instituted and implemented forced busing to desegregate the city's schools.

Judge Wendell Arthur Garrity Jr., who lived in Wellesley, MA, a wealthy suburb, administered the controversial school desegregation plan. Boston's white residents resisted the plan causing racial violence and boycotting of several schools. This resistance lasted for about two years. It was not until 1988 that Garrity transferred back to the Boston School Committee full control of the desegregation plan.

Desegregation affected the white school-age population. Their attendance declined from 75% in 1964 to 64% in 1970, then to 57% in 1973 (before the court order) and to 47.8% in 1975 after the court ordered busing. Of the 100,000 students enrolled in the Boston Public Schools, during those years, attendance fell from 60,000

---

405 Mastroianni, B. (2016). Feds: Apple has unlocked iPhones "many times" before, *CBS News*. Retrieved from http://www.cbsnews.com/news/feds-apple-has-unlocked-iphones-before/

to 40,000.[406] At the same time, Dr. Christine Russell, a Boston University research scholar, found desegregation to be only one of many factors in school attendance. *"White families, she thought, sought the larger homes and house lots and social amenities of the suburbs."*[407]

The negative consequences of desegregation forced Roxbury High School closed, and South Boston High School plunged into receivership to survive. It was a doomed pairing from the start, pitting groups of youth from three white housing projects in South Boston against another group from three minority housing projects in Roxbury.

The positive results of desegregation include: the desegregation of the teaching staff, an increase of bilingual staff, the closing of antiquated, unsafe school buildings, and the decrease in minority student suspensions. An increase in participation of universities and cultural organizations, and a reduction in the role played by patronage in obtaining employment developed into another constructive outcome. A 1973 decision by the Boston Teachers Union not to buy tickets to Boston School Committee member's parties and testimonials, as had been the custom, defined this action.[408] Fittingly enough, the time for cash filled envelopes for elected officials ended.

The Nurses, the Boston School Committee and the Union

Mr. Louis Vangel, BTU Business Agent, and Fred Reilly, BTU President, said at a meeting on November 2, 1966, the negotiations for school nurses didn't go well. Reilly stressed when the school nurses want an additional benefit in their contract, such as an extension of sick leave, or for a study year's leave with pay, they should contact the BTU, not the School Hygiene office. As noted earlier in this chapter, the nurses starting salary in 1966 was $4,980, which Vangel considered ridiculous. He compared it to the $6,300 starting salary for nurses at Boston City Hospital. He said nurses should have a phone for private and confidential conversations, and they

---

406   Delmont, M. Retrieved from https://www.theatlantic.com/politics/archive/2016/03/the-boston-busing-crisis-was-never-intended-to-work/474264/

407   Cronin, J. *Reforming Boston Schools, 1930-2006: Overcoming Corruption and Racial Segregation.* (2008). New York, NY. Palgrave McMillan. P. 114.

408   Ibid. P. 123.

should request the Legislature file a law to direct the Board of Education to certify nurses as Health Education Teachers. Nurses were not on tenure. He emphasized that after four years of employment, they should be on tenure, following the same path as the teachers. They should spell these issues out in a contract. Teachers received tenure in 1952.

The BPSNC (they had started to use BPSNA, ending with Association instead of BPSNC, C meaning club) sent a letter to all school nurses on 11/17/1966, notifying them they were in the process of negotiating their first contract with the BSC to improve their professional standing. The letter contained the bargaining points they considered important and asked school nurses to review the document and add anything else they considered relevant. Also, they requested the nurses to send in any factual data they had concerning the items. The following is a list of the items.

1. Salary $6,300, 9 steps at 400, double step at tenure $10,300
2. Tenure clarified
3. Title
4. Hours defined
5. Sabbatical leave
6. Duties defined
7. Meetings for the department on in-service days
8. Working conditions
9. Daily reports
10. Seniority
11. Student observers
12. Transfer policy
13. Grievances
14. Qualified first aider
15. Full-time nurse, Junior and Senior High, telephones
16. Home visiting policies
17. Attendance at conventions
18. Credit for outside experience
19. School nurse at interviewing of applicants during exams
20. Educational reimbursement
21. Parking permits
22. Mileage allowance
23. Standing orders
24. Provisional nurses

25. Retired nurses for substitute work
26. Reinstatement in the department of nurses, those who have transferred to other school departments
27. Rating qualifications stabilized
28. Mail at school or home
29. General aides
30. Rotation of duties of supervisors

During their March 1, 1967 meeting, the issue of a lack of funds for substitute nurses brought about the cancellation of an important meeting of the nurses Bargaining Committee with Attorney Schroeder, a representative of the BSC. Nurse Supervisor Mrs. Holthaus called the cancellation. The nurses unanimously agreed upon two courses of action in the future: first, nurses in the districts would cover for each other, and second, the BPSNA would pay substitutes from the BPSNA treasury.[409]

I am at a loss concerning some of the negotiating items. These were obviously unchartered waters for them. One of the negotiating items was covering for each other in schools. Nurses' agreeing to cover for each other set an unsafe precedent. The critical issue here is the safety of the students. How many emergencies can one nurse cover? At that time, each nurse had between three and four schools. In that case, a nurse would be covering six to eight schools. How many risks are they taking? Under these circumstances, who is the winner, and who is the loser? They made another agreement to pay the substitute nurse out of the BPSNA treasury. Were schoolteachers doing this? Absolutely not.

In 1967, they would drop the requirement for a college degree for a school nurse, which in no way would raise their professional status, nor put them on the same educational level as teachers.

The school nurses were ill-advised. To my way of thinking, they should have crusaded for hours and duties defined, standing orders, transfer policy and grievances, a full-time nurse at Junior and Senior High Schools, telephones, and home visiting policies. Advocating for more consistent and unvarying policies, procedures, and record keeping would have benefited the nurses more in the long term. What agenda items would my readers have advised them to pursue?

---

409   Boston Public School Nurses Club Minutes

Immunization Laws

The immunization law, initially written in 1855, was rewritten again in 1967 to explain further the meaning of "duly vaccinated." In 1967, it specifically mentioned vaccinations, including diphtheria, pertussis, tetanus, measles, and poliomyelitis vaccination. The sentence ends with the phrase "and other communicable diseases as may be specified from time-to-time by the department of public health." (Acts, 1967, Chapter 590, Section 15). In other words, the Department of Health could add other disease vaccines when needed. If students did not have these vaccinations, they were excluded from school, another responsibility of the school nurse. The Legislature updated this law over concerns for public health disasters due to contagious diseases.

The nurses faced new situations in the decades to come in the form of transfers, loss of leadership, and students' complex health issues. How they met these challenges and with what kind of impact will be followed in the ensuing chapters, bearing in mind these words from Ecclesiastes 3:1 *"For everything there is a season, and a time for every matter under heaven. We do what is suitable to the season. What is suitable to one time is inappropriate to another."*

Twentieth Century Milestones Affecting School Nursing (Continued)

1970 - Trials of Computerized Axial Tomography (CAT) begin.

1972 - The U.S. elected Richard Nixon as President of the United States for his second term.

1973 - The United States Supreme Court declares abortion is a constitutional right in the landmark decision on the Roe v. Wade case.

1974 - Boston school desegregation begins.
U.S. President Richard Nixon resigns from office after the Watergate Scandal. Vice-President Gerald Ford becomes the next U.S. President.

1975 - The Vietnam War ends.

1977 - MRI (Magnetic Resonance Imaging) Scanner is first tested.

1978 - The first test-tube baby is born.

Chapter 15

School Health Restructures in the 1970s

In 1970, a Brookings Institute study rated Boston as one of the most distressed cities in the country. Boston began to take steps towards its transformation after being referred to as a "Basket Case" in the second half of the 20th century. As historians at the Massachusetts Historical Society explained, "there is no doubt that the Boston Redevelopment Authority, politicians, and community activists had leading roles" in starting Boston's journey to become a world-class city.[410] Indeed, they did. As a result of the citizen's opposition to urban renewal, political activists like Mel King, new immigrants, and old-time residents preserved and improved the city.

In 1974, Arthur Fiedler and the Boston Pops began their annual tradition of a concert and fireworks show on the Fourth of July; Kip Tiernan founded Boston's Rosie's Place, the first homeless women's shelter in the United States, and Boston school desegregation began. Plywood Palace became the first name of the troubled, glass John Hancock Tower built in 1976. To the owner's dismay, the windows popped out, and the building swayed in the wind. Nevertheless, after endless repairs, it remains the tallest building in New England. First Night began, and the development of the Faneuil Hall marketplace became a reality. The John F. Kennedy Library was dedicated at Columbia Point in 1979, gazing at the blue-gray expanse of gentle swells in Dorchester Bay, acknowledging JFK's love of sailing. Raymond Flynn became Boston's Mayor in 1984, succeeding Kevin White.

---

410   From Basket Case to Innovation Hub. *MHS Miscellany*, 108, 8.

Part 1 The 1970s - Teachers Strike

The year 1970 started with fireworks when the teachers staged a one-day strike; the first teachers strike in Boston's history and the sixth in the state since the Massachusetts legislature granted collective bargaining rights to teachers and other public employees in 1965. We discussed in previous chapters how school nurses strived for the same salary schedule as teachers. Therefore, whatever transpired with teachers, likewise applied to school nurses.

The teachers voted on March 22, 1970, to boycott classes to force the Boston School Committee to offer them higher salaries in the Fall of 1970. As has been pointed out in Chapter 14, teachers and school nurses received a starting salary of $7,000 (See charts in Chapter 14). School Superintendent William H. Ohrenberger persisted in keeping the 194 public schools open for the 92,000 Boston school children and directed teachers and other employees to ignore the strike vote.

In a separate development, Union President John P. Reilly rolled out his plans: 1) Teachers and other staff were to picket in front of their schools for an hour before school and an hour after classes. 2) Then they were to meet at a downtown hotel for a series of speeches, 3) Followed by a march to school department headquarters, and from there, 4) A protest rally at City Hall. Ohrenberger stated the Boston Teachers Union (BTU) encouraged schoolteachers to engage in unprofessional conduct. He believed in the collective bargaining process and claimed the Boston School Committee (BSC) negotiated in good faith. On the other hand, Mayor Kevin H. White proposed some alternatives with the BSC on how to deal with the budget gap. Suffice it to say, the climate was anything but copacetic.

The Boston Globe newspaper ran a picture of the strikers marching to City Hall on March 24, 1970. The 42 degrees temperature on this day brought a chill to the air. A long line of mainly men and some women, stretching several blocks marched about four abreast in the street. The three-man group leading the procession carried a union banner. Marchers looked professionally dressed, wearing long coats, storm coats, neckties, a few hats, kerchiefs, and scarves. Just between us, looking at the picture, they looked like an orderly group. Emergency vehicles drove slowly on the other side of the street. Passersby watched from the sidewalks. Were school nurses marching in these ranks? We could see women in the lines, and those could be school nurses, as all the school nurses at that time were women.

The BTU represented 4,200 permanent classroom teachers and 200 other employees in higher job categories. During the bargaining sessions, either side could reject the proposal of the other. A group of young teachers requested to add some additional demands such as more school nurses, librarians, remedial reading teachers, and the replacement of old equipment. However, the rank and file voted against the proposal because "it's detailed demands would tie the hands of negotiators."[411]

The strike lasted 13 days. This long walk-out hit the high schools hardest, where 83 percent of the teachers, 1,011, and 73 percent of the students, 13,565, stayed home.[412] Parents did not know whether to send their children to school or keep them home. Some working parents sent their children to school; only later, the school returned them home because of the lack of teachers. BSC lawyers claimed the strike failed to comply with both the state collective bargaining law and the current union contract. The stinging consequence for participation in the strike resulted in the loss of those absent day's pay.

When both parties agreed with a proposal that unresolved issues in the dispute submit to binding arbitration, the teachers' strike ended in a state of uneasy harmony. The law counsel for the BSC, Herbert Gleason, did not accept this approach to settling the strike. He claimed, "it is not possible for public officials to enter binding arbitration on an open-ended and undefined mater." Not surprisingly, BTU attorney, Albert Goldman, disagreed and said other states set precedents permitting arbitration with public officials. Both the BTU and the BSC hoped they settle the unresolved issues before the dispute went to arbitration. That is to say, if they could resolve the disagreement on whether they could enter into mediation.[413]

Again, the question is quite simply, did school nurses join in the picketing and protests? What effect, if any, would this unlawful behavior have on their professional nursing license? Was there any person who would stand in the nurse's shoes offering

---

411 Van Dyne, L. (1970, Mar 23). 1-Day Strike Voted By Hub Teachers. *Boston Globe (1960-1985)* Retrieved from https://search.proquest.com/docview/375431028?accountid=9675

412 Van Dyne, L. & Davis, J. (1970, Mar 25). Teacher strike: 56,400 Pupils Miss Classes. *Boston Globe (1960-1985)* Retrieved from https://search.proquest.com/docview/375420097?accountid=9675

413 Davis, J., & McCain, N. (1970, May 20). Teachers' strike ends with arbitration. *Boston Globe (1960-1985)* Retrieved from https://search.proquest.com/docview/504806462?accountid=9675

first aid, treatments, hearing and vision tests, teaching good health habits in the classroom, and encouraging and stimulating the development of social and emotional skills? In answering the question, we must assume though the newspapers did not mention the school nurse's involvement in picketing and protests, a percentage probably joined in. It is possible they attended after school meetings, joined in the preschool picketing, did nothing, everything, and had divided loyalties.

However, we have no records to sustain this premise, specifically, because there were no Minutes from April 1970 until they commenced in a notebook on March 29, 1972. Perhaps more nurses in the high schools joined in as compared to the elementary schools since the young, male, high school teachers evolved into the union's most militant members. At the same time, if the nurse did not sign in at her school assignment, she would be looking at a smaller paycheck.

On August 25, 1970, shortly before the opening of school, the BSC approved the teachers' contract, amidst the tirades of Chairman Joseph Lee denouncing teachers as "not respecting children, the laws, God or themselves." Did he mean to include nurses also? Later during the meeting, he resigned his chairmanship, and along with Committeeman John Kerrigan, refused to sign the recommended contract in protest. The other committeemen declined to accept his resignation. Accordingly, Lee agreed to stay on as acting chairman until January 1971.[414]

In negotiations, the BTU asked for a beginning salary increase from $7,000 to $7,800 and a maximum higher than the current $11,300. The BSC countered with an offer of a minimum of $7,600 and a maximum of $12,600. Subsequently, after the results of binding arbitration, they settled for a starting salary of $7,600 and a maximum of $12,900. The new arbitration package also required non-union teachers to pay an agency fee to the union. For the first time, this salary schedule integrated school nurses with teachers in Group I (See the Salary Schedules in Chapter 14). As has been pointed out earlier, above all, the school nurses wanted to be on the same par as teachers, and at last, they accomplished their goal.

Mayor White refused to fund three of the items of the arbitration package but

---

[414] McCain, N. (1970, Aug 26). Boston School Committee OKs teachers' contract. *Boston Globe(1960-1985)* Retrieved from https://search.proquest.com/docview/503718934?accountid=9675

agreed to underwrite the new earnings of the teachers and others represented by the BTU. This contract propelled Boston teachers into being the highest paid in the state.

More than likely, the same was true for school nurses. Nevertheless, in comparison, the Massachusetts Nurses Association (MNA) negotiated a new contract for staff nurses at Boston City Hospital in 1969, awarding them a starting salary of $140 per week, amounting to $7,280 annually. The Boston public health nurses who also worked in the parochial schools received a similar contract.[415] This amount was close to the $7,600 awarded to the Boston school nurses. Do readers recall from Chapter 14 the discussion regarding the unification of the public and parochial school health programs? Supporters of unification claimed the religious school health program was inexpensive to administer compared to the Boston public school health program. The Boston public health nurses received a hefty raise in salary, increasing the parochial school health service budget, not making it any more desirable to acquire.

Not to be surpassed, staff nurses at Boston's Peter Bent Brigham Hospital ratified a contract negotiated by MNA in 1969, giving them the highest starting salaries in the state. Staff nurses' wages started at $152 per week, a total of $7,904 a year.[416]

Mayor White, a fierce adversary, also recommended they cut in half the $1.6 million the BSC voted to give to administrators not covered by the BTU contract. Additionally, he proposed to fund the arbitration package with the $1.2 million not paid to employees during the 13-day strike.[417]

Another obstacle put before them stemmed from a bill on Massachusetts Governor Francis Sargent's desk. This bill would make contracts binding between school committees, cities, and other groups that voluntarily enter into such agreements. The BSC would have to honor the accords when the Governor signed it

---

415 News. (1969). *The American Journal of Nursing*, 69(5), 913-1071. Retrieved from http://www.jstor.org/stable/3453899

416 At Press Time. (1969). *The American Journal of Nursing*, 69(10), 2047-2048. Retrieved from http://www.jstor.org/stable/3453996

417 Brody, J. (1970, Sep 01). White trims $2.6m in teacher package. *Boston Globe (1960-1985)* Retrieved From https://search.proquest.com/docview/503642564?accountid=9675

into law (Brody). Indeed, they accepted the settlement. Moreover, the BSC heeded the requests for more nurses and increased the number of full-time nurses to 76. As of January 1, 1971, they would add five more nurses, making a total of 81, in contrast to the 75 plus school nurses on board in 1969.[418]

Governor Sargent signed the bill as mentioned above in November 1973. This law overhauled municipal employees' collective bargaining agreements in Massachusetts. The law repealed existing laws at the time. For instance, they made strikes by municipal employees unlawful, and replaced it with an act giving employees the right to self-organize and also join, form, or assist other employee organizations for collective bargaining.[419]

School Nurse Workforce Issues

The BSC brought a reorientation to their relationship with the school nurses by recognizing the Union as the exclusive bargaining representative for all school nurses in the school nurse unit. Up until that time, the school nurses were just a tag-along on the teachers' contract since they had none of their own. Finally, after the Union and Union Negotiating Committee received the requested suggestions of what nurses needed to improve their working conditions and other concerns, accordingly, a contract emerged with the assistance of collective bargaining. The agreement covered safety concerns, equal school assignments, parking permits, reimbursable carfare, student nurse internship, promotions, transfers, and grievance procedures. The following is a summary of the school nurses' first agreement called Eleven Articles of the School Nurses Contract covering September 1, 1970-August 31, 1971.

The agreement defined their working conditions:

- The SN shall not be required to remain in a building after administrative personnel has left.

---

418   *Proceedings of the School Committee, City of Boston 1970*. P. 241. Retrieved from https://archive.org/stream/proceedingsofsch1970bost#page/34/mode/2up/search/nurse

419   Massachusetts General Laws. Retrieved from Chapter 1078: 1124-1138
http://archives.lib.state.ma.us/actsResolves/1973/1973acts1078.pdf
http://hdl.handle.net/2452/16629

- School nurse's assignments as to numbers of pupils should be equal. (An) unequal assignment may be grieved. Nurses traveling between schools shall be given parking permits. A list of assignments shall be made available to school nurses or the Union when requested. School nurses traveling between schools shall be reimbursed (their) car fare.

- Student nurse observers as part of their clinical training, can be assigned to school nurses that agree to have them. In turn, the colleges and hospitals sending these student nurses will be requested to supply <u>appropriate</u> lecturers for the School Nurse In-Service Programs.

- Nurses meetings shall be held on the established In-Service Day for teaching staff.

- When promotions and transfers are available, a circular will be sent to all School Nurses notifying them of these vacancies. This circular shall include all qualifications, requirements, duties, salary, and other pertinent information. All applications must be in writing to be considered. If there is a change in qualifications for any position, notice must be given to personnel at least six months in advance.

- The rules of seniority apply to all transfers and assignments. All requests for transfer shall be made to the Chief Supervising Nurse.

- A "grievance" is described as when there is a violation, misinterpretation, or inequitable application of one of the provisions of the agreement; and a person has been treated unfairly or inequitably, which is contrary to established policy affecting employees. This shall only apply to conditions where the BSC has the authority to act. The grievance procedure contains many steps. Both sides should meet with the view to arrive at a mutually satisfactory resolution of the complaint. A Union representative can also represent the school nurse. If the parties don't agree with the corrective action requested, the grievance can be further appealed. Grievances can be filed for assignment size, salary reasons, and for school nurses improperly denied a leave of absence. The Union can submit a grievance that still remains unresolved for arbitration. Both parties will agree to and will abide by the final decision by the arbitrator.

- The Union has responsibilities to accept all eligible persons in the school health unit, regardless of race, color, creed, national origin, sex, or marital status. Members of the Union Negotiating Committee will be released from their schools with pay, also providing substitutes to cover their assignment, for the time spent in negotiations. The Union may secure authorization for payroll deductions of Union dues. There will be no Union Activity on school time.

- When new issues arise, which are proper subjects for collective bargaining, the BSC has agreed that it will make no changes without prior consultation and negotiation with the Union. The Union and the BSC have agreed that differences between the parties will be settled by peaceful means. The Union and any employee in the school health unit will not engage in or be involved with any strike, work stoppage, or any concerted refusal to perform routine work duties.

- The BSC concluded that this collective bargaining was a new field for them. They sought to address the issues of compensation and working conditions for the school nurses. They hoped that "through this partnership with the Committee, which enables them to bring to bear on the growing problems inherent in the advancement of education, their intimate knowledge, and experience on matters of professional concern." The Committee <u>finished</u> by reminding the school nurses that they have complete authority of the policies and administration of the schools as required by law.[420]

These guidelines offered the nurses some concrete steps to take in the performance of their daily commitments. Hopefully, principals and the teaching staff were made aware of them. As an example of one of the tenets of the contract, for at least ten years, I received senior student nurses from Boston College William F. Connell School of Nursing during their community health experience at the Thomas Edison Middle School in Brighton. In return, I received an annual letter from the academic dean, allowing me to use their library as an adjunct instructor.

Annie McKay, our first school nurse in Boston, Massachusetts, received car

---

[420] *Proceedings of the School Committee, City of Boston 1970*. P. 294-298. Retrieved from https://archive.org/stream/proceedingsofsch1970bost#page/34/mode/2up/search/nurse

fare from the Instructive District Nursing Association when she travelled between her schools in the South End. For that reason, I think they should continue the practice. Additionally, the contract did not elaborate on how they would equalize the assignments. Eventually, they accomplished this goal using a complex formula.

After they developed their first contract, I wonder if they permitted themselves some thoughtful reflection. Did the school nurses dance with joy or sigh with relief after long and arduous sessions with the Boston School Committee? To be honest, we will never know, but they probably did both. Over time, teachers have long overshadowed the school nurses in the school system, and now the nurses received past-due recognition. Fittingly enough, when thinking about their future, they can ponder advice from Winston Churchill: "It is always wise to look ahead, but difficult to look further than you can see."[421]

Causes for Concern

Headmasters and principals finally became proactive on behalf of the school nurse and school physician assignments. Headmaster John C. Tragakis of the Boston Trade High School, at 550 Parker Street in Roxbury, sent a letter to Chief Supervising Nurse Louise B. Holthaus on September 19, 1972. He commented his school nurse also serviced the Ira Allen School, located at 540 Parker Street, now part of Wentworth Institute of Technology. His concerns revolved around student safety and welfare since his school was the only one in the system that had 12 fully equipped industrial shops operating all day from 8:10 AM to 2:45 PM, which contained heavy machinery and power tools.

Though the distance between the schools was not great, Tragakis strongly believed he needed a nurse full time on his premises due to the dangers inherent when students learned the mechanisms of heavy machinery. At that time, cell phones were only in a technology developer's imagination. Communications depended on the ability to locate the nurse in the other school, and then request her to rush pell-mell to their building.[422]

Another principal, James D. Supple, of the Dever School, 325 Mt. Vernon

---

421 Retrieved from http://www.brainyquote.com/quotes/quotes/w/winstonchu129821.html
422 Nurses 1957-1974, *Boston Public Schools Health Services Collection*, Box 2.

Street, Dorchester, wrote to Dr. Richard J. Gorman, Director of School Health Services, on June 23, 1972. His comments centered around the increased caseload of his nurse Helen Burke, at the Dever-McCormack Schools, especially regarding case conferences of children in Special Needs Classes, and routine record keeping. Recently, he remarked, a constant influx of children arrived from the rural south and rural Puerto Rico needing health services, while at the same time, Columbia Point Health Center reduced their services. In his opinion, Mrs. Burke required more assistance, perhaps a medical aide. He was pleased not only with her work in the health office but also in the field of community relations and coordinating with local organizations to provide services in mental health and well-child health supervision.[423]

Earlier, another letter found its way on January 26, 1971, to the Assistant Superintendent's office from Ralph E. Mann, Principal at the Andrew Jackson School, revealing another concern. According to the letter, a school doctor assigned to make daily visits to the Commonwealth Development Kindergarten Unit had not arrived at the school in several months. Two months ago, Principal Mann inquired about obtaining a substitute. School Health Services told him they would look into it.

Additionally, another situation developed at the Andrew Jackson School. Principal Mann asked for advice about the infrequent visits of his school nurse. The nurse assigned to his Kindergarten Unit every Monday and Thursday last visited the school at the end of November. As a result, the school did not receive any regular well-child health checkups, nor immunization follow-ups. She responded to the teachers' call for health records during two short visits. One key aspect of this dilemma stemmed from the lack of communication between all those concerned. School Health Services needed to sit down with both the school nurse and the principal to determine their needs and the school nurse's assignment. We will see how they addressed these problems.

The Boston School Committee (BSC) still awarded School Nurse Certificates in 1972. As you may recall, registered nurses received a certificate after taking a competitive school nurse exam, making that person eligible for a school nurse assignment. For unknown reasons, the BSC postponed the test for nurses, as reported in the Boston Public School Nurses Minutes at their December 5, 1973,

---

[423] Ibid.

meeting. President Marie Rubico, at their January 2, 1974, meeting, reported the Boston Teachers Union intended to file a grievance on the action of the BSC in postponing the exam. Unfortunately, nothing ever came of that.

All of this occurred amidst the disturbing decision to yet again, transfer School Health Services to the Department of Health and Hospitals. The Mayor's committee called the School Health Services Task Force, a joint project of the Office of Commissioner of Health and Hospitals, Leon S. White, and the Boston School Committee recruited a new member, Dr. Gorman, Director of School Health Services. Dr. Gorman related this information at a Nurse Faculty Senate meeting. The Task Force's goal was to restructure School Health Services under either the BSC or Health and Hospitals.[424]

Dr. Gorman responded in 1974 to references from Health and Hospitals that school health resources included duplication, inadequacies, and were too costly. He expressed how the schools had utilized outpatient clinics at the large city hospitals and the new community health centers. Staff from the community health centers replaced some School Health Services doctors. As an example, the New England Medical Center (Floating Hospital), now known as Tufts Medical Center, assumed control of health services at the Quincy and Lincoln schools. As you may also recall, the Quincy school was one of Annie McKay's schools, Boston's first school nurse.

A common misconception was that school physicians were required to visit their schools every day. This was not the case, said Dr. Gorman. School enrollment determined the frequency of visits. He further explained small schools with only 200 to 300 pupils should receive visits two to three times a week, whereas a doctor should visit larger schools with 500 or more students daily.[425]

In his letter to the BSC, Dr. Gorman brought up the subject of using nurse practitioners, a sensitive area with school nurses. Nurse practitioners hold advanced nurse degrees and are licensed to perform primary care, including sports physicals. Naturally, the school nurse questions whether if the school has a nurse practitioner, they would also require a school nurse? "The use of school nurse practitioners in school systems to eventually replace school physicians has been gradually

---

424 *Boston Public School Nurses Club Minutes*, January 16, 1974

425 Task Force on School Health Services 1973, *Boston Public Schools Health Services Collection*, Box 2.

(occurring) across the country," Dr. Gorman related. He further explained they looked at similar programs in Denver and San Diego that developed into successful courses. As a result, the BPS placed a nurse to work as a nurse practitioner in one of Boston's high schools and started to train another nurse to do the same. The nurse practitioner course ran full time for four months and required extra funds. He hoped more of Boston's school nurses would avail themselves of this opportunity.[426]

Immunization Laws

The Immunization Laws were noted in Chapter 5 and Chapter 14, (*Massachusetts General Laws*, (b) Acts, 1967, Chapter 590, Section 15). The laws were rewritten again in 1979. A new law M.G.L. c.76, s.15 in 1979 reinforced and put teeth in the 1967 Immunization Law by requiring a physician's certificate for children admitted to Kindergarten including dates of immunization against mumps and rubella after September 1, 1979. This requirement would apply to all grades the following year. It assisted nurses in stressing to parents and administration that the school principal would exclude their children from school if they did not have the specific immunizations.

Part 2 - Doctor's Inquiry

The Boston School Committee (BSC) scheduled a hearing in 1976 about the school doctors: namely, who they were and what they did for the children of Boston. They considered a proposal to abolish the civil service position of school physician. Chapter 1 of this book relates the story of the beginnings of School Health Services in the United States. You will recall that Boston, Massachusetts, in 1894, was the first city to implement the health supervision of school children.

Mayor White and the Boston City Council cut $20 million from the BSC budget. School physicians cost $350,000 annually. To be precise, that is one-tenth of one percent of the city budget, not one-tenth of the budget. These amounts look trivial when you consider the big picture. Further, Mayor White generated a message to Boston residents declaring the School Department was responsible for the $59 increase in city taxes,[427]

---

426   Ibid.

427   School Doctor's Inquiry. P. 52. *Boston Public Schools Health Services Collection*, Box 2.

Imagine you attended the inquiry, which transpired in a crowded, stuffy room, at the end of summer, on August 16, 1976, an 80-degree day. The clock struck 11:45 AM. It was hot outside, probably inside too. Participants looked at their watches with furrowed brows, raised their heads to look at the massive wall clock, pulled at their shirt collars, and periodically left the hearing to grab a cigarette in the corridor.

Eighteen doctors assembled at the beginning of the hearing to hear their fate. The BSC called Assistant Director Dr. Fischer to testify first. Dr. Fischer recounted his 28½ years as a school physician. He conceded he consulted with children from the same families, because many of them had no contact with a physician other than with the school physician.[428]

In 1976, Dr. Fischer continued, 73,000 students attended the Boston Public Schools, plus faculty and ancillary staff amounting to 11,000. If any of these people came to the school doctor, he/she was obliged to treat them. Each doctor performed about 1,500 physical evaluations for the school year. The doctor conducted physical exams on students entering school as kindergarten children, in grades one, four, seven, and ten, for students in high school that participated in the athletic programs, and newly arrived children at the BPS. They conducted assessments of the children selected for the 766 programs (special needs), including the required physical, psychological, and neurological sections of those examinations. Independent contractors charged $300, but the school physician did not charge for this.[429]

The panel asked a question about why parochial schools don't often call for 766 evaluation exams. Dr. Fischer answered, "I believe I am correct when I say that it being a private school, very often private schools don't get involved in 766. If they have a problem child, either physical or moral or mental or anything, that child usually winds up in public school anyway. They don't keep them."[430]

He continued to explain just what the school physician does. Children who have not received the required inoculations are immunized. They check on children with disabilities every year. However, they don't treat or prescribe medications

---

428   School Doctor's Inquiry. P. 27. *Boston Public Schools Health Services Collection*, Box 2.

429   School Doctor's Inquiry. P. 24. *Boston Public Schools Health Services Collection*, Box 2.

430   School Doctor's Inquiry. P. 26. *Boston Public Schools Health Services Collection*, Box 2.

for them, but they advise parents on what to do. Doctors generally discover these conditions in the first year or two of school. School physicians have seen students with the following deficiencies: about 100 with circulatory disorders, 280 with intestinal disorders, gastrointestinal disorders consisting of ulcers and colitis, and kidney diseases; 105 cases of cerebral palsy; 153 cases of Grand Mal epilepsy, hyperactivity, paralysis; Petit Mal epilepsy 134 cases, and 1,009 cases of asthma.[431]

Additionally, they continuously looked out for infectious diseases during sick call and were responsible for keeping their eye open for anything unsanitary in the school cafeterias. Furthermore, they identified child abuse, drug use, and malingering students, to name a few. They advised the nurse and the principal regarding ill children attending school.[432] Other questions arose concerning the length of time a doctor spent in the school, about a half-hour, and the time spent performing physical exams, about two hours. At times, the school nurse was not there to assist because many visited two to four schools.

Now the BSC requested to interview other physicians who came to the hearing. In the beginning, 17 or 18 doctors arrived at the meeting, but at that late hour, only five remained. They called upon Dr. Marcus W. Berman, MD, about the follow up of students with a deformity such as a systolic murmur, a heart condition. In that case, he reported, the doctor wants a further evaluation of the child, sends a note home, and looks for a return letter.[433] "As to whether the nurse keeps a file on it, I am not quite certain, but I have asked in the past, and the nurse tells me she is having difficulty." The school nurse phones the house and will make a home visit to encourage the parent to follow-up, he related. A parent or guardian will take the child to the clinic; however, "we have had very, very poor response from parents or guardians."[434]

The hearing turned to the subject of school clinics. At the time of the inquiry, two clinics operated, one at the Quincy (one of Annie McKay's schools) and the other at Blackstone School, and both had health centers attached to the schools. Dr. Fischer related he visited both clinics and asked the physicians there to take over the care of

---

431   School Doctor's Inquiry. P. 32. *Boston Public Schools Health Services Collection*, Box 2.

432   School Doctor's Inquiry. P. 29. *Boston Public Schools Health Services Collection*, Box 2.

433   School Doctor's Inquiry. P. 94. *Boston Public Schools Health Services Collection*, Box 2.

434   School Doctor's Inquiry. P. 99. *Boston Public Schools Health Services Collection*, Box 2.

the children in those schools. As soon as the clinic physicians heard they would receive the going rate of $35.00 a day for school doctors, they refused. If these children walked through the doors to their clinic, they would see them. Then, they would charge at least $10-12 for each inspection, physical examination, and immunization calling them third-party payments. By the end of the year, that added up to a large sum of money. Dr. Fischer stated, in his opinion, the cost was prohibitive for the city.[435]

Now the genie was out of the bottle. The latest buzzword was third-party payments; a word guaranteed to spark conversation and fuel emotion. Third-party payments and reimbursements to schools for health services provided in schools would possibly finance school physicians and school nurses. These additional dollars would solve this dilemma. The BSC noted welfare families comprised 40 percent of the school children attending the BPS. They posed a hypothetical question stating if these same indigent children went to Health and Hospitals and received similar services like those provided by Boston school physicians, would Health and Hospitals receive reimbursement through Medicaid by a state or federal agency? Dr. Fischer answered, "Yes, I think they could." However, Dr. Fischer replied, "They (the BSC) do not have that right."

School Committee members and Dr. Fischer then bantered over a memo he sent to the BSC a few years back where he did make mention of a possibility of third-party payout, but they took no further action. School Committee members voiced how they knew they should be paying more money to the school physicians.

At that time in 1976, Boston employed 50 school physicians for 161 schools, though all schools did not receive coverage. Dr. Fischer reported 10 or 15 small schools received no services. He revealed the budget did not allow him to hire anyone. In any case, if a principal requested a doctor, he would find someone to go out.

If we could be in that hearing room, I think we would hear a collective sigh as BSC members again questioned if they abolished the school physician position, would the children ever return to receiving reasonable medical care? They contemplated if their actions eroded the rights of children. For the time, 1976, they were doing a fair job. Collectively, they in all likelihood looked at each other, and another member, Miss Sullivan, said what they all thought.

---

435   School Doctor's Inquiry. P. 47. *Boston Public Schools Health Services Collection*, Box 2.

"Is this Committee going to have the dubious distinction of being the first city in the country of taking away the doctor from the children? Is it really enough to say: Let the mayor (Mayor White) handle it?... because he's the one who is pressuring us?"[436]

I wonder if the BSC was conversant about the school physician's history. To recapitulate, in the United States, Boston first led the way in 1894 to improve the health care for school children by implementing the medical inspection of students in schools using physicians. Now, in 1976, some 82 years later, school doctors teetered on the chopping block.

School Committee Member, Mrs. Palladino, expressed her opposition to any reduction that would directly affect kids in school and agreed if it were not for the school doctors, many of the children would never see a physician. She continued that the school system contained a poor population where the parents at times did not follow-up on notes sent home by the school nurse. Frequently, the notes requested the parent to take the child to a doctor because he/she failed a vision or hearing test. For this reason, she would not vote for a budget reduction. "Our kids get very little at this point, and if you don't have a healthy body, you can't have a healthy mind."[437]

Consequently, they summed up by saying they postponed their decision until the end of the school year. In the ensuing time, they planned to study and give careful consideration to other alternatives in the best interest of children.

Despite making their decision, other members of the audience still waited to testify, hoping to influence them further. Edward J. Doherty, representing the Boston Teachers Union, stepped forward, giving evidence to retain school physicians.[438] Mr. Doherty outlined the numerous reasons school physicians were essential to the school health program. They performed school physicals for the child who does not have a private doctor. The 766-assessment process for children (special needs), and the competitive sports programs required a physical exam. Schools were given a window of 30 days to complete the 766 process, and hospitals and

---

[436] School Doctor's Inquiry. P. 112. *Boston Public Schools Health Services Collection*, Box 2.

[437] School Doctor's Inquiry. P. 114. *Boston Public Schools Health Services Collection*, Box 2.

[438] School Doctor's Inquiry. P. 116. *Boston Public Schools Health Services Collection*, Box 2.

clinics frequently were not able to offer appointments within that period. Without the school doctor performing the necessary review, many of these students would not be able to participate in the sports program. It would affect the immunization program because the school nurse administers immunization under the supervision of a school physician.[439]

Following Mr. Doherty's remarks, he introduced a group of Boston Teachers Union members that studied the issue of third-party payments. They called themselves the 766 Task Force. This group articulated that since the 766 statutes became law in 1974, mandating the schools to provide a service, like a physical evaluation, it should have included the school's eligibility to develop into a Medicaid provider. They asked if the service was reimbursable, could the school receive the reimbursement or even apply for it? During the discussion, the BSC decided the Boston Schools would contact the Secretary for Administration and Finance and request a ruling on whether the Boston School Department could submit an application and receive a medical provider number. At last, they concluded to postpone their decision about the termination of the school physicians until June 30, 1977.[440] The doctors received a second chance.

Consider for a moment remarks made in a Carnegie Corporation Report, Turning Points, 1989. "School systems are not responsible for meeting every need of their students. But where the need directly affects learning, the school must meet the challenge. So, it is with health." Would the Boston Public Schools comply with these guidelines?

Medicaid Reimbursement

Reimbursement of school-based health care directly to schools developed into an immense challenge that remains unresolved in 2020. However, different people see an event in different ways. As noted in earlier chapters, in 1965, lawmakers passed Title XIX of the Social Security Act giving birth to Medicaid, a federal medical assistance program to benefit the poor. Basically, within some federal guidelines, the plan reimburses health care providers for services rendered to the poor, so income is not a barrier to receiving health care. Amendments added in 1967 to Title

---

439   School Doctor's Inquiry. P. 116-118. *Boston Public Schools Health Services Collection*, Box 2.

440   School Doctor's Inquiry. P. 124-128. *Boston Public Schools Health Services Collection*, Box 2.

XIX authorized the Early Periodic Screening, Detection, and Treatment (EPSDT) to provide continuous health supervision for children covered by Medicaid. Under the program, benefits included a standard health test, immunization, well-child health supervision, and dental care services.[441]

By 1988, federal law amended the regulation to allow Medicaid payment for services provided to children under the Individual with Disabilities Education Act (IDEA).[442] The state Department of Welfare, now known as the Division of Medical Assistance, DMA, recognized school districts as Medicaid providers. Since 1994, Massachusetts has allowed school districts that became Medicaid providers to receive 50 percent federal reimbursement for qualified services provided to special needs students who receive Medicaid. The law required these students to be enrolled in special education programs, as prescribed by an Individualized Education Plan (IEP). This assistance was available to cities, towns, and regional school districts.

The main problem with this arrangement centers on the fact the reimbursement does not go to the schools directly, but for the most part, the city or town receives the payment. This arrangement will be further explored in an upcoming interview with K. Marie Clarke in Chapter 16.

School Nurse Meetings

The school nurses now met in a small conference room at the Boston Teachers Union at 180 Mt. Vernon Street, in Dorchester. The union hall's property overlooks Dorchester Bay. On a cold winter's day, the wind from the water whips you around and can freeze you on the spot. During 1974 the Union increased its presence with the school nurses. This relationship was warranted, as they were dues-paying members of the BTU.

The Boston Public School Nurses Association (BPSNA) reported they held no meetings because they were so busy between September 1974-May 1975, probably due to desegregation and forced busing. They managed to meet during the spring

---

441 Kort, M. (1984). The Delivery of Primary Health Care in American Public School, 1890-1980. *Journal of School Health*. 54(11) 456.

442 *American Speech-Language-Hearing Association Medicaid Toolkit*. Retrieved from https://www.asha.org/Practice/reimbursement/medicaid/Medicaid-Toolkit-Schools

and sent out a letter on April 9, 1974.[443] This letter requested support from State Representative Melvin P. King, social activist, for the nurse certification bill and to vote favorably for House Bill 1194.

The House bill deals with Section 53, 53A, and 53B of Chapter 71 of the General Laws and requests to insert the word "registered" before the word "nurses" wherever it occurs. The bill, petitioned by the Massachusetts Teachers Association, concerned the employment of registered nurses in the public schools. It required nurses working in public schools to be registered nurses as opposed to nurses and/or practical nurses. The school nurse certification bill remained in committee.

House Bill 1194 passed and became Chapter 0411 of the Acts of 1974. The bill did not apply to nurses currently employed by a town, city, or district. Therefore, this new law did not affect communities that hired practical nurses before this law became effective. Practical nurses' education generally covers one year and can be hired for a smaller salary than an RN. For the first time, a school nurse was required to be a licensed registered nurse. This law resulted in a major change to the previous law passed in 1921. See the image on the next page. Chapter 7 covers how the 1921 bill passed. I applaud the BPSNA's involvement and advocacy in 1974.

ACTS, 1974. — CHAPS. 411, 412.   283

Chap. 411. AN ACT RELATIVE TO THE EMPLOYMENT OF REGISTERED NURSES IN THE PUBLIC SCHOOLS.

Be it enacted, etc., as follows:

SECTION 1. The first sentence of section 53 of chapter 71 of the General Laws, as appearing in the Tercentenary Edition, is hereby amended by inserting after the word "and", in lines 2 and 9, in each instance, the word:— registered.

SECTION 2. The first sentence of section 53A of said chapter 71, as so appearing, is hereby amended by inserting after the word "school", in line 5, the word:— registered.

SECTION 2A. The second sentence of said section 53A of said chapter 71, as so appearing, is hereby amended by inserting after the word "or", in line 2, the word:— registered.

SECTION 3. Section 53B of said chapter 71, as so appearing, is hereby amended by inserting after the word "and", in line 3, the word:— registered.

SECTION 4. This act shall not apply to any person employed as a nurse by a school committee of a city, town or district prior to or on the effective date of this act.

Approved June 25, 1974.

---

443 Boston Public School Nurses Club Minutes: 4/9/1974

On the other hand, not holding meetings at any time emerged as a bad practice. How could they present a united front when they were not aware of what was happening with their colleagues? By May of 1975, the nurses' and teachers' contract went to arbitration. The union advised they accomplish all their nursing business through a faculty senate. They decided the faculty senate should meet monthly or whenever a problem arose.[444] Now one can see how the BPSNA evolved into a social organization, and the faculty senate developed into the group that appropriately addressed their business decisions. For instance, the BPSNA planned a demonstration of Elizabeth Arden's "Red Door" beauty products at their meeting.[445]

Subsequently, the BPSNA Executive Board sat down with their Chief Supervising Nurse, Miss McLaughlin, to discuss pertinent items of interest to the Boston Public School Nurses Association.[446] A list of the topics discussed included: 1) School Nurses Examination. They received information there would be no nurses' examination in 1975. The BSC reported they received a letter from the Department of Health and Hospitals requesting the postponement of the examination schedule, and the note listed their reasons. They referred to the letter as Item 3(a).

On more than one occasion, I searched for the phantom letter regarding the examination's suspension at Boston City Archives but was unable to locate the document. I wonder what the message contained. Were Boston City Hospital nurses required to take an exam? No record lists that as a requirement. As far back as December 2, 1964, the Director of School Health Services forwarded a letter to the Assistant Superintendent of Schools, Mr. John M. Canty, stating the difficulty in recent years in recruiting nurses to take the exam needed for the appointment. Also, they found it even more arduous to find substitute nurses. For these reasons, the Director requested permission to increase the daily wage of both substitute nurses and vision and hearing testers from $18 per day to $20 to match the usual going rate of hospitals.[447] Whether these observations entered into the decision to postpone the exam remains unclear.

---

444 *Boston Public School Nurses Club Minutes:* 11/16/1976

445 *Boston Public School Nurses Club Minutes:* 3/6/1978

446 Boston Public School Nurses Club Minutes: May 19, 1975

447 Letter: Dr. Gorman to Dr. Canty. December 2, 1964. *Boston Public Schools, Department of School Health Services Collection*, Box 1 07-079, Folder Associate Superintendents

In the meantime, the nurses directed letters to Dr. Gorman, the Boston School Committee (BSC), Superintendent Marion Fahey, and the Board of Examiners, urging the reinstatement of the examination. The Executive Board of the BPSNA sent a letter to the BSC recommending new school nurse applicants have a current Massachusetts license as a registered professional nurse, a BS Degree in Nursing with experience in public health nursing, or pediatrics, or have a School Nurse Practitioner, or Pediatric Nurse Practitioner Certificate.

Other topics discussed were: 2) Nurse attendance at workshops or conventions; 3) In-service Meetings; How often to have them, and should they have speakers? Would there be monthly Executive Board Meetings with the supervising nurse and how to relay this information to the BPSNA?; 4) Transfers: Miss McLaughlin would seek clarification from the Superintendent's office regarding seniority and assignment of nurses to districts. Because many schools closed due to desegregating the schools and forced busing, district communities might change.

They continued their discussion: 5) Immunizations; They suggested when nurses administer immunizations, the tray should have a vial of adrenalin, and a supervisor or backup nurse should be present. The group considered new guidelines for giving vaccines. Adrenalin was needed when and if a patient developed an allergic reaction called anaphylaxis. That is a severe allergic reaction that comes on rapidly and may cause death. Epinephrine (adrenalin) is considered the drug of choice for treating anaphylaxis. Notice they did not mention Sabbatical leave during the meeting. From 1976 through 1977, they looked at their school nursing practices again and planned to incorporate these procedures and policies into a booklet for permanent reference.

K. Marie Clarke, at this time, was president of the Boston Home and School Association. Marie, both a Boston parent and a nurse, but did not work for the BPS. Early on, she demonstrated her leadership ability that plainly developed during the ensuing years. She proposed some negotiating items with the City, including "the number of nurses will be increased as of 9/1/1976 so that there will be at least one nurse for every 450 pupils; in no case will a nurse be assigned to cover more than two buildings." She wanted the BSC to provide a substitute for an absent nurse. Although the number of 450 pupils per nurse was unrealistic, it was an excellent negotiating item to start with and work on from there.

The Boston Public School Nurses Association (BPSNA) sent a letter to Union officials thanking them for obtaining justice for 14 provisional nurses unjustly fired on September 8, 1977. The BSC reinstated them.[448] Unfortunately, the *Minutes* don't reveal the reason for their firing. However, the BPS had a practice of sending out dismissal notices to all provisionals in June. That gave the BPS the option of rehiring them in September. On the other hand, the fired provisionals could collect unemployment during the summer months.

The negotiating teams reached a contract settlement that spanned the period of September 1, 1976 to August 31, 1978. The main thrust of the agreement consisted of job security, stating any teacher, or nurse, with tenure or permanently appointed should continue to be employed. Regarding staffing: No provision of the agreement required the School Committee to hire any particular number, or type of teachers, or other personnel. In other words, they were not going to fire anyone, but on the other hand, they were not going to hire anyone either.

Members of the Home and School Association met with a group of school nurses on 12/8/1978. They informed the nurses of a new rumored restructuring of School Health Services. The school nurses shared their concerns regarding the lack of a qualified medical director and the elimination of chief supervising nurses and nursing supervision. Home and School Association stated they stood 100 percent behind school nurses. They drafted a letter to School Superintendent Robert Woods, President David Finnegan of the Boston School Committee (BSC), and BSC members voicing their concern over the elimination of School Health Services and the possible transfer of nurses. The coverage period of the previous contract expired.[449]

In the meantime, the Nurse Faculty Senate addressed the BPSNA about these new rumors of the elimination of school nurses and possible transfer of School Health Services to local health centers.[450]

The Home and School Association followed up on their promises. Subsequently, they sent a letter to the Boston Public School Nurses Association (BPSNA) stating

---

448   Boston Public School Nurses Club Minutes: 9/10/1977

449   *Proceedings of the School Committee, City of Boston 1972*. Retrieved from https://archive.org/stream/preceedingsofschl1972bost#page154/mode2up/search/clarke

450   Boston Public School Nurses Club Minutes: 12/12/1978

they conferred with Boston School Committee President David Finnegan and Superintendent Robert Wood, receiving assurances they would not terminate school nurses. Also, the BSC planned to retain a professional medical person, i.e. pediatrician, to oversee school health services. Everyone agreed on the need for upgraded school health services. Also, the Home and School Association discussed the perception among many school nurses that school nurse caseloads were unequal. They recommended every high school and middle school has a full-time nurse, and no nurse has more than three elementary schools.[451]

The BPSNA promptly sent a thank you note to the Boston Home and School Association saying, "there are no greater voices than those of concerned parents and friends of our school children."[452]

Marguerite McLaughlin retired in January 1979, becoming the last supervising nurse for several years.

Ed Doherty, Executive Vice-President of the BTU, met with the Nurses Faculty Senate and informed them of the following: 1) Nurses are entitled to and should have substitute nurses if they are sick, starting on the first day of their illness; 2) Provisional nurses who have completed their third year of service will receive annual salary step raises; 3) The Faculty Senate should take a position on seniority for nurses for job security and transfer purposes.[453]

The BPSNA did meet and voted all permanently appointed nurses should supersede provisional nurses in seniority rights.[454] This situation comes into play when the administration places a new nurse in a vacant position to fill in for an absent nurse. If the "sick" nurse does not return, the new nurse would remain in that position until the end of the school year. At that time, administrators would post the job, and a permanent nurse could apply for that position. The principal has no other choice but to hire a permanent nurse.

---

451   *Boston Public School Nurses Club Minutes*: 12/21/1978

452   *Boston Public School Nurses Club Minutes*: 1/11/1979

453   *Boston Public School Nurses Club Minutes*: 10/16/1979

454   *Boston Public School Nurses Club Minutes*: 10/29/1979

The Boston school nurses survived another decade filled with challenges, successes, and failures that bound them together. The BTU's role expanded to include the school nurses in their deliberations, protecting them from an outside takeover. They advocated for the successful passage of a bill requiring registered nurses in public schools. The school doctor's situation remained uncertain. Despite their pleas, the appointment of a replacement-supervising nurse continued unheeded. There was no one at the helm. Like it or not, they were pursued by technology that advanced in leaps and bounds beyond the average person's understanding. The 1980s awaited them. They might take note of these words from tennis star Serena Williams who said, "At any age, I see the finish line. And when you see the finish line, you don't slow down. You speed up."[455]

---

455   *Vogue*. (2018, February). p 172.

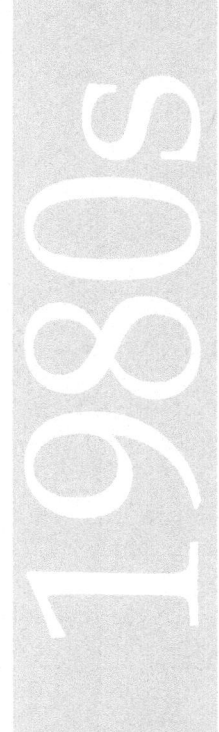

Twentieth Century Milestones Affecting School Nursing (Continued)

1980s - National League for Nursing (NLN) publishes a credential document and establishes recognized standards for all nursing professionals.

1980-1990 - Continued innovation in medical research/technology and specialization.

1980 - Postural Screening of school children required by law.

1981 - First HIV cases identified. Personal computers introduced.

1982 - National League of Nursing endorsed the baccalaureate degree in nursing as the minimum preparation into professional nursing practice.

1983 - First bill passed authorizing nurse practitioners to write prescriptions in long-term care facilities and for specific patients at home. This is the first time registered nurses are allowed to write prescriptions. Limited prescription writing authority is granted to midwives.

1983-1990 - Causes of HIV/AIDS identified, treatments defined.

1984 - First public use of the Internet.

1987 - American Academy of Pediatrics supports professionally prepared school nurses in schools.

Chapter 16

Boston Public School Nurses in the 1980s

Part I

Revered American poet Robert Frost wrote about a path he did not follow in "The Road Not Taken." He wrote, "Two roads diverged in a wood, and I-I took the one less traveled by."

Robert Frost's poem referred to decisions he contemplated when deciding which road to take. In comparison, on January 20, 1981, the school nurses developed a plan for School Physician Services. Boston, the first city in the nation to employ school physicians to implement the health supervision of school children in 1894, now contemplated dismissing their school doctors because of the high cost. They cost the city 1/10th of 1 percent of the school department's budget. A pittance. The school nurses program contained five possible paths for Superintendent Paul Kennedy to follow, as outlined below:[456]

1) Leave the school physicians as is, at no change in cost of $115,812

2) Use the process of attrition to gradually reduce the number of school physicians, and then go to services, like community health centers. Due to several unknowns, such as the number of retirements every year, or the termination date, at times, disruption of services might develop. No change in cost

---

[456] Boston Public School Nurses Club Minutes: January 20, 1981

3) Contract out minimal health services to community health centers following termination of school physicians, the same price. They would do sports physicals, Chapter 766 examinations, exams for excessive absences due to unexplained illness, emergency care, first aid, assist the school nurse, and assist in the formulation of health education program planning within the school. Same cost

4) Contract full health services to community health centers, cost to be determined. In addition to the services mentioned above, this would include the traditional physical examinations for students in Grades I, IV, VII, and X according to Section 57 of Chapter 71 of the General Laws of the State of Massachusetts

5) Contracting individual physicians to perform mandated duties

We all face crossroads, so many choices. A decision was imperative. The school nurses judged to support Option 5, contracting with individual physicians, who may or may not be current school physicians to do the necessary legally mandated tasks. Shortly after that, the Nurse Faculty Senate sent a letter to Superintendent Kennedy supporting Option 5, saying it consisted of the most cost-efficient, practical method of providing health services for students. They added they were anxious to assist, in any way including advisory, in finding a solution to the problem.[457] Therefore, the school nurses felt secure enough in their position to offer the Superintendent their advice.

This chapter will follow the Boston school nurses in the 1980s. We will watch them become more proactive than in previous years. With the assistance of the Boston Teachers Union, they fought for issues important to them, for example, a superior school health service for Boston Public School students and families. Most importantly, though Boston had no practical nurses on their staff, they fought the pressure from other municipalities to allow licensed practical nurses to administer medications in school. We will follow them as they advocated for a nurse supervisor, dealt with a job freeze, substitute nurse issues, equity in assignments, not to mention coping with children admitted to school without or incomplete immunization records, whether to employ nurse practitioners, and new computer technology. Along the way, they discovered new ways to advance their scope and practice and promote legislation towards this goal.

---

457 Boston Public School Nurses Club Minutes: January 27, 1981

Inside Boston Politics

For a moment, let us look at the city. Raymond Flynn succeeded Kevin White as Boston's Mayor in 1984. Boston's economy fluctuated with the nation's and the rest of New England. Starting from 1983, Governor Michael Dukakis presided over six years of Massachusetts' strong economic growth and prosperity called the "Massachusetts Miracle." Consequently, a recession followed this period in 1989. As a result, the recovery in the 1990s showed a structural change. Boston depended less on manufacturing and industrial jobs. Instead, the city relied on vocations in financial services, healthcare, education, and other professional and business service industries.[458] This change left the nurses in a strong position since they represented health care in the education system.

Other Developments

In the meantime, several developments continued to evolve. The Nurses Faculty Senate (NFS) reminded John J. McDonough, President of the Boston School Committee (BSC), in a letter that they had no nurse leader or Senior Nurse Coordinator since January 1979, when Marguerite McLaughlin retired. The note summarized their situation by emphasizing the staff nurses had no one to go to for direction, advice, or counsel: "Directives from administrators have been ambiguous, inconsistent, and at times non-existent, which leads to fragmented services or duplication of efforts."[459]

On a similar note, Roma L. Vangel, Chairperson of the Nurses Faculty Senate (NFS) sent a letter to the BSC in May 1980, of course on BTU stationery, reminding them they have not appointed any new school nurses since October 1975, due to the suspension of a qualifying examination after December 1972. That means Boston did not employ any new nurses for five years. Despite the Massachusetts Miracle, at their meeting on 12/18/1980, the NFS revealed the hiring freeze adopted by the city affected the selection of a nurse supervisor.

---

458 Lewis, G., Avault, J., & Vrabel, J. (1999). History of Boston's Economy Growth and Transition 1970-1998. Retrieved from http://www.bostonplans.org/getattachment/ea39b8db-1a8e-49b4-ab1c-94832c84c56d/

459 Boston Public School Nurses Club Minutes: February 12, 1980

Issues

Over the next few months, the school nurses continued to address the earlier noted broad workforce issues, such as substitute nurse coverage, transfer policy, and the discrepancy of school hours in nurses' assignments. Additionally, their concerns embraced the District V School Health Plan, the certification of school nurses through the Department of Education, and the nurse practitioner program. Other problems concerning them included analgesics given in school, ordering first aid supplies, House Bill 4250 (School nurse reimbursement for services), the orientation of new nurses, and the job search for a new director of nurses to start July 1981. All qualified nurses were encouraged to apply for this position.[460] The problem of students admitted to school without properly documented immunizations persisted.

Several of these issues deserve further explanation. At the time, Northeastern University offered an eight-week pediatric nurse practitioner course from July 1982 to September 1982, followed by a year of preceptorship with several weekend workshops adding another eight weeks. The program costs $500 per semester, totaling $1,500. Indeed, a bargain. However, the role nurse practitioners would play within School Health Services remained unclear. Would the school department employ them, or would they be employed by a community health center that managed a school clinic? If a nurse practitioner worked in the school, would they additionally need a school nurse? School nurses reviewed these various scenarios over the next few years, looking for equitable solutions. Dr. Gorman's discussion of this issue is reviewed in Chapter 15.

Pertaining to analgesics given in school by the school nurse, they agreed a 3" by 5" card would serve the purpose, and to update the information on it annually. This card contained the parent's permission to give an analgesic in school. Was it the actual permission slip with the parent's dated signature? That is unclear, as was the existence of "standing orders." For a nurse, a "standing order" is a prewritten medication or treatment order and specific instructions from a licensed medical practitioner to administer a medication or treatment order in clearly defined circumstances. They are often based on national clinical guidelines and customized to specific populations.[461]

---

460   Boston Public School Nurses Club Minutes: February 24, March 3, 12, 1980

461   UCSF Center for Excellence in Primary Care Standing Orders. Retrieved from https://cepc.ucsf.edu/standing-orders

The school department's doctor in charge did not have MD after her name but a Ph.D., Dr. Audrey Fisher, Ph.D., Senior Advisor, Community and City-Wide Health Services. Union regulations required the nurses to meet with her once a month. How could the school nurses give an analgesic without an updated standing order from an MD? Subsequently, the school nurses and administration developed higher quality protocols and a procedure manual.

Nurses having an assignment with both early and late start schools arose as another issue. Schools started at a variety of different times, beginning from 7:25 AM to 9:00 AM. Their day finished from 2:00 PM to 3:00 PM. Frequently, they arranged these timetables to accommodate bus schedules. However, what resulted were schools left uncovered at the beginning or end of the day. In an emergency, the school would call another nurse in the district who would, of course, have her own schools to cover. If that nurse was unable to respond, the school would call 911 if needed. The Nurse Faculty Senate (NFS) urged school nurses with these assignments to write Dr. Audrey Fisher explaining their situation. Dr. Fisher stated she would attempt to make adjustments for the following year.[462] They needed someone more in touch with their work environment.

One year later, the NFS discussed this again, saying no policy existed for school nurses covering for one another. Weighed down with excessive assignments, and school coverage issues, the Boston school nurses tried another gutsy tactic. On January 27, 1981, they requested the BTU attorneys respond to the following questions:

1) Is the School Department required to provide reasonable school assignments and nurse/pupil ratios to allow the completion of the legally mandated procedures as first aid, student inspections, immunization survey-immunizing-related tasks, vision and hearing testing, physical examinations which include obtaining consents, scheduling, and assisting; core evaluations comprising attending, interpreting medical data, and sociological assessment as required; weighing and measuring, "paperwork" related to all above tasks, parental contacts, referrals, and follow-up as needed?

2) Is the School Department required to provide continuous coverage during school hours?

---

462 Boston Public School Nurses Club Minutes: March 18, 1980

a) Currently, schools are in "limbo" when: the assigned nurse is absent, administration does not provide a substitute, and another nurse called the "back up" is called in an emergency. It is not unknown to have the assigned nurse and the "back up" nurse absent simultaneously, leaving two school assignments (2-8 schools) without nursing coverage.
b) A disparity exists in the opening/closing times of schools in the same job, leaving either am starting or pm closing time when a particular school(s) is/are uncovered.
c) "Back-up" nurse's assigned schools have different hours than schools she is "back up" for duplicating or compounding the problem (b). In c, the variations may be 15 minutes to one hour, 15 minutes.

3) How should the NFS proceed to:
   a) Prevent the burden of liability from falling on the school nurse when tasks are unfinished due to excessive caseload.
   b) Secure equitable manageable assignments.
   c) Safeguard continuous coverage for all schools.

The Union responded to this query by sending a letter to the Boston School Committee (BSC) on 5/7/1981, informing them the insufficient number of school nurses employed has resulted in and continued to result in inadequate school coverage and at times, no coverage during school hours. They requested the BSC review the matter and employ sufficient nurses to comply with standards of the Massachusetts School Nurse Organization of 600 pupils to 1 nurse, rather than the approximate 1,000 to 1, which was in effect in the Boston schools. Also, the Union advised them to complete this before a tragedy occurred, possibly followed by parental litigation.

The BSC approved the orientation of new nurses and planned to begin in September 1981. Therefore, counter prevailing forces again interrupted the plan because no orientation existed when I started working in School Health Services in 1986.

Legislation

House Bill 4250, 1981, pending in the legislature, permitted a licensed registered nurse performing procedures such as immunizations, hearing tests, and first aid in a school the ability to file for third-party payments from sources like Blue Cross, Blue Shield, if health care providers considered such procedures and treatments reimbursable when performed by other licensed personnel in different settings. If passed, the money collected via reimbursement could provide funding to employ school nurses. Sadly, the bill did not pass.

House Bill 250, 1980, referred to the certification of school nurses. A groundbreaking advancement occurred in 1997, when a similar bill finally passed, Chapter 0220, Chapter 71, Section 92. This bill allows a school nurse employed by a school district to apply for a standard certificate as a school nurse.[463] This bill elevated the school nurse to the same level as a schoolteacher.

A Conversation with Dr. Lamb

The issue of the school health program was of particular importance to school nurses concerned about its future. The Nurses Faculty Senate (NFS) invited Dr. George Lamb, MD, Director of Parent and Child Services, Boston City Hospital, May 6, 1980, to their meeting to discuss the future of the school health program. Dr. Lamb formed the School Health Advisory Committee to give him advice related to his role as Chief Medical Consultant to the Superintendent and the Boston School Committee. He offered insightful responses to questions posed by the NFS.

In his opinion, the school health program leadership needed a person or persons with management skills more than medical or nursing expertise. Dr. Lamb preferred district management of the health program rather than central control. He suggested some management techniques in the form of team nursing within districts with cross-supervising by nurses, linkage of district areas with schools of nursing for supervision of the health program, nurse or doctor as part-time consultants for each region in the management of the health program, and establishment of protocols with the schools (i.e.-positive strep throat treatment, analgesic management). In addition, he would place more emphasis on health education, health counseling, and preventive medicine in the health program. For instance, examples of team nursing within the district would have Allston supervising Allston, and Roxbury supervising Roxbury.

Dr. Lamb had other suggestions for the Nurses Faculty Senate (NFS) to deliberate regarding the management of the Boston School Health Program: Look for and contact successful school health programs in the U.S., write up plans on how to implement the school health program at the district level, consider trying a pilot program, and

---

463 Massachusetts General Laws. Retrieved from http://archives.lib.state.ma.us/actsResolves/1993

think about involving a consultant with experience in public health and management in the establishment of a school health program. On leaving, he conveyed if the NFS presented a plan he considered viable, he would endorse it before they brought the project to the administration and the Boston School Committee.[464]

As you know, we were not there, but the nurses must have pondered his suggestions and proposals, wondering how relevant they were, and how to grow amidst the constant flux of change. But Dr. Lamb's recommendations were not to be taken lightly nor dismissed. He held an influential position. Don't be surprised if we hear from him again.

Meeting with Superintendent

Marie Clarke, the former chairperson of the Home and School Association, joined the Boston Public Schools Health Services as a school nurse in 1978, and was elected chairperson of the Nurse Faculty Senate in 1981. Both Clarke and another nurse, Roma Vangel, met with Acting Superintendent Joseph M. McDonough in 1981. They requested the school department seek external foundation funding to provide certification in physical assessment/nurse practitioner status for a specific number of BPS nurses annually. McDonough endorsed this idea and directed John Diggins, Senior Advisor in Student Support Services, to work with nurses to develop a proposal for funding.

On the other hand, McDonough adamantly denied a request for more nurses, though he made a firm commitment to recommend 75 nurses for 1981-1982. Regarding hiring a nursing supervisor, he said, "Tell me how to do it. Shall I eliminate one or two nurses to fund a nurse supervisor?" He emphatically repeated the BPS had no additional money to hire a supervisor. Despite Dr. Lamb's opinion, in contrast, they emphasized only a competent administrator with medical knowledge would meet their requirements.

The budget for 1980-81 funded $5,000 for Dr. Lamb as the medical advisor. Superintendent McDonough expressed surprise when told Dr. Lamb would be away for three months with the World Health Organization. They desperately needed someone for the entire year. Subsequently, Dr. Michael Grady, MD, replaced Dr.

---

464   Boston Public School Nurses Club Minutes: April 14, 1980

Lamb as medical coordinator in February 1982.[465]

Contracted Medical Services

By September 1981, the Superintendent and the Boston School Committee (BSC) decided to partner with neighborhood health centers to resolve the school physician dilemma. We don't know how the school physicians received their dismissal information. Back in 1976, the BSC called Assistant Director of School Physicians, Dr. Fischer, to testify first at the school physician inquiry. We can imagine how Dr. Fischer felt as he walked away from the students and the job he loved after 33 years of dedicated service. If only we had the opportunity to wish him well.

A key aspect of the new plan consisted of enlisting school nurses as area chairpersons for each of the nine school districts. The school nurses agreed they should support and promote a primary health care center for all students as the optimum goal. After discussing ways of improving existing school health services, they suggested the following:[466]

- The urgent need for a Nurse Director/Coordinator/Coordinators,
- Uniformity of procedures,
- Orientation for nurses hired within the past five years,
- Upgrading of existing school health rooms,
- Implementation of scoliosis screening (postural screening),
- Assignment equity:
  - 800 pupils/nurse Elementary level,
  - 600 pupils/nurse Middle level,
  - 1,000 pupils/nurse High School level,
- The development of a nurse-assessor form for use at 766 full core conferences (special education),
- Improvement of In-service Education Programs

The contract for medical services outlined the school department's expectations of the city's 22 community health centers and nine major hospital programs concerning their roles in providing school health services. In short, they must have

---

465   Boston Public School Nurses Club Minutes: 6/18/1981, 2/24/1982

466   Boston Public School Nurses Club Minutes: 10/22/1981

the ability to collect and bill from Medicaid and private insurers, work with school staff, and perform physicals with the assistance of a Boston public school nurse. The physical examination must include a hematocrit (blood test), urine analysis, and T.B. (tuberculosis) test. They need to perform routine physicals for any student referred by the school nurse for the following reasons: new "enterers," as school nurses refer to new admissions to the school, excessive absences, suspected health-related problems, return to school after an illness, any suspected handicapping condition, sports physicals, working paper certificate physicals, and 766 examinations for core conferences (special education). Also, when requested, they should provide emergency medical services, and when asked, provide consultation with the school nurse. See the following image - Parental Request Form.[467]

---

467 Boston Public School Nurses Club Minutes

Concerning billing, the BPS required community health centers to present to the school department the number of students seen, for what reason, and the billing category for each visit, whether under Medicaid, a private insurer, or Boston Health Plan. Further options open to school districts included the health provider supplying materials needed for collecting urine and blood samples.

School nurses should not involve themselves with collecting any third- party payments, i.e., social security numbers, Blue Cross-Blue Shield numbers, Medicaid numbers, and place of employment for the clinics.[468]

Staff Reductions

As so often occurred in previous years, once again, a budget crisis loomed on the horizon. On the advice of Superintendent Robert R. Spillane, the Boston School Committee reduced Assistant Supervising Nurse Shirley Erickson to Group I on the Salary Scale. They then reassigned her to school nurse rank on June 8th, 1982.[469] She was the last assistant supervising nurse. We met Shirley in Chapter 14, where she described her nursing career and family. Due to these budget cuts, after serving as an assistant supervising nurse for six years, the BSC appointed her to the nurse position at West Roxbury High School. Endings can be new beginnings. Shirley served West Roxbury High School for another ten years.

At the same time, the Superintendent additionally recommended both teacher layoffs and a list of administrators that included demotions, reassignments, and terminations.

Incomplete Immunizations

The Nurses Faculty Senate (NFS) made a bold decision during their meeting on January 3, 1983 when they convinced the BTU to file a grievance on behalf of the NFS because of students' incomplete immunizations, in violation of the State Statute, Chapter 76, Section 15 of the General Laws of Massachusetts. Students remained in school regardless of immunization requirements. When students changed schools, their health records did not always arrive at their new school. The wording of

---

468 Boston Public School Nurses Club Minutes: 1/11/1982

469 Proceedings of the School Committee, City of Boston 1982. P. 139. City of Boston Archives.

the grievance recommended informing parents of immunization requirements, requiring immunization records upon admission to a school, and enforcement of the exclusion policy when students did not provide immunization records. Additionally, the grievance proposed adding funding to develop a computerized record management system established in cooperation with the NFS, similar to ones piloted at the Jackson Mann Elementary, Lewenberg Middle, and Roxbury High School during the 1980-1981 school year.

The NFS strongly suggested all nurses keep an up to date list of students without records or immunizations, and to document their efforts to bring these students into compliance (i.e., note home with date, conference with parent and date, meeting with principal and date, action taken, etc.). They requested that nurses send to the NFS the number of students without records and the number of students needing one or more immunizations.

Waivers

School Health Services applied for and received waivers from the Massachusetts Department of Health for the school years 1981-1982, and 1982-1983 eliminating the need for a physical exam, except for referrals, new admissions, handicapped cases, 766 (special education) cases, and sports. The waiver added the following nursing duties:

- Graphing all students' height and weight,
- Health history and BP (blood pressure) for grades 1, 4, 7, and 10,
- Postural screening grades 5 – 9,
- Vision & hearing screening 1, 4, 7, 9, and 10.

Dr. Grady, Director of School Health Services, wanted the nurses' input regarding the waivers. In all probability, they received the exemption due to the nurses' large caseload and lack of physicians during the transition period. The Nurses Faculty Senate (NFS) objected in 1983 to School Health Services receiving a waiver requiring physical assessments in grades 4, 7, and 10. The school nurses felt the need for closely monitoring the health and safety of their students.

Other Points at Issue in 1983

During their meeting on 1/12/1983, the nurses pointed out their lack of supplies. They made plans for their February in-service meeting where they were to adjourn to groups by school level to exchange ideas and mutual concerns and submit nominations for Team Leaders.

Melanie Barron, Director of the new School-Based Management Project, sent a disturbing letter to all headmasters and principals on February 4, 1983, advising them how to develop alternative delivery strategies within their budgets, which they were to decrease by ten percent. The School-Based Management Project Director suggested they could accomplish nursing services in other ways than the existing system. They proposed clerical personnel or parents could maintain health records, and a community health agency could monitor student's health problems. She requested principals and headmasters to submit all of their cost comparisons and a timeline for their implementation. Their responses should include the reassignment of existing personnel, scheduling of training for volunteers, and the names of outside agencies they considered to replace existing staff.

This proposal was the coup de grâce - another threatened job loss. Surely, it must have created stress both individually and collectively as a group. Perhaps they made a vow this would never happen to them again. Will they draw a line in the sand? We are more committed to some vows than others. Let us continue to follow them as they respond to the latest threat.

K. Marie Clarke, Chairperson of the NFS, responded quickly to this latest threat to their existence. They reached out across the gaps that divided them from the administration to begin a dialogue. The NFS sent a copy of the letter to all Boston school nurses, strongly suggesting they meet with their principals and community superintendents. They should point out, optimistically, what their caseloads were, their mandated duties and responsibilities, and the many jobs not known or understood that nurses perform.

The school nurses' approach to this pending job loss involved requesting meetings with Melanie Barron, Director of the new School Based Management Project, and Rosemary Rosen, regarding their letter proposing alternative health delivery strategies. Also, the nurses sent a letter on March 25, 1983, to Ms. Rita Walsh Tomasini, Chairperson of the Boston School Committee's Budget Committee. In the letter, K. Marie Clarke called the termination of any Boston public school nurses an unsound, unrealistic proposal. She stated that 32 of 75 nurses carried caseloads exceeding a manageable level (800 to more than 1,200 students in one to three buildings). The letter included an outline of legal requirements and nurses' obligations, pointing out due to the excessive caseload and their increasing duties, this "frequently prohibits the completion of the legally mandated procedures."[470] See the images on the following page. The suggested reduction in nursing staff would render the state mandate screenings an impossible task. Also, she added the school nurses now had a plan to present to the Boston School Committee and Rosemary Rosen that would improve health services and reduce costs.

> **POSITION PAPER - BOSTON SCHOOL NURSES FACULTY SENATE**
>
> In order to understand more fully the extent of the health services that are rendered by the Boston School Nurses, it is necessary to consider the present day environment of both the schools and of society as a whole. The nurse's role has become more important and involved for many reasons:
>
> 1. Increase in number of children from unstable family backgrounds.
> 2. Children from homes where alchohol and drug abuse exists.
> 3. New enterers from outside cities, states and countries.
> 4. Non-English speaking children.
> 5. Early sexual activity resulting in pregnancy and/or venereal disease.
>
> Some of the procedures that the Boston School Department is legally mandated to provide (Chapter 233, Sec. 75), and performed by nurses are:
>
> 1. Physical examinations for new enterers, K1, 2 or Grade 1, Grades 4, 7, 10 with follow up of defects/abnormalities.
> 2. Immunization surveys, immunizations, and immunization-related tasks - consents, records, etc.
> 3. Annual vision and hearing screenings, with referral and follow up.
> 4. Identification, documentation and reporting of the neglected and abused child.
> 5. CORE Evaulations - attending, interpreting medical data, sociological assessments as required.
> 6. Emergency health care, first aid and related tasks
> 7. Weighing and measuring
> 8. Screening programs for early detection of communicable diseases such as pediculosis, tuberculosis, ringworm, impetigo, etc.
> 9. Administration of prescribed medication with parental consent.
> 10. Early Childhood screenings.
>
> In addition to the above mandated duties, the school nurse also acts as:
>
> 1. Health Educator
> 2. Resource person to the staff, students and parents
> 3. Medical liaison for school, home, and social agencies
> 4. Confidante and advisor to student on many family, personal problems
> 5. Coordinator for other valuable programs such as scoliosis and lead screenings, dental inspections.
> 6. Advisor for modifications to educational programs for health reasons.

Continued on the next page

---

[470] Boston School Nurses Position Paper - Boston Public School Nurses Club Minutes

> -2-
>
> 7. Make home visits
>
> 8. Assess and evaluate the nursing needs of children who are multi-handicapped, and require special services. These would include children with colostomies, amputations, prosthesis, seizure disorder, diabetes, problems of incontinence.
>
> The health of a school age child has a vital impact on his educational program. The current educational philosophy is that all children be mainstreamed into the regular classroom whenever possible. Therefore, many more children with physical handicaps are now present in our schools, and this necessitates the supervision of their medical needs by a qualified registered nurse.
>
> The school nurse is an integral part of the educational team. Her responsibility is to the child and the school department; she has no conflict of interest. The School Department should not have personnel working in the schools who are not subject to school department accountability. The school nurse is the most logical and desirable professional to assume the responsibility for coordinating the health care of the students. The most economical way to provide these mandated health services is the maintenance and improvement of the current School Health Services.

In the meantime, during the spring Nurse Faculty Senate (NFS) meetings, they discussed the evaluation criteria for nurses and the development of a nurse questionnaire. The nurses and Dr. Grady met with the city's public relations personnel to publicize immunization requirements. They advised headmasters and principals to appraise school nurses only on their administrative skills, for example, does the nurse arrive at her assignment on time, and not on her nursing proficiency.

The NFS asked nurses to return the newly developed eight-page questionnaire giving their best estimate of the kind of problems they dealt with by May 2, 1983. For the first time, the Nurse Faculty Senate (NFS) planned to compile statistics indicating the types of issues encountered by school nurses. Hopefully, the questionnaire would demonstrate the frequency, age group(s), and what action they took to resolve the problems identified by the survey. They said every nurse needed to respond to this survey so they could compile study data demonstrating the outcomes impacted by school nurse interventions.[471]

Dr. Lamb's Follow up Critique

In 1983 Superintendent Robert R. Spillane requested the opinion of Dr. Lamb, Director of the Department of Health and Hospitals, regarding the status of Boston's School

---

471 Boston Public School Nurses Club Minutes: 4/13/1983, 5/2/1983, 5/11/1983

Health Services and what was needed. Dr. Lamb responded by sending a three-page letter on August 26, 1983. He pointed out the school health program held no document that included its goals, objectives, and policies. "Further," he explained, "there are about 65-70 school nurses of variable quality interpreting and providing school health in various ways without professional supervision and without consistent, quality on-going education." They did not establish any professional supervision or evaluation of the contracts for medical services. He continued, referring to "haphazard" school health records," which were not in compliance with state immunization regulations. An essential component of the health screenings consisted of the follow-up of the positives discovered in the screening programs. Still, Dr. Lamb said he was unsure if they did sufficient monitoring. His suggestions to improve the school health service included the following:

- Need for school health administrator,
- Need for professional guidance and supervision,
- Development of policy and procedure manual,
- Improvement of forms,
- Improvement of data collection and analysis,
- Standardization and improvement of emergency care,
- Review and modernization of health education and education about health,
- Development of a health advisory council or revitalization of the Boston Child Health Task Force,
- Improvement of in-service programs for health professionals,
- Attention to safety in schools-around asbestos, air, playgrounds, etc.
- Plan for use or non-use of nurse practitioners in schools,
- Method to evaluate services in future,
- A decision regarding contractual possibilities for the school health program,
- Allocation of resources.

Dr. Lamb hoped his overview was helpful and would move them forward. He conducted a thorough review.[472]

At their November 30, 1983 meeting the NFS discussed Dr. Lamb's letter. Was it a wakeup call? We don't know what they said, but K. Marie Clarke expressed, "We are all busy and have family responsibilities: We all must take some responsibility

---

472   Department of Health and Hospitals Letter, Boston Public School Nurses Club Minutes: 8/26/1983

for furthering our profession." She asked them to serve on the Nurses Faculty Senate and for more nurses to attend meetings as was so often requested in the past.

They did step up to meet these challenges. Joan Sheehy volunteered to be the editor of a newsletter. They found a physical assessment course costing $272, and films "Am I Normal" and "Dear Diary" were available for nurses to use in sex education classes. The NFS encouraged nurses to support each other in the absence of a nursing supervisor/coordinator, and each of the nine districts should meet as a group to discuss their mutual concerns.

I can't help but wonder if the school nurses recalled the suggestions Dr. Lamb offered at their meeting with him in 1980, three years before. Looking back, he acknowledged their need for supervision, but he believed that person only needed management skills, not a nursing or medical background. Who would oversee their nursing expertise?

Since the Superintendent deleted the assistant nursing supervisors in 1982, no management personnel existed to represent the nurses. Medical Director, Dr. Grady, worked only part time for School Health Services. Team nursing with cross supervising by other staff nurses had no power, no authority to bring someone up to standards. Approaching schools of nursing for the supervision of the health program would give authority to an outside agency that had no connection with the city schools. Collaboration with schools of nursing, offering their student nurses public health and community health experience was a positive move. Dr. Lamb's other suggestion of involving a consultant with expertise in public health and management establishing a school health program seemed redundant because he took on that role.

Nonetheless, the NFS recognized their need for stronger protocols and uniform documents used by all of the Boston school nurses. Unfortunately, the Boston Public School Nurses Club Minutes never mentions the eight-page questionnaire composed in the Spring of 1983 again nor the results. More than likely, only a few were returned, and not enough to offer possible solutions. At the same time, they should be given credit. They were on the right track because superintendents and school committees, whether located in urban or rural communities, respect numbers. Data collection paints a picture of what is happening. It provides evidence of the costs and benefits of school nursing programs and assists the administration in making decisions about the school health services. Collecting data proved to be crucial. However, that will come later.

All in all, 1983 proved to be a challenging year.

A decade later in 1993, under the direction of the Essential School Health Service grants, Boston School Health Services developed a program concerning team nursing and cluster leaders within districts. Anne Sheetz, the Director of School Health, Massachusetts Department of Public Health, established the Essential School Health Service grants available to school districts throughout the Commonwealth. The tobacco tax initially funded the grants. This plan strengthened the school health program's administrative infrastructure. It mandated having a school nurse leader, implemented a tobacco control and cessation program, linked the school health program with local health agencies, and developed a data collection system. As you can see, the new plan significantly complied with Dr. Lamb's suggestions and vision for an improved School Health Program.

1984

The year 1984 dawned, holding more promise when Dr. Grady arrived at their meeting, bearing good news. He informed the Nurses Faculty Senate (NFS) that the school budget now included a nurse supervisor. Though he warned them, in all likelihood, it would be cut, he encouraged them to seek support from the Boston School Committee.[473]

At their March meeting, the NFS filed a grievance for two issues: a medical contract evaluator and computerization of records. The school nurses considered the job description in the medical contract incomplete. Secondly, the Boston School Committee added computerization of health cards to their workload without allocating added time to accomplish it. By May, they accepted the School Department's settlement offer and started data processing immunization records.[474]

As the year progressed, Dr. Grady and members of the NFS met with Ken Caldwell, from Human Services, regarding the need for a nursing supervisor. Unfortunately, Ken Caldwell relayed they would not hire a nursing supervisor in the coming year due to a "no expansion policy."

---

473   Boston Public School Nurses Club Minutes: 2/8/1984

474   Boston Public School Nurses Club Minutes: 3/14/1984, 4/11/1984, 5/9/1984

During the new 1984-1985 school year, K. Marie Clarke, chairperson of the NFS from 9/1980 - 10/1984, relinquished the position to Carol Almeida, co-chaired with Mary Ellen Flynn Monahan. Clarke reviewed the problems the school nurses encountered, which included: computerization of medical records, medical supply problems, and lack of a nursing coordinator/supervisor. She encouraged nurses to become involved, support and assist the newly elected officers.[475]

After that, Marie became the Medical Contract Evaluator overlooking the contracts with health centers, with a desk at Boston Public School headquarters on Court Street. In this capacity, she sent a letter to Kenneth Caldwell, Senior Officer, Student Support Services, recounting the problems the school nurses confronted, and again, outlining the need for nursing supervisor/coordinator. Additionally, she reminded him of the decentralization and reorganization of the management structure that occurred in the late 1970s that eliminated the medical management personnel at the central level. This decentralization and reorganization removed an administrator to present and document the needs of school health services to other administrators, especially important when developing and justifying a budget.

Clarke continued although the law required vision and hearing screening, many nurses did not have this equipment, and therefore could not perform these screenings. New nurses did not receive any orientation or monitoring by a nursing supervisor. Record management developed many problems where each nurse had developed her system, style, and abbreviations for recording a student's medical information on the health card. Confusion existed among the nurses regarding where to note confidential information such as pregnancy, rape, and venereal disease. Besides, transferring health records was another area where school nurses practiced no uniform method and terminology.

Over the years, Clarke noted, nurses created their own medical forms, which they used to communicate with parents and health care providers. Instead, they should have standardized forms included in a policy manual. They could use these uniform documents to gather statistics, monitor health programs, and pinpoint areas that needed attention. She continued on for the need of a policy manual showing clear medical directives regarding the management of emergencies, medication administration, first-aid, and exclusion and readmission criteria. "Serving as a

---

475   Boston Public School Nurses Club Minutes: 11/8/1984

guide for nurses and others, the manual would clarify duties and responsibilities, foster accountability, and aid in the orientation of new nurses."

The end of the 1986 school year saw a Nurse Faculty Senate (NFS) meeting with guests Dr. Michael Grady, MD, John Diggins, and Ken Caldwell, Senior Officer, Student Support Services. Pauline Shanks and K. Marie Clarke requested more time to complete a Policy and Procedure Manual. The subject of the nurse supervising position surfaced again, and Ken Caldwell explained the salary levels for this position came under the domain of the Personnel Department.

At this meeting, they discussed another sensitive subject, the hiring of LPN's (Licensed Practical Nurse). The NFS vehemently opposed this because of the LPN's education and the added responsibility of an RN (Registered Nurse) supervising the LPN. An LPN's education required one year of classes at an approved school, whereas RN's needed at least two to three years of preparation at an approved school before they could sit for the registered nurse exam.

A discussion of contractual violations emerged regarding nurse practitioners replacing physicians in contracted schools. Dr. Grady planned to call Dr. Linda Grant and explain that nurse practitioners would not be allowed to work in schools because it violated the medical contracts.

At this point, we hope Kenneth Caldwell, Senior Officer, Student Support Services was more aware of the challenges the school nurses faced. Surely, he would listen to their concerns and commit to working on solutions. Let us take some time and make a private visit to K. Marie Clarke.

A Lobster Lunch with K. Marie Clarke

My GPS rejected her address. MapQuest lost me on the street in Dedham. K. Marie Clarke, RN, was not at her best giving directions. In other words, I found myself adrift on a rainy day in heavy traffic. A policeman working a construction site kindly redirected me, and I was on my way again. We were communicating by phone, and Marie was standing out in the rain in the parking lot, anticipating my arrival.

At last, we connected. Marie is an attractive woman of medium height with silver-gray hair. She lives in a convenient, senior citizen apartment complex. Later that day, her screened-in porch served as the backdrop for our pictures. After some time, Marie's white, fluffy cat settled down on the couch, indicating I passed her inspection.

The interview began by asking Marie how she first became involved with the Boston Public Schools. Marie explained she lived in West Roxbury. Because her children attended the Boston Public Schools (BPS), she became active with the City-Wide Parents Association. Consequently, she rose to become their President and, in that capacity, appeared before the Boston School Committee (BSC) many times on several education issues. During that time, Judge Garrity, who administered the BPS's desegregation plan, appointed her as a member of the Committee to Recommend Guidelines and Qualifications for the Position of Superintendent of Schools during February and March 1972.[476]

Marie paused for a moment before she talked about how she became an employee of the BPS.

"I was recruited … The school nurse at the Joyce Kilmer School, Annette Carol, went to the same nursing school as I did. She was a lovely woman, a good nurse. She encouraged me to put my name in. I finally did, and the next day I received a phone call."

"They needed a substitute nurse. I never expected to be called and was not that enthusiastic. My youngest child was in middle school in 1978, [but she accepted]. I had four schools, the Randall G. Morris School, Kilmer, Bates, and Beethoven Schools, all elementary schools in West Roxbury. It was an easy commute for me. When you are handling four schools, you cannot do a proper job."

Marie recalled her experiences with children and staff in the BPS.

"It was my first year on the job." The Morris School called her to see a

sick child. She said the principal was a lovely man and kept the child isolated while waiting for her to arrive. *"*

"I actually saw Koplik spots [pre measles sign] inside her cheek. I explained to the principal that the child had to be isolated because she was highly contagious. The child lived

---

476 Proceedings of the School Committee, City of Boston 1972

in the projects on Washington Street. She was in first grade. He [principal] would have to round up the parent. It was my second day on the job. I was replacing someone [school nurse] who had fallen at the Bates School. She never came back. I will never forget those spots."

This student's story begs the question of why the child attended school without having the measles vaccine. Having reviewed the immunization laws in Chapters 5, 14, and 15, there is no reason to repeat the rules again. Marie Clarke's student probably attended school before the 1979 immunization law, which required that a child must have proof of immunization against mumps and rubella. To my way of thinking, the school most likely admitted the child under the promise from the parents they would complete the child's immunizations.

We stopped for a few minutes while Marie recollected her first year on the job amidst all the uncertainty.

"I had absolutely no orientation. Nothing. No job description. I had a short interview with my supervisor. I can't remember her name. She asked to see my [nursing] registration. ... The nurse that I was replacing called me several times wanting me to check the health records for immunizations. I was brand new. I didn't know what I was supposed to do. I didn't know what to look for. ... But I didn't know what was required."

"All they asked me for was to see that I got my Bachelor of Science degree after I became a school nurse. I started my Master's program, but I was a married woman with three children. My husband was tired of going places by himself, so I dropped out of the Master's program. I took the exam to be a certified school nurse and got a very good grade."

Marie continued. *"Then I was transferred to Jamaica Plain, District 2. What a nightmare that was. I had three schools on Main Street, a lot of drugs in the area. I had the David Ellis, a big elementary school, over 400 students, the Henry Higginson in Roxbury, and the Roosevelt Middle School in Jamaica Plain. That middle school is not there anymore. ... I had all my stuff [equipment] in a nice bag. They [school staff] told me to get rid of my bag and get an old ratty bag because it was not a good area. ..."* [Muggings, crime].

"We were given an impossible task to provide what we were supposed to provide given the number of students we had, and then, of course, if somebody, the faculty, or an adult became ill while visiting the school, you were stuck with them too." In Marie's words, the assignments were *"unmanageable."*

She further commented, "*I had three schools, but two large busy schools, with multiple languages, and a middle school with all the problems of adolescence. ... Everybody had monumental assignments. ...I used to bring the records home with me. We never had the time during the school day. I would bring them home to check the immunizations. By then, I knew what was needed. I knew what, was what. ...In the Theodore Roosevelt Middle School, I saw my first case of genital herpes ... Then I was excessed from District 2. I was thrilled. I had a smaller assignment, but not really. I had a middle school and an elementary school in the Field's Corner, Dorchester area, now an elementary school.*"

"*I'm surprising myself remembering this.* [They were the] *Lucy Stone Elementary School, and the Oliver Wendell Holmes* [Middle School]" ...

"*I had a diabetic child at the Henry Higginson Elementary School. I was assigned there one day a week. The principal was extremely cooperative. The child had to have a dipstick in the urine every day before lunch. ...We arranged for his teacher, and he had a man teacher... to do this. He said I didn't have to come over there every day for that. I made up a notebook. He* [the teacher] *would escort him to the bathroom in the nurse's room. The little boy would go in and void in the container. The gentleman would test with the dipstick test; if it was abnormal, he was to call me. Fortunately, the child was always in* [the] *normal range. He was a little boy, not beyond second grade ...I also had another diabetic at the other school too.*"

Additionally, Marie referenced some of the special programs she developed. "*Although the Holmes was a middle school, there were 16 and 17-year olds, and possibly even an 18-year old. There was a substantially separate boy's class.*"

The staff asked her to conduct sex education classes on adolescent development.

"*I got a couple of movies for boys and girls. The principal gave me free rein...They were so glad to have someone do it* [the class]. *I got a couple of films. I don't remember where I got them. I didn't have to pay for them. One was "Am I Normal" for the boys, about normal growth and development, including the wild erections adolescent boys get. I developed an AIDS Education program.*"

Other programs that she developed included a six-week class about the treatment and prognosis of cancer, when she found out several children had relatives dying of cancer. She received parental permission to hold the class. After completing the course, the students went further and distributed pamphlets from the American Cancer Society to the entire school and staff. She said, "*I don't know if it did any good, but it made the kids feel better.*"

Similarly, she discussed her duties at the O.W. Holmes School. "*My caseload was such that I went to the principal and asked for clerical help. He would give me someone one hour a week to record, or especially when I was doing vision and hearing tests, I always asked. I couldn't do the job right and spend my whole day on paperwork. He knew I did time teaching in the classroom. If there was something that I needed and it was reasonable, I asked.*"

"*I was there [for]14 years at the Holmes. It was a long time. We had 51A's, the same thing everyone had* [51A's are calls made to the Department of Child Welfare when there is suspicion of child abuse or neglect]. *We had cases of venereal disease and cases of pregnancy. When I was out sick, we had a sub who rode a motorcycle to work, who was a real hippie. I know she referred a girl for an abortion. I wouldn't have done that. There was a special needs girl that had a pregnancy.*"

Marie said the girl was delighted. Her mother would raise the child, even though she [her mother] had 12 children.

Do you think the nurses were respected? How did the staff regard the school nurse? Did you receive respect and recognition?

"*I did. I always received a gift on nurses' day. I remember one of the teachers came in with a little plaque. … I was easy to get along with.*"

Did you give many medications? "*There were not many meds to give.*"

At this point, we took a break and had the delicious lobster salad lunch she ordered from her building's restaurant. What a pleasant surprise that was, and unexpected. Shortly, her cleaning lady arrived, so the remainder of the interview was interspersed with the growling noise of a vacuum.

After lunch, Marie resumed our discussion about her career in the BPS and chatted about her time at the busy Ohrenberger School, after the BPS closed the Holmes School for renovation.

Continuing, she talked about another service she provided to the school. She started doing throat cultures when she was at the Theodore Roosevelt School, on

School Street, in Jamaica Plain. She picked up the culture swabs at the State Lab in Jamaica Plain. She was able to do this on her way home, and the State Lab called the school with the results the following day.

As a result of doing throat cultures, "*I actually excluded the principal. There were several cases of positive strep in the school. He asked me to check the classes. The throat culture came back and said he was positive, and I excluded him. He was astounded. I said, 'You can't stay, you are contagious. I am very sorry, but that is the rule.'*"

Were there technology dependent children?

To illustrate, Marie recounted her situation at the Ohrenberger. "*At the Ohrenberger, I had 25 multi-handicapped children with all types of treatments, including one with a tracheotomy, one with a gastric feed, and another one with grand mal seizures.*"

These medical conditions required her knowledge and mastery of complex medical technologies and regimens, as well as her use of clinical judgment to ensure student safety and satisfactory outcomes.

Another example of her wellness programs involved organizing a health fair in partnership with Faulkner Hospital. She relayed she was able to accomplish that because she had a smaller caseload instead of the previous four schools.

Marie cited another example of the types of problems school nurses faced. "When a child comes from an unstable situation, the problems are different. ... In one week, we had seven students who had witnessed a murder." The BPS's bused these students into the Shaw from another community.

"*They came to school, and they were hysterical. It was a horrible week. Every day there was something. Years ago, the nurse could do nothing more than the vision and hearing tests and not much else, I am sorry to say. They handed out band-aids, checked head lice, and heights and weights. Now you can use your medical expertise to create other programs, to deal with other situations. When I think of all I dealt with all those years. This has been good for me. It has brought back many memories, dealing with problems. It will get me going on my own book.*"

Members of the Nurses Faculty Senate (NFS) at the October 3, 1980, elections elected Marie as a representative, and then chairperson. Marie commented, "*The president at the time, I just didn't feel the nurses were well represented. She had personal problems. ... She was highly respected. I don't think I should criticize her. She is dead now. I thought there was room for improvement."*

Marie presided as chairperson of the NFS until June 1984. *"I went to contract negotiations. ... I don't know what it is like now, but I thought the nurses lacked something to join together and speak up for what they needed in order to do their work properly. They were just coasting along. It seemed to me there was no cohesiveness in the group."*

"Then they said they were going to develop the [supervisor] position again. Carol Almeida became the supervisor [in 1987]. Having been downtown [school headquarters] for a few months, I found there was no direction there to try to improve the school health program. None."

While Marie chaired the NFS, the nurses ended up in arbitration between the Boston Teachers Union (BTU) and the Boston School Committee (BSC) regarding the number of schools in their assignment. *"In a separate development during one of our dark times in 1992, we couldn't see our way forward. Commissioner of Public Health, Judith Kurland, presented a new proposal to Boston School Superintendent Lois Harrison-Jones and the Boston School Committee of transferring school nurses and School Health Services to Health and Hospitals. They promised the School Department a saving of one million dollars. In return, Health and Hospitals would receive schools Medicaid reimbursement money. Then President of the Boston City Council, Thomas Menino, supported this proposal."*

Though the Superintendent said she was undecided about this offer, on May 29, 1992, all 86 Boston school nurses received termination notices. Before this action, the Superintendent did not attempt to negotiate this change with the Boston Teachers Union (BTU).

First and foremost, under this new arrangement, the Boston Public Schools required school nurses to reapply for their jobs. In their new positions as employees of the Trustees of Health and Hospitals, which was supported by grant money, they would be ineligible to continue in the state pension system. If the Trustees of Health and Hospitals allocated no grant money for nursing positions, they would scrub the jobs. It was a dire situation. Where should the school nurses place their faith, their hope, as they tried to turn away from despair?

Though Marie knew our history, most of the other nurses did not, and certainly not the BTU. The Boston School Committee employed the school nurses, not the mayor; therefore, the mayor could not fire us. Armed with this new evidence, our BTU lawyer convinced the Superior Court to issue an injunction prohibiting the transfer until the outcome of contractual grievance-arbitration proceedings at the State Labor Relations Commission.

To further explain, the day before school opened in September 1992 the BSC rehired 53 nurses. This number of nurses represented a 40 percent decrease in nursing staff. In the legislature, pending legislation which would allow Massachusetts schools to bill for reimbursable medical services directly. The law passed, and Mayor Flynn, before he resigned from his office to become the United States Ambassador to the Vatican, signed it allowing Boston schools to become health care providers. This permitted schools to collect Medicaid funds. However, these dollars go directly into Boston's general fund, not to the schools. In the case of a small town with a regional high school, the dollars directly go to the school system. As a result, Health and Hospitals no longer expressed an interest in acquiring Boston School Health Services.

As an example of how Boston collected from the nurses' work, Marie related,

"I had a diabetic (a person with diabetes). I had to do blood tests and gave insulin every day. The city bills for that. The city used the money they received from that to hire police officers. However, it saved our jobs."

Perhaps Marie's historical research was not the primary consideration in this case, but it did act as a deterrent. As has been pointed out time and again, one must know what has gone on before, and how the past informs the present.

How did you get substitute nurses?

"I think sometimes they didn't call for them."

She was right. Frequently, principals would instead hold that money to cover an absent teacher.

Did they have Para's then (nurse assistants)?

"No."

Were nurses working in other school systems on the same level as the teachers?

"I knew a school nurse in Dedham. I couldn't believe the pittance she made."

Were the BPS nurses involved in the Massachusetts School Nurse Organization?

"Not formally. I think I called them (MSNO) several times for information and had I continued working, I probably would have joined them. They were trying to raise the salaries of the school nurses around the state. That was their main goal. The BPSN had accomplished that many years before."

What is your perspective on school nursing now?

"I have been away from it for a number of years. I saw a big change during the time I worked. Records were computerized. I don't believe anyone had four schools. Most people had two or three. We were successful in winning the battle to hire more school nurses, reduce the caseload so that we could do more of a meaningful job. I think there was more recognition of our role that the nurse was a person qualified to deal with emergency situations. I know my principal paid far more attention to me. I could pretty much design and implement a program usually as a result of the situation in the school."

The Massachusetts School Nurse Organization honored K. Marie Clarke with the Massachusetts School Nurse of the Year Award in 1994 in recognition of her impressive career. See the image to the right - K. Marie Clarke holding a gift she received at retirement.

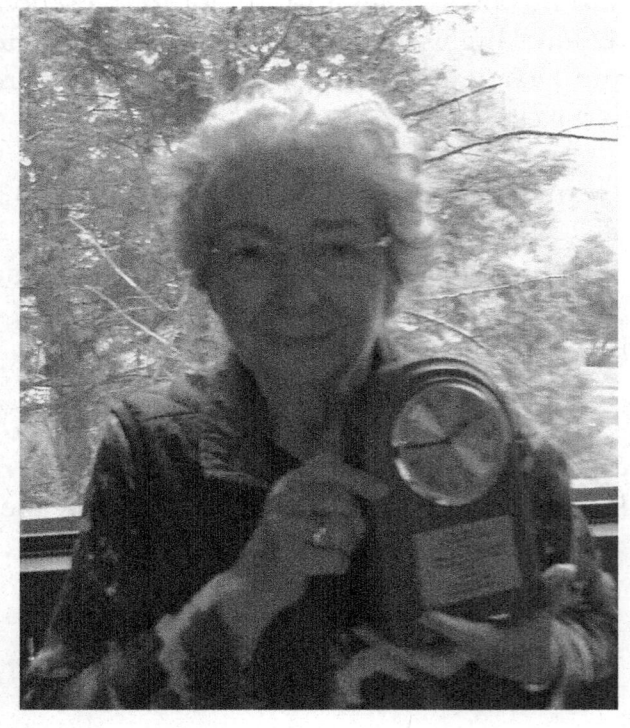

School Based Health Centers

The concept of on-site student health clinics came to the forefront of the Nurse Faculty Senate (NFS) meeting on 12/3/1985.[477] The question asked of all headmasters and principals of all middle and high schools centered on whether they had any interest in having a health center in their building. Though the *Minutes* were not clear on who presented this proposal, it was probably Ken Caldwell, with the approval of the Superintendent. At an earlier NFS meeting, Carol Almeida reported on "Clinics in Schools Study."[478] How the school nurse would fit into this new model had neither been explored nor defined. If nurses wanted more information about school-based health centers, they were to contact Carol Almeida.

A nurse practitioner, who is required to have advanced degree beyond a registered nurse, would run the school-based health center. They provide primary health care, could diagnose and treat illnesses, and prescribe medications. Ideally, they work with the school nurse, school staff, parents, and the student's primary care provider. They do not replace them. Frequently, the local community health center sponsored the school health clinic.

School nurses had visions of the nurse practitioner commandeering their health office and duties. By springtime, the Boston Teachers Union (BTU) fired a letter off to John A. Nucci, President of the Boston School Committee, supporting the Boston school nurses in their opposition to the proposed school-based health clinics. While the nurses agreed there was a disproportionate number of adolescent problems they should focus on, such as the high incidence of teenage pregnancy, school dropouts, drug and alcohol abuse, and psychosocial issues, they advocated a different approach. Instead of offering additional physical health services to the schools in the form of school-based clinics, they recommended spending the money on providing comprehensive counseling and preventive education at all school age levels.[479]

---

477   Boston Public School Nurses Club Minutes: 12/3/1985

478   Boston Public School Nurses Club Minutes: 10/1/1985

479   Boston Public School Nurses Club Minutes: 4/16/1986

Their other objections included:

- The city's 22 neighborhood health clinics and nine hospital-based programs already enrolled many of the students. The school nurses offered to survey how many students previously enrolled in the above-mentioned programs.

- At this point, the administration required comprehensive consent from parents. However, it did not stipulate a parent should be notified of a pending medication or treatment, leading to the disenfranchisement of parents.

- Class time lost while in the school clinic,

- How long would the funding last?

- School-based health centers close during school vacations, evening, and the summer, causing fragmented health care. The backup clinic might be geographically distant from the student's home, leading to a loss of continuity of care.

- Possible duplication of some of the mandated state programs as vision, hearing, scoliosis and blood pressure screening, physical exams, and immunizations.

- What are the parameters when prescribing analgesics and birth control pills?

- The Administration did not clarify the details of staff qualifications and staff requirements. They questioned the need for a nutritionist, health educator, and an outreach worker.

- Some existing programs, for example, Family Planning Perspectives, as yet had never been evaluated. (This makes it appear the school sanctioned sexual activity).

Some of their objections sounded similar to Dr. Lamb's problems with the school nurses, as in no evaluation of current programs. By December, the NFS proposed making a presentation to the Boston School Committee and a letter campaign to all BSC members reiterating their objections to the recommended school-based clinics.[480] The following month, the BTU declared support for the nurses in opposing the proposed school-based health centers, the School Health Project of the Boston Student Service Collaborative.

Since I don't want to leave readers wondering about the sketchy future of school based clinics, School Nurse Supervisor Rita Laughlin, presented to a joint meeting of school nurses, student support coordinators, and nurse practitioners, in November 1993 the history of school health services since 1991-1992. During this talk, she said school-based health clinics started offering services to students in April 1993. She described the relationship as a "shotgun marriage" since she admitted they made mistakes in the past. Rita said, *"With collaboration, with sharing, with trust, we have the potential of offering a working model of a successful School Health Clinic."*

In this writer's opinion, school is where the high-risk students are, and they are the least likely to use traditional health services. Finally, and perhaps most importantly, on-site school health centers benefit students because they treat pupils for minor illnesses, which may improve their general health as well as their school attendance.

PART II - 1986-1987

Among other issues, the Nurses Faculty Senate's (NFS) priority for this school year focused on attempting equity in school nurse assignments. In this era, 38 of the 75 nurses carried caseloads of 700 to more than 1,200 students among one to as many as three school buildings. The nurses found these caseloads to be exceeding a manageable level.

With three busy schools, how could a nurse respond when a student presents with a life-threatening allergy? Was there someone at the school who could administer the life-saving drug epinephrine if the nurse was not present? Anne Sheetz discussed this in an article about school nursing. Boston schools had been fortunate in not having any deaths as a result of anaphylaxis, but other states had not fared that well. However, it is important to note, 20-25 percent of persons receiving epinephrine from a school nurse did not have a known life-threatening allergy.[481]

480   Boston Public School Nurses Club Minutes: 12/9/1986
481   Sheetz, A. H. (2015) Focus on School Nursing. Massachusetts Report on Nursing 13(3), 8-9.

As a result of her significant assignment, one nurse decided to file a grievance, citing uneven assignments, as well as favoritism, with nurses switching individual schools. Her responsibility included three large elementary schools as compared to another nurse in the same district who only had one middle school. A grievance process arbitrated by the Union resolved the issue, resulting in a mutually satisfactory resolution of the complaint.[482]

In the meantime, nurses Pauline Shanks and K. Marie Clarke continued to labor at completing a Policy and Procedure Manual, another request of Dr. Lamb's. Dr. Grady and Ken Caldwell made arrangements for more release time for these nurses to finish the needed manual.

The Nurses Faculty Senate (NFS) consistently had meetings with Dr. Grady and Ken Caldwell discussing such issues as the nurse supervising position, hiring LPN's (Licensed Practical Nurses), and nurse practitioners in schools. Dr. Grady reported he supported the position of supervising nurse. It was heartening to see he backed up the nurses' view of installing a medical person instead of a business manager. When considering LPN's, they would cost the city less, but the LPN had less education than an RN. The NFS opposed this proposal, additionally because of the added responsibility of an RN supervising the LPN. The issue of nurse practitioners in schools replacing physicians violated the current contracts.[483] If they were to go forward with the school-based clinics presided by nurse practitioners, this was another aspect they would have to resolve.

The Massachusetts State House presented other diversions in the form of Senate Bill 270 which deleted the word "registered" preceding the word "nurse" in line 12 of the bill, allowing a "nurse" to give psychotropic medication in schools (a psychotropic drug is any drug capable of affecting the mind, emotions, and behavior). School nurses feared this was another maneuver to assist in the use of practical nurses and health aides in the schools. The NFS urged school nurses to call their state representatives and senators and oppose the change of "registered nurse" to "nurse."[484]

---

482   Boston Public School Nurses Club Minutes: 1/15/1987

483   Boston Public School Nurses Club Minutes: 4/9/1986

484   Boston Public School Nurses Club Minutes: 12/2/1986

The NFS mailed their letter to the Chairman and Members of the Joint Committee on Education at the State House opposing any change in the current requirement that a registered nurse or physician only administer psychotropic drugs in the public schools. Their letter pronounced, "In addition to their potential for abuse, these drugs have possible adverse reactions and interactions that require monitoring of the student. The registered professional nurse, by her education, training, and experience, has the medical expertise to recognize and deal with changes in a students' clinical status that may signal pending medical problems or toxicity. Furthermore, the Department of Public Health is eager to eliminate certification of psychotropic drugs, which would reinforce the state to continue to require that the medications only be administered by a registered nurse or a physician"[485]

However, the LPN's were persistent. The LPN Association filed another bill to allow LPN's to give psychotropic drugs in school. The Department of Public Health supported their request. Kathy Kelly, a former president of the BTU, read the letter the BTU sent on 4/6/1987 to the Chairman and Members of the Joint Committee on Education supporting the school nurses' position. At this point, the Chairman and Members of the Joint Committee reinstated the word "registered" into the bill. The rewrite of the law did not pass.[486]

Following up again on Dr. Lamb's improvement suggestions, the school nurses investigated their counterparts' duties in other cities. This research showed New London, Connecticut, had a school nurse supervisor. Moreover, New London sent each nurse to school for six weeks to obtain their nurse practitioner license at the cities' expense.[487] Boston school nurses were many steps behind with such a plan since they were still trying to traverse this new space of nurse practitioners.

Nurses experienced more support when Superintendent Dr. Laval S. Wilson continued to include nurses on the new Student Support Services and Student Support Teams in middle and high schools as part of his Adolescent Issues

---

485   Boston Public School Nurses Club Minutes: 4/14/1987

486   Boston Public School Nurses Club Minutes: 4/14/1987

487   Boston Public School Nurses Club Minutes: 1/15/1987

recommendation of the Boston Education Plan. The NFS sent him a letter praising him for his proposal.[488]

New England Surprise; they canceled their November Nurses Faculty Senate meeting due to snow. Finally, at their 12/3/1987 meeting, the Boston Public School Nurses Club Minutes state they will invite Carol Almeida to their next meeting on January 7, 1988. Carol Almeida endured the grueling application process and won the school nurse supervisor position, surpassing other applicants.

A Chat with Carol Almeida Fortes

I met Carol Almeida Fortes at the Lawler Library in New Bedford, Massachusetts, on a warm, sunny day in August 2015. Finding a secluded table for our interview in a busy library, we sat down to begin our discussion. Carol is an attractive African American woman, married, retired, of medium height, with dark hair. During our conversation, she was quick to laugh and seemed to enjoy relaying her experiences. Carol became my former nursing supervisor when we were both employed by the Boston Public Schools.

Education

Carol reminisced about her early school years in New Bedford, Massachusetts in the 1960s. All of her teachers told her she was not college material and not qualified to go to college. When she failed French, New Bedford refused to give her permission to go to summer school and moved her into business courses. These courses did not meet the college entry requirements. Her family then left New Bedford and moved to Boston where she attended the Jeremiah Burke High School for grades 10-12. Still, the school staff did not change her school program to include college entry subjects. She reflected she didn't receive proper direction. As a result, she did not have the required courses to attend a school that would lead her to become a registered nurse. Consequently, she attended Chelsea Soldier's Home School of Nursing, Chelsea, Massachusetts, at Quigley Memorial Hospital and became a licensed practical nurse (LPN). A stipend of $25 per week proved to be a bonus.

---

488   Boston Public School Nurses Club Minutes: 10/1/1987

"I was fighting for whatever I wanted to do, starting in high school," she remarked. After graduation, she worked for six years at Quigley Memorial Hospital, taking courses at night to prepare her to enter a school of nursing for her RN. At that time, in 1968, the state offered a program where one could work 20 hours a week, receive full pay, and go to school for your RN. To accomplish this, Carol had to switch days with her co-workers. However, her supervisor there disapproved of these changes, forcing her to decide to leave Quigley.

Undaunted, Carol took a job in labor and delivery at St Margaret's Hospital, Dorchester, allowing her to complete her courses at night. In the meantime, she applied to nursing schools at Boston University, Boston College, and Northeastern University. Northeastern, in 1969, offered her full tuition, a free ride with room and board included. Who would turn that down?

The three-year program at Northeastern would only give her an Associate degree, whereas the five-year program awarded a Bachelor of Science degree. Associate-degree programs, created during the 1950s, prepared entry level nurses. Five years loomed like an eternity for Carol, but a school administrator said, "We can see you are very motivated. You can stop at any time and come back and finish."

Thus, Carol applied and was accepted into the five-year program. She continued to work at a nursing home while attending Northeastern because she needed the extra money. Indeed, one cannot anticipate and prepare for every eventuality fate throws in your path. During the Northeastern program, Carol became pregnant. The relationship did not work out.

Her friends said, "Are you going to quit?" After mulling over the pros and cons of her situation, she replied, "No."

Later in the pregnancy, she became sick and applied for public assistance. Looking back, she admits she did not reveal that to a lot of people. The year 1974 dawned, and with her family's help, a determined Carol graduated with a BSN from Northeastern.

Nursing Positions

After graduating, Carol went into community health nursing at Harvard Street Neighborhood Health Center, working at their obstetrics-gynecology clinic. Instead of working in the clinic, she preferred to be in the community making home visits. So, after 18 months, Carol switched to following up tuberculosis and neonatal cases in Beacon Hill, Roxbury, and the South End. When following up on new births, she could start in a housing project with a teenage mother, then end up visiting Beacon Hill, where they would have the china laid out for her with tea and cookies. They were fun visits.

Nonetheless, as a single mother with a child to support, she needed a job that offered her benefits. After that job in 1988, she taught students studying to be licensed practical nurses (LPN's) for the City of Boston. She loved working with the students. Unfortunately, she disliked correcting their math homework at night.

In 1980, her brother told her about a posting for an RN involving team-teaching basic skills for 9th graders at Boston's Hubert Humphrey Center, now Madison Park Vocational and Technical High School. It was a new exploratory program where you would have ninth graders for three weeks to teach them hand washing, heights and weights, nutrition counseling, and field trips to neighborhood health centers.

Since she only had one week to get her application in, Carol immediately called her former boss, asking for help updating her resume. After putting her daughter to bed that evening, Carol spent the night on her typewriter, and delivered the application the following day. She received a call for an interview, one of the last meetings to be held. Carol subsequently got the job.

One of the subjects the she taught was hand washing using a petri dish and swab technique, usually on a Friday. When students returned on Monday, they were amazed to see the plates full of bacterial colonies, demonstrating that hand washing is a simple technique proven to reduce disease transmission. Unfortunately, a handful of months later, the administration cut the job.

Boston Public School Nurse

In the meantime, by 1980, Carol had been applying to the Boston Public Schools for a school nurse position for several years. The staff acknowledged her paperwork was in order but kept asking, "Would you like to be a substitute?" Being a sub was an excellent way to get your foot in the door, so to speak. However, at that time, a sub position would not offer her the benefits she needed, so she declined.

Another opportunity developed in September 1981, when she visited her daughter's school to review her case with the school nurse. Her daughter wore a Milwaukee brace (a back brace used in the treatment of spinal curvatures in children). This school nurse, Carol thinks it was Joan Sheehy, revealed substitutes currently covered three school nurse positions.

"Tell John Diggins that I recommend you," Joan declared.

Immediately, Carol proceeded to the central office and spoke with John Diggins, the Director of Guidance and School Health. At first, she said he told her there were no positions available, but when Carol responded with Joan's information, he recanted and thought about a job in Charlestown. Then he said he couldn't send her there.

"I will go anywhere," was her retort.

She speculated if he lied to her. After a few minutes of deliberation, he said he would send her to the Charles E. Mackey Middle School and Copley Square High School, each having 500 students.

"Is the procedure manual at school?" Carol asked.

Diggins responded by saying he planned to send her for one week with high school nurse Barbara Banks who would teach her all she needed to know. That encompassed her orientation. While observing with Barbara Banks, Carol asked for a procedural manual, but of course, none existed. At that time, she became acquainted with the staff at School Health Services: Dr. Michael Grady, MD, who worked only a half-day a week, John Diggins, and a secretary, Barbara Knolton, comprised the staff. Note, the workforce did not include a nursing supervisor.

School Programs Developed

While at Mackey Middle School, Carol developed a student weight loss program. The school doctor would evaluate the pupils with their parent's permission. Due to the school's limited, available space, they met on the auditorium's stage. Carol taught them about nutrition, healthy eating, the benefits of exercise, and how advertisers try to trick them into buying unhealthy food. Participants would do exercises together on the stage. Their homework goal consisted of maintaining their weight, though if they lost weight, that was even better. The program ran 12-15 weeks. Carol followed the 6th grade group for three years and wrote a summary of the program. She said colleagues encouraged her to submit it for publication, but she never followed through with their advice.

Unfortunately, Carol Almeida developed shingles after five students with chickenpox languished in her office for several hours. Ms. Almeida still remembers some of the students and the problems they faced. One such case involved a boy who always had a cold and frequently ended up in the emergency room. She documented all of his symptoms, his visits to the health office and told his mother to give it to his doctors. Since he saw different doctors each time he went to the emergency room, and before the computerization of medical records, they were never able to pull it all together. Consequently, the mother brought in Carol's report on her next visit to the emergency room. From that report, his doctors concluded he had cystic fibrosis.

Another girl frequently visited the nurse's office. Her teachers said, "She comes to class full of energy, does her work, and then is exhausted."

At age 18, this young woman received an uncertain diagnosis. Unfortunately, she never received a lot of parental support. Carol wrote up all of the girl's medical history and told her to give it to her doctors on her next visit. The young woman called her from the hospital a few days later.

"They are trying to figure out if I have lupus or syphilis," she exclaimed. "They can't believe you did all this work." Ultimately, the young woman received a diagnose of lupus erythematosus, an autoimmune disease. Carol kept in touch with her after graduation. Sadly, her former student passed away at age 25. Health providers acknowledge that a good history is 90 percent of a diagnosis.

In 1985, Copley Square High School received grant money for teachers to attend the University of Massachusetts at Amherst for their advanced degree at a reduced cost. The program enabled her to obtain her Master's in Education degree.

Carol's courses included counseling and group dynamics, subjects that would help her to deal with people. The program's Amherst, Massachusetts, location required class attendance from 7-9 PM once a week. This time frame necessitated an overnight stay at the school before her early morning drive to work the following day.

Position Posting

Meanwhile, the Nurses Faculty Senate requested the Boston School Committee multiple times over several years to assign a new supervisor after the former nurse retired. The BSC finally, in 1986, posted the school nurse supervisor position. Carol continued she was "shocked" the posting only required a bachelor's degree. All other department heads, such as psychology and guidance, required a minimum of a master's degree.

She became aware another well-qualified school nurse who did a lot for the nurses and fought a lot of their battles competed for the opening. Though Carol claims she had little interest in the position, the other minority nurses urged her to apply. She applied for the position and got the job.

After a while, Carol and Medical Director Dr. Grady had a conversation about her selection for the post. She related Dr. Grady said he discussed it with his wife, and after reviewing Carol's resume, he decided she was the better-qualified candidate.

Carol the Supervisor

Dr. Grady requested Carol to go out in the community to visit schools, support the nurses, and continue work as an administrator as well. Therefore, her schedule included visiting schools two days a week and spending three days in the central office. If a school nurse developed a problem on one of Carol's office days, she took the T (public transportation) to connect with the nurse.

After Carol's experience as a new school nurse, it comes as no surprise that the development of a policy and procedures manual became one of her priorities. She formed a committee, including Phyllis Paisley Lomax, Jackie Harrington, and others. The committee completed it within 18 months. More than likely, they based it on the procedural manual prepared by Pauline Shanks and K. Marie Clarke in 1986. Once it hit the printing press, Carol delivered it to the Massachusetts Department of Public Health School Health Unit, where they expanded it further.

In the meantime, other school departments from all over the state heard about the manual and requested copies. Carol said School Health Services ended up mailing copies to all those who sought it. At that time, in 1990, Ann Sheetz emerged as the Director of the Department of Public Health School Health Unit.

As a supervisor, though the school department aimed for nurses to have a degree, Carol also hired nurses who only held an RN. Carol favored those nurses with a strong medical, surgical background, and pediatrics. Nurses of color amounted to 12 percent of the workforce when Carol became the supervisor. She made it her goal to double that number, considering the majority of the students were also minorities. When Carol attended school, she said she did not have a teacher of color until 7th grade, and once again in high school. Because of her asthma, she frequented the nurse's office.

"I never saw a minority nurse ever. They were nice. They all did their job. But…"

Carol observed a certain attitude during department head meetings. For example, a principal might ask, "Why do you want to know that?" There was a pervasive, "Just do it," because I said so, kind of attitude. Administrators believed the principal should be in charge, and during a medical emergency, the principal should be the one to call 911.

Carol would often point out, "The kid or staff person needs emergency care. The school nurse doesn't have the equipment to take care of them. The nurse will inform the principal she has called 911 and to expect the arrival of the fire department and or other emergency personnel."

Again, Carol would tell principals, if they were having problems with their nurse, don't call their supervisor (the principals), call her. She promised to come out to the school, sit down with the nurse, and figure out what was going on. Over time, Carol explained, the principals trusted her. They would call her to review their concerns, and collaboratively, try to work it out.

"They had no concept of school health. Principals were used to being in charge," Carol claimed. "I emphasized to the nurses: you have to clarify to the principal what we need to do, why we are doing this, and why we can't do that."

Two principals confirmed to her, "Every time I have a conversation with you, I learn something I didn't know about health."

Carol asserted, "That is my job. I am a nurse, and I am an educator."

School-based health centers provided other services for Boston students, for example, physical exams, and treatment. Carol found being the liaison between the BPS and community health centers and hospitals turned into a memorable experience. She worked to bring the two agencies together. Realistically, she reported some of the nurses were skeptical about having a school-based health center, but most were happy with the concept. Like everything else, some experienced growing pains, but it developed into a collaborative effort.

Another of Carol's accomplishments included joining the Army Reserves in 1990. Even though she considered herself too old, unbeknownst to her, there was a need for more nurses before the onset of Operation Desert Storm and Desert Shield. She went through the officer's training in San Antonio, Texas, that included head nurse training, emergency room, disaster training, and ICU (intensive care unit) training. She didn't do well in the 110-degree heat, and decided to resign her commission as captain, but valued the entire experience.

Carol remained as a school nurse supervisor until 1992. Simultaneously, the BSC drastically cut funds to School Health Services, and Medical Director, Dr. Grady, left his position. Unfortunately, the BSC downsized nurses from 90 to a total of 50. Dr. Grady considered it an unsafe environment and advised Carol to find another post as soon as possible.

During the first two weeks of school, in September 1992, two nurses totaled their cars while on duty because of the stress of having to cover three to four schools. Principals called the central office, demanding to know why the nurse was not there giving the noon medications?

"The nurse cannot be in four places at once. She will start at 11 and do the rounds," Carol answered.

Of course, all of the sick children would be waiting for the nurse when she arrived to give the medications, thus delaying her arrival at the next school.

Other Plans

Listening to the advice she received, Carol decided to take an unpaid sabbatical, which allowed her to later return to her position. She indicated that was the last year leaves of absence were allowed. Carol accepted a nursing position with the pediatric and adolescent clinic at Tufts Medical Center to upgrade her nursing skills.

Returning to the Boston Public Schools

In 1993, Carol returned to the Boston Public Schools. While on her sabbatical, Carol relayed that Dan Schwartz revised the nursing supervisor's job description to make it a strictly administrative job. Rather than endure a stressful situation, plus a very long commute from New Bedford, she asked for a staff nurse position. Hyde Park High School became her new assignment. She remained there until December 2003, when she retired after a long nursing career.

The Future of School Nursing

"I think a lot of the things we were trying to do, like the supervisor position, the number of kids (number of schools each nurse has), when I returned in 1993, they are finally doing it. They (cafeteria staff) were taking the junk out of the cafeteria, like chips …We, as nurses, see these overweight kids; doctors were not addressing it." The dining hall director would tell you about the "junk food. That is how we fund the program," but it is not healthy food for the students. Carol insists, "I think every school should have a nurse; kids have problems; they need some place to go."

Regarding computer programs, Carol said she fought for them since she was a supervisor, but when she retired in 2003, they had not acquired them. (At last, in 2007, School Health Services adopted the SNAP electronic health record to assist school nurses in their daily work.) Additionally, she points out she does not know how nursing is now, but, "they have sicker kids, special education kids who previously had never lived that long. Now there is abuse, a lot of drugs, alcohol babies, and homelessness."

Carol emphasized the school nurse cannot do everything, for example, teaching hand washing techniques, sex education, and performing the vision and hearing testing, when you have kids coming in and out of the office with problems. A nurse's aide, she argues, would be helpful doing heights and weights with the nurse supervising.

Carol Almeida Fortes had many unique opportunities to target nursing interventions as well as policy decisions to move Boston school nursing forward during her career. Her contributions included offering much needed support, direction, organization, and cohesiveness to the school nurses, not only with a procedure manual but also by working collaboratively with administrative staff. She collaborated with the neighborhood health centers and hospitals to provide the groundwork for school-based health centers at the schools. Perhaps, most importantly, as a result of her own experiences, she empathized with Boston students and encouraged the employment of more minority nurses.

My interpretation of the controversy regarding the school nursing supervisor's position is candidates with advanced degrees received the nod over those that did not have such a degree. When returning after her sabbatical, she decided to take a staff nurse position. I commend her for being the perfect gentlewoman, by not interfering with the current administration at that time. After her retirement, she endured several serious illnesses which limited her healthy tomorrows. She passed away March 5, 2020.

A New Start

At long last, the Boston school nurses had a new school nursing supervisor. This was what they strived for since Marguerite McLaughlin retired in January 1979. We don't know what was said. Were they euphoric? Perhaps their new situation would resemble what Robert Finch referred to in his book, "The Outer Beach: A Thousand-Mile Walk on Cape Cod's Atlantic Shore." He deliberated about the seashore and living with change. "With each night tide, it wipes out our history, providing us with a clean slate in the morning, our sins, and soiled lives washed clean."[489] They stood on the precipice of a clean slate, a fresh start.

Many supervisors, or Assistant Medical Directors as per the name change, followed Carol Almeida, such as Rita Loughlin, Debra Fox, Anne Sullivan, Arlene Swan-Mahoney, Susan Fencer, Maureen Starck, and Mary Jane O'Brien, to name a few, who all in their unique way, advanced the role of school nurses and at the same time, improved student health and academic achievement.

The train has arrived at one of its last stations. It signals the end of our journey with the Boston Public School Nurses during their formative and sometimes

---

489   Finch, R. (2017). The Outer Beach A Thousand-Mile Walk on Cape Cod's Atlantic Shore. New York: W.W. Norton & Company.

turbulent years. I hope you appreciated my narrative of the Boston Public School Nurses, the dilemmas they faced, why they made their decisions, and perhaps shined a fresh light on their story. Additionally, I wish my readers gained a better understanding of school nursing, have picked up some information that will benefit themselves, and enjoyed the trip through Boston's history. At this point, we can permit ourselves some thoughtful reflection. I think their political activism, finding a leader at various times that understood their challenges, reaching out to the communities they served, and most important, their resilience and commitment to their cause helped them achieve their goals for school nursing practice.

Knowing the history of school nursing, new school nurses can stand proud of the roles their predecessors played in promoting and advancing the health of this country's schoolchildren. Above all, it will motivate them to continue this legacy. As noted in the Introduction, the available *Boston School Nurses Minutes* ended in 1988. Hopefully, sometime soon, more recent *Minutes* will be located, and I know some excellent hands will write the next chapter of our storied legacy. Stay on board. The next chapter tells the story of the formation of the Massachusetts School Nurse Organization (MSNO).

SECTION III
LOOKING FORWARD

Chapter 17

The First Twenty Years of MSNO 1970 – 1990

On a chilly, overcast, spring morning, Jonathan Rich wheeled his mother, Martha Bears Rich, accompanied by her family, to the podium of the Simmons College graduating tent for the Nursing Pinning Ceremony on May 17, 2018. The College's School of Nursing and Health Sciences were honoring Martha, Class of 1944 at Simmons, for her passion and love of nursing. Foundress of the Massachusetts School Nurse Organization (MSNO), she retired in 1988 from her full-time position as Sharon High School's school nurse.

Founding and Early History of the MSNO

The Massachusetts School Nurse Organization (MSNO) is a professional organization for Massachusetts school nurses. Its membership encompasses nurses from all areas of Massachusetts, including small towns, big cities, rural, and urban areas. Sometimes, with only one school nurse in a town, or maybe two, they found themselves out there on their own with little support. But, whether in a small town or big city, it became crucial to have an organization where school nurses could receive support from others on policy, procedures, and status within school systems.

Early Efforts to Organize

An earlier group called the School Nurses Association of Massachusetts (SNAM), made itself known to the Boston School Nurses Club in 1958, as earlier noted in Chapter 10. Several years later, they also approached Martha Rich, who served as the first president of the current MSNO, from 1970-1972. But as Martha related in a personal interview in 2011, she thought the SNAM group consisted of older nurses from New Bedford and Fall River who were reaching retirement age. Therefore, she felt they didn't have the energy to move forward at the rate she and her colleagues considered necessary to form a new strong, and vibrant organization.

Martha Rich spoke about the early days of the National Association of School Nurses (NASN) in an interview.[490] She related that in July of 1968, a national organization, known as the National Education Association (NEA), established a Department of School Nurses that allowed school nurses to become an affiliate of it. The Department's mission then was "to improve the quality of school nursing, to upgrade the skills of school nurses, and to further the abilities of all children to succeed in the classroom.[491]"

By 1969 the National Education Association set up a fact-finding meeting in Philadelphia, which was attended by about 200 Massachusetts school nurses. As a result, these Massachusetts nurses decided to affiliate with the Department of School Nurses, which then would become their national organization. In 1970 the Department of School Nurses elected Sally Williams as their first president. Consequently, they formed committees, developed policies, and elected officers. Each state then launched its state organization under the umbrella of the Department of School Nurses.

However, yet another organization emerged in May 1967, called the National Council for School Nurses, and held its second annual business meeting at the American Association for Health Physical Education and Recreation (AAHPER) convention. In addition to electing officers, they published *The School Nursing Monograph No. 1*, dealing with solutions to critical health needs with implications for school nursing, and *New Dimensions in School Nursing Leadership*. These documents contained the proceedings of the first national leadership conference for school nurses held August 3-5, 1968 in Washington, D.C. School nurses from 38 states attended this meeting, an impressive number.[492] Therefore, two different groups

---

490   D.Keeney, personal communication 2011

491   *Our History*. In National Association of School Nursing. Retrieved from https://www.nasn.org/nasn/about-nasn/about/our-history

492   *NCSN Action*. (June 1969). Retrieved from http://www.tandfonline.com/doi/abs/10.1080/00221473.1969.10610545?needAccess=true&journalCode=ujrd18(NCSN

competed to represent school nurses. However, the stronger National Education Association with its Department of School Nurses eventually won the challenge.

As members of the Department of School Nurses/NEA assembled in 1978 in Dallas, Texas, they voted to break away from the NEA and changed their name to the National Association of School Nurses (NASN). The following year, in 1979, they incorporated as NASN, consequently becoming independent of the NEA. NASN today represents the largest association of school nurses and serves as the center for all the state organizations.[493]

MSNO Comes to Represent Massachusetts' School Nurses

In the same interview with Rich (M. Rich, personal communication 2011), she described how they founded the current MSNO. The Massachusetts Nurses Association (MNA), came to one of the school nurses' early meetings in 1970 and implored them to join their organization. On a good note, MNA promised to help them obtain salary increases. However, any interest in joining disappeared when the president, in front of a group of 50 nurses, said of the school nursing profession, "Get a real job." Not surprisingly, after that disparaging remark, school nurses decided they would pursue an organizing effort on their own and formed the Massachusetts School Nurse Organization (MSNO).

As a result, Martha Rich became the first president of MSNO on February 25th, 1970. During another personal interview, in June of 2010, Ms. Rich described her first year as establishing the infrastructure of the organization and the second year as president. After that, she stepped down and assumed the immediate past president position, a more supporting role, and then spent another year as National Director, their representative to the national organization. Martha Rich rose to become president of the Department of School Nurses, from 1976-1977, later to become known as NASN.

Usually, the association met once a month at the home of one of the directors, or sometimes in one of their schools. They held conferences in the spring and the fall, and depending on the program, would have about 35-75 school nurses in attendance.

---

493   *Our History*. In National Association of School Nursing. Retrieved from https://www.nasn.org/nasn/about-nasn/about/our-history

The Board communicated with their membership by telephone and regular mail. Since they didn't know the names nor the number of school nurses in the Commonwealth, as there was no master list, they contacted all school superintendents to locate their school nurses. While a good idea, the effort required a lot of work.

Martha Rich cited the main goals of the organization at that time as: a) improving the status of school nurses employed within educational systems, b) improving salaries, c) improving educational background standards among school nurses, and d) developing standards for certification, requiring a BS or BA degree for entry level positions. In 1970, Ms. Rich said, "a large percentage of school nurses had only an RN degree and little or no education or experience in schools." As to the amount of time she spent on MSNO work, Ms. Rich said she didn't recall, but remembers her children saying, "Where are you going tonight, Mom?"[494]

Unfortunately, the minutes from those early meetings have not survived. The one thing Ms. Rich regrets was not furthering her education to obtain a master's degree. Ms. Rich is happy now that the history of MSNO is recorded and saved, because as she observed, the newer members of MSNO should know what happened in the early days (M. Rich, personal communication, June 26, 2010).

Recollections from The Wet Towel

In the early 1970s, MSNO published a newsletter two to three times a year named *The Wet Towel*. (As an aside, what did they think when they gave it that name? How did the title relate to school nursing? They explained a nurse frequently soothes discomfort by placing a cold, wet towel on the patient's forehead. Armed with that clarification, it is debatable whether that title raised the status of school nurses among nurses in other fields). We will follow MSNO's activities and accomplishments through various articles in *The Wet Towel* as they established their organization, and promoted issues that were important to school nurses, students, and their families.

MSNO divided the membership into six geographic regions across the state. Each area had a chairperson, and the individual regions met every few months, sometimes at a restaurant or one of their schools. Their agenda usually consisted of

---

[494] Keeney, D. (2010, September). Conversations with former presidents of MSNO. An interview with former president Martha Rich. *Massachusetts School Nurse Outlook*, 16,17.

the chairperson updating their members on MSNO's current issues, sharing their everyday problems, and generally, had a speaker.

The annual membership fee in 1977 amounted to $27 annually, a combination of local, state, and national dues. By 1984, they would increase their dues to $50.

See the image below - Membership Application (For state dues only). Photo courtesy of McAuliffe MSNO Album.

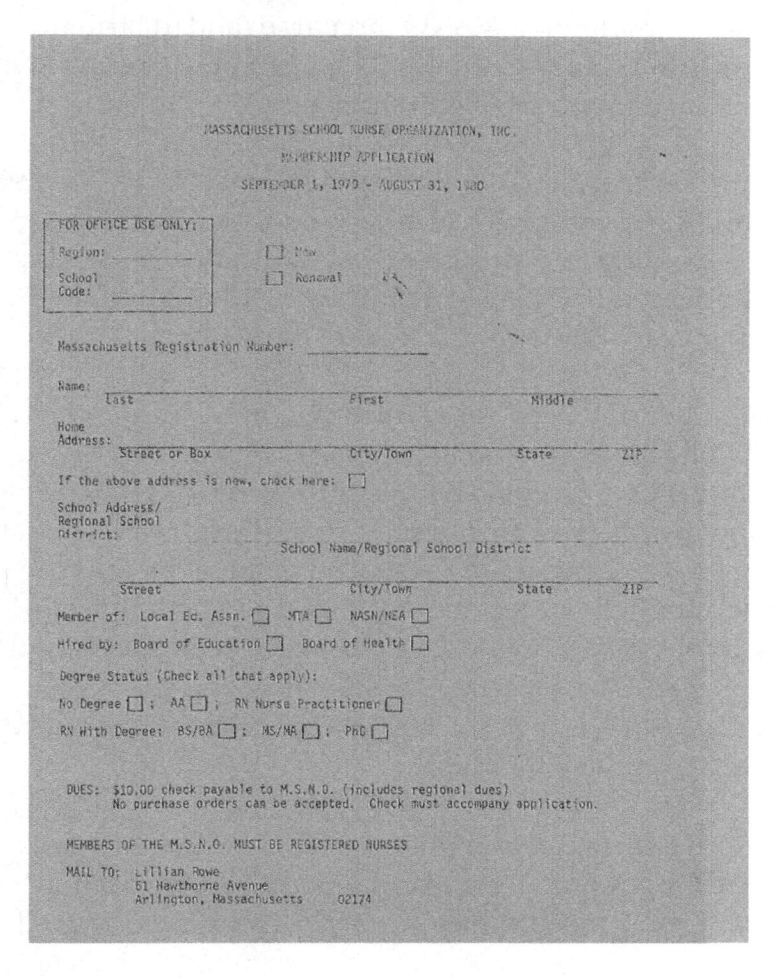

Legislative Activities

From the beginning, MSNO played an active role in lobbying state legislators for causes that were important to them. *The Wet Towel* related in May 1980 then Governor King signed into law the program of postural screening for school children in grades

5-9, amending Chapter 71 of the General Laws. This program of spinal screening detected curvatures of the spine. The bill also included mandates for hearing and vision screening.

Early Efforts at Certification

Considering some other events in the early years of MSNO, the founding president, Martha Rich, filed the first state certification bill in 1971 for school nurses. Finally, and perhaps most importantly, MSNO prepared and distributed a booklet of guidelines for school nurses. Certification sought to elevate the standards, state-wide, of school nurses and school health services.

The Massachusetts Teachers Association filed Senate Bill 250 in 1980 petitioning Boards of Education to grant certificates to school nurses. This legislation didn't pass. School nurses continued their pursuit of certification during the presidency of Nancy Miller, who served from 1984-1986. They would grandfather current nurses but in the following year's, they would require nurses to hold a BS degree.

Miller expanded on the need for certification in a letter to the membership in *The Wet Towel*, March 1985. She announced the Massachusetts Teachers Association at their annual convention accepted MSNO's proposal to recognize school nurses as full dues paying members of their association. MSNO was also in the process of writing regulations to certify themselves as school nurses by the year 1987. Setbacks occurred, as Nancy pointed out when they found the Massachusetts Department of Education refused to certify school nurses. Instead, the Massachusetts Department of Education suggested they become school health educators. As a result, though enormously dismayed, nevertheless, they soldiered on and proceeded to look in other directions to accomplish their goal.

The outgoing president, Nancy Miller, added in her commentary to *The Wet Towel*, June 1986, the continuing saga of the need for certification, in spite of the MTA's refusal, saying a nurse's education is different as compared to a teacher's instruction. In other words, all nurses were not required to have a college degree. Undaunted, the Executive Board persevered, just like the Red Sox baseball team, and sought out the legal expertise of Marie Snyder, who was both a nurse and attorney. She declared they could self-certify the members of MSNO through testing and evaluation, and then repeat the process every five years.

Administering Drugs

As late as 1984, to give psychotropic drugs within Massachusetts' schools, each request required approval by the State's Psychotropic Drug Program, Maternal and Child Health Services. These approvals created a volume of paperwork for school nurses. Compounding this, these were difficult times as administrations cut back school nurse positions. Yet, on the other hand, the State talked about expanding the role of the school nurse and increasing their academic preparation.

The headlines of *The Wet Towel*, December 1986, highlighted the issue of the administration of psychotropic drugs by a "nurse" rather than by "a registered nurse" to public school children. New legislation, Senate Bill 270, proposed to amend the Massachusetts General Laws, Chapter 71, Section 54B, purporting to reduce the amount of paperwork for the schools and the Massachusetts Department of Health. The Senate passed this bill, the Joint Committee on Health Care rendered it a favorable report, and the Massachusetts Department of Public Health supported it.

However, MSNO did not support this legislation, since a "registered nurse" was the only nurse that had the "educational background and skills" to administer psychotropic drugs in schools. MSNO advised its members to contact their state representatives and voice their opinion (Wood, 1986). Chapter 16 also discussed this issue. Faced by strong opposition, the bill didn't pass.

Other Activities:

Awards
In 1982, NASN established the "Lillian Wald Research Award" named after the founder of the first in the nation school nursing services in New York City, as noted in Chapter 1. NASN designed this award to encourage research in the field of school nursing.

Technology
The Wet Towel announced changes to its publication in 1984. MSNO planned to publish the newsletter quarterly, and allowed the Massachusetts Teachers Association (MTA), to mail it four times a year at a significantly reduced cost. It generally ran four to six pages long, but sometimes eight. Unfortunately, it could not accept photographs because the technology of the time could not incorporate them.

The first mention of computer technology appeared in the June 1984 issue of *The Wet Towel*. Arlington Adult and Continuing Education advertised their computer course for school nurses as a resource for improving nursing organizational skills. Hopefully, as of 2020, every school nurse has the use of a computer and computerized health records.

School Nurse Image

Then MSNO President, Nancy Miller, in September 1984, sent a letter out to all members announcing a strategy on how school nurses could obtain the recognition they wanted and deserved, and how their voices could be heard. She suggested they should become politically active to achieve visibility, send pictures of what they did to their local newspaper, and reminded them one person in every forty-four was a nurse. She was right on target.

Many schools participated in fluoride mouth rinse programs to prevent dental caries. The school nurse would bring the paper cups filled with the fluoride solution to the classroom. See the image below.

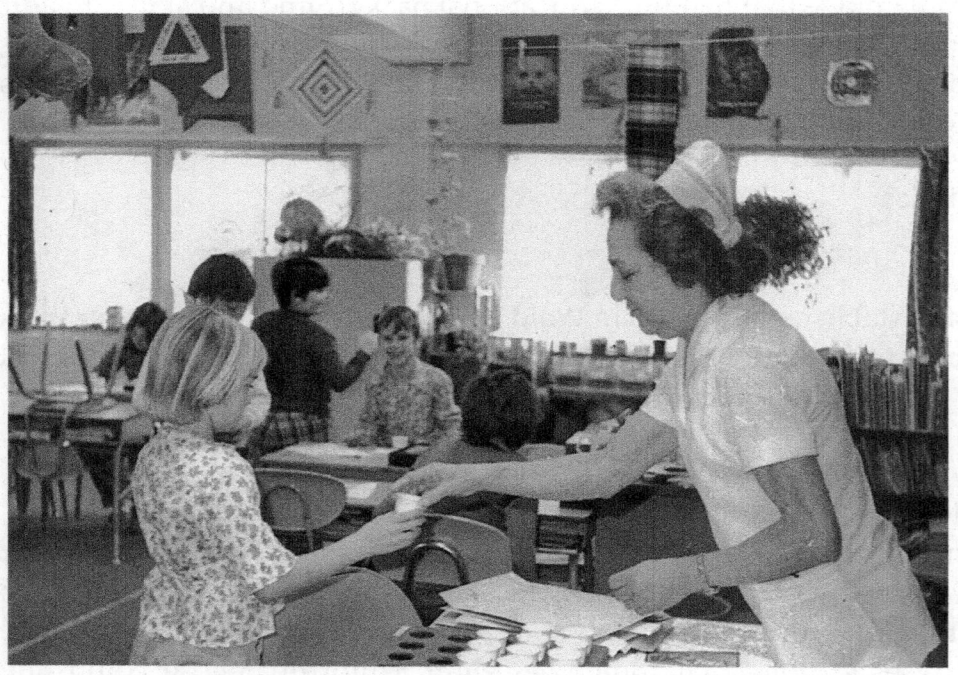

Fluoride Mouth Rinse Program. An unidentified school nurse dispensing the fluoride mouth rinse in an unknown school. Photo courtesy of McAuliffe MSNO Album.

Advocacy-1980

The State Department of Health sent a letter dated March 12, 1984, from Commissioner Bailus Walker and John Lawson, Commissioner, Department of Education, to all School Superintendents. The message reported as part of fundraising activities, schools sold students foods containing high amounts of sugar. It goes on further to explain studies have linked the consumption of high sugar content foods with health conditions such as obesity, dental caries, diabetes, heart disease, and other chronic health problems. Furthermore, as these health conditions have affected Massachusetts's school children, they have ignored the most crucial fact. A proper diet could prevent these disorders.

The letter continued to remind the Superintendents, Chapter 71, Section 1 of the General Laws required students to take health classes, including instruction in nutrition, health, and wellness. A second reminder stated the "Federal State Regulations of the School Lunch Program forbid the sale of candy and non-nutritious foods during the school day," and required they credit income received from the sale of all foods to the school lunch account and program. This letter prompted schools to change their ways to stay in compliance with the law.

It was not until 2010 that the Massachusetts Legislature passed "An Act Relative to School Nutrition," Chapter 0454, banned the sale of salty and sugary snacks and high-calorie sodas in public schools. It arose while the state battled a rising tide of childhood obesity and other chronic health problems. The Massachusetts childhood obesity rate data in 2007 identified 34 percent of 10-13-year-old's as overweight/obese and 25 percent of 14-17-year-old's as overweight/obese.[495] Over the long term, positive results have emerged as a result of these initiatives, leading to *The Boston Globe* headline October 17, 2013, "Obesity Rate Decreases for Mass. Children." "You get rid of sugary drinks from schools, improve the quality of school lunch, promote regular physical activity, and children's body weight responds" pointed out Dr. David Ludwig, Director of the New Balance Foundation Obesity Prevention Center at Boston Children's Hospital.[496]

---

495 Daigneault, J., Rasche, C.H., Hines, D., and Rios, H. (2014) *Massachusetts Family Impact Seminar*. Child And Adolescent Obesity in Massachusetts: Opportunities for Effective Policy Interventions at the State Level. Retrieved from https://www.purdue.edu/hhs/hdfs/fii/wp-content/uploads/2015/07/s_mafis05c02.pdf

496 Lazar, K. (2013, October 17). Obesity rate decreases for Mass. children. *The Boston Globe*, p. A16.

Conferences

MSNO regions continued to hold conferences throughout the state, covering a variety of subjects. Topics included: Premenstrual syndrome; "Pathways for Children," dealing with the care and education of chronically ill children; The Role of Nutrition in Preventing Disease, presented by the Dairy Council; "Role of the School Nurse as Child Advocates"; "Management of the Child with Asthma in School"; "Anxiety Disorders in Children: Implications for School Adjustment"; "A Neurological Exam"; "Empowering Self and Assertive Skills for School Nurses"; and "Children's Rashes." MSNO regions designed these programs to better prepare school nurses, add to their competent professional assessment, and improve practices that impact school health.

At a MSNO Region III meeting, held at Marconi's Italian Restaurant, Ashland, on October 9, 1984, while reading the meeting's minutes, then President Nancy Miller, met some unexpected opposition on several new proposed initiatives. Since not all of the attendees were MSNO members, they questioned why there was no discussion beforehand about the increase in dues, and why was joint membership with NASN necessary. As Nancy dutifully pointed out during the heated, insightful dialogue that followed, the main reason for connecting with NASN was to work towards school nurse certification becoming federal law.

This law would cover not only Massachusetts, but all states, requiring the same qualifications regardless of state affiliation, and grandfathering in those nurses currently employed as school nurses. Also, she answered someone from the region should attend the executive board meetings, for the district to receive the designated funds. Apparently, this ruffled those in attendance, because instead of following their planned program, they abandoned their speaker on "ENT Assessment" and continued with a debate on whether members belonging to both MSNO and MTA suffered from duplication of dues.

Later Activities

The Wet Towel account, of May 1985, from President Nancy Miller, disclosed a steering committee gathered to plan the fall conference. Both the physicians from the Massachusetts Society of Eye Physicians and Surgeons and MSNO nurses agreed pre-kindergarten students, in addition to the test for vision acuity, should be checked for amblyopia as well. (Amblyopia, sometimes called "lazy eye," is a condition where the vision in one of the eyes is reduced because the eye and the brain are not working together properly). They would work together to make these changes in the state health department regulations.

MSNO encouraged school nurses to give testimony at the Massachusetts State House regarding the law known as Chapter 766, which guaranteed all students, ages 3-22 who had special needs, were entitled to an education. As can be noticed, MSNO encouraged school nurses to be politically active. Meanwhile, Nancy Miller and President Elect Ann Lowry planned to attend the Massachusetts Teachers Association Convention in Boston. They would make more inquiries about nurses' status within MTA and the issue, as mentioned earlier of MTA dues.

A report from Joan Piacquadio, school nurse at Lee High School, summarized her attendance at a Massachusetts Teachers Association (MTA) Summer Leadership Conference held August 12-16, 1985, at Williams College, Williamstown, Massachusetts. Since she was required to sign up for a tract, she chose the Communication Tract, which consisted of instruction in designing newsletters. This developed into an opportunity she could not let slip away. Moreover, she said the entire conference highlighted political action, the use of the media, and personal appearances on television.

She emphasized school nurses should take a more active role in their local unions. When they did this, she felt they would find they gained more equality and professionalism, something which many nurses reported currently missing. On the other hand, she looked forward to a time when the MTA would include a tract at their conference called "School Nursing Issues." Joan set an example on how to use currently available resources to make changes.[497]

As 1986 emerged, MSNO, with Ann Lowry as president, hosted a five-day NASN (National Association of School Nurses) Convention in Boston. Amidst a flurry of sessions, keynote speakers, and meetings, 836 school nurses attended, representing 47 states and the territory of Guam, 100 percent more than attended the previous year's conference in Denver. Not until 2006, would MSNO's attendance be again equaled.

During 1986, MSNO meetings took place at the MTA Central Regional Service Center, 48 Sword Street, in Auburn, starting at 5:30 PM. The scholarship committee encouraged members to nominate MSNO members for the Massachusetts School Nurse of the Year award and would submit that year's winner to NASN as

---

497   Piacquadio, J. (1986, November). MTA Summer leadership. *The Wet Towel*, 3.

Massachusetts's nominee for School Nurse of the Year.

The Wet Towel, in January 1986, announced they planned to elect their officers for the first time by a mail-in ballot system. Another change arrived in December 1986, when *The Wet Towel* reported they would mail the newsletter by first class mail with the MTA logo emblazoned on the envelope.

Head Lice Checks

The National Pediculosis Association thanked MSNO for encouraging Governor Dukakis to proclaim September 1985 as a pediculosis prevention month. (Pediculosis is the medical term for lice infestation. Lice are blood-sucking bugs that live on the scalp, in the pubic area, or on clothing. They spread by crawling from the infected person to another person through close physical contact.) School nurses can recall, as I can, performing classroom head lice checks, after one student in the classroom reported having head lice. See the image below.

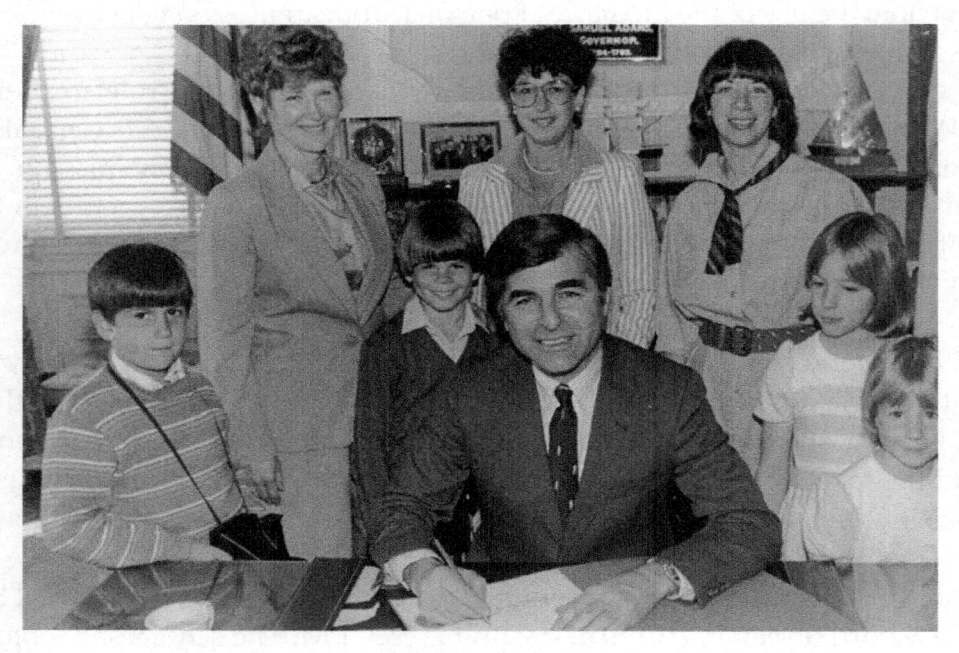

Michael Dukakis, then Governor of Massachusetts, proclaims September 1985 as "Pediculosis Prevention Month in Massachusetts," the first state to do so. Pictured are from the left, back row, Anne Kinsley, MSNO, Deborah Altschler, and Leslie Kenney of the National Pediculosis Association - front row Gov. Michael S. Dukakis and young friends. The photo is courtesy of McAuliffe MSNO Album.

Certification Exam

Jackie Mawhinney, NASN Director, reported NASN asked each state to send in fifty questions to use on the certification exam. Focusing on the process of credentialing school nurses, the Professional Testing Corporation announced it would offer the first Certification Examination for School Nurses on August 9, 1986, in approximately 42 test sites around the country. "With the advancement of nursing and the development of specialty groups, school nursing has developed its standards of school nursing practice and designed an evaluation guide for self and peer review." The Professional Testing Corporation further stated their main objective was to promote the delivery of safe and effective care in schools and was an indication of current competence in a specialized area of practice.

Educational Standards

The Education Reform Bill turned into another subject of interest. In 1986, MSNO members reported their unions told them, even though they ratified School Reform Bill 188, nurses were deliberately omitted from the language because nurses were not eligible. For a second time, the MSNO Executive Board sought out the council of Marie Snyder on how to bring school nurses up to the same level as educators. Snyder mentioned nurses were given entrance to their profession by State Board Certification, and simultaneously to this requirement, they had to be certified by their professional organization, including identifying graduate course work.

Outgoing President, Nancy Miller stated further in a 1986 message,

> *"It is becoming more obvious that certification through ANA or NASN is going to become a reality and a requirement for employment in the school. Presently employed school nurses were being grandfathered into the system. This certainly was a step in the right direction. An RN who graduated 20 years ago or graduated with no college background, certainly did not have the qualifications to fill the challenging job of a school nurse."*

She again encouraged school nurses to contact their MTA bargaining unit and express their grievances about being left out of the language in the MA Education Bill.

The question of what the proper preparation for school nursing and general nursing as well, came up again, as it would many times in the ensuing years, in a

"Letter to the Editor" of *The Wet Towel*, December 1986. In a poignant letter, school nurse Helen Zekanoski, RN, from Blackstone-Millville Regional Junior-Senior High School outlined how President Nancy Miller's comments offended her. Miller said nurses without a college background were not qualified to be school nurses.

Nurse Zekanoski went on to describe her education from a diploma school (three-year hospital program). Further preparation included a four-year stint in the U.S. Air Force Nurse Corps during the Korean War, marriage, and raising a family of five children. During this time, she continued to work in nursing. She argued other school nurses had similar backgrounds and were busy raising their families and saving money for their own children's education. Likewise, she felt they were interested in maintaining and updating their skills because she met them frequently at continuing education programs, which was a requirement to maintain a nursing license in Massachusetts. Ms. Zekanoski contended the most critical qualification for school nurses was not necessarily a bachelor's degree. On the other hand, she reflected, school nurses should have a bachelor's degree to put them on the same par with educators to receive equal salary benefits. "But to state that diploma graduates with no further formal education are not qualified to be school nurses is an insult."

School-Based Clinics

The School Nurse Organization of Washington State sent a letter to MSNO in 1986 requesting their assistance on how school-based clinics were run in Massachusetts since the Washington legislature considered placing ten school-based clinics in Washington. They voiced their concerns as they already provided the services outlined for the program or were available within the community. "It is perceived by many school nurses in our state as a threat to the future of school health services," wrote Shirley Carstens, Chairperson, SBC Study Committee. She requested they forward a 12-question questionnaire to those school nurses in Massachusetts who currently had a school-based clinic. The responders should return them to Carstens. There was no further reference to it again. In Chapters 15 and 16, Boston school nurses exhibited their reluctance to have school-based clinics. Apparently, they were not the only school nurses harboring those feelings.

Bargaining Table

"School Nurses Belong at the Table," ran as an editorial in *The Wet Towel*, September 1986, by Jean Wood. It referred to the collective bargaining table for better salaries and benefits for school nurses. At the time, the maximum wage for school nurses frequently fell below the starting salary of inexperienced teachers armed with nothing more than a bachelor's degree. Nurses paid the same dues as educators, but often they were the last items that were negotiated on the contract schedule and were frequently traded off. "The unique contribution of school nurses lies in our ability to provide professional health care and guidance and to coordinate the resources of the school, home, and community as these pertain to the total health of the students. Healthy children learn better," wrote Jean Wood.

Moreover, the Massachusetts Department of Education, the Massachusetts Department of Public Health, the Massachusetts Nurses' Association and the Massachusetts School Nurse Organization recognized school nurses as professionals, then, why were they not adequately represented at the bargaining table? The editorial encouraged school nurses not to be afraid to ask questions of their bargaining committee and find out why school nurses were an afterthought. Was it deliberate or an oversight?

Finally, A New Newsletter Name

By September 1986, *The Wet Towel* searched for a new moniker, saying that its name had outlived its usefulness. The new name, they suggested, should portray the school nurse "as capable and dynamic- a name that will project a positive image."

Excerpts from More Than Band-Aids

We will follow MSNO from 1987 as they rolled out a new name for their newsletter, continued to strive for school nurse certification, fought to promote their specialized branch of nursing, and became more politically active. MSNO had dedicated and talented members to produce a newsletter, and of course, they were all volunteers.

More Than Band-Aids, the name of MSNO's new news bulletin, made its debut in the summer of 1987. According to the editor, members submitted many new names, but the organization chose the submission from school nurse Helga Kohnfelder, employed by the Longmeadow School Department. Her reasoning for the name was "to remind school nurses of the diversity of their roles and the value and importance of their work."

Perhaps MSNO also chose this name because they struggled with school committees during negotiations to receive the same financial compensation as teachers with similar education and experience. Their job expertise was not recognized nor respected, and this continued to be a frustration for many more years to come.

Gradual Peer Recognition

On the positive side, the Massachusetts Department of Education amended Chapter 766 regulations to include school nurses in team evaluations. It stated a registered nurse might represent the physician in the case of a comprehensive health assessment. Chapter 766 referred to the Massachusetts special education law, initially issued in 1974, which guaranteed the rights of all young people with special needs (age 3-22) to an educational program best suited to their needs. Educators conducted Team Evaluations and Annual Reviews to develop an ongoing individual education plan to ensure an appropriate education. This law preceded the federal education law of 1975, the Education for All Handicapped Children Act, and served as its model.[498]

At its annual convention in May 1987, as also reported in the summer 1987 issue of *More Than Band-Aids*, the Massachusetts Teachers Association (MTA) issued a statement saying they supported school nurse certification. MSNO Past President Nancy Miller, current President Ann Lowry (1987-1989), and President-Elect Anne Kinsley, also attended that convention. MTA wrote that nurses, as professional members of the educational organization, should be included in master contract agreements along with other professional members of the school system. They further urged that newly employed nurses possess a bachelor's degree, which should be a requirement for entry level certification, and encouraged the Massachusetts Department of Education to establish a process of certification for school nurses. These suggestions and resolutions would eventually become part of the school nurse certification process in Massachusetts. They were strong words of support.

Meanwhile, the President of the Massachusetts Nurses Association (MNA), lawyer and nurse Marie Snyder, filed a bill for the 1988 legislative session to amend teacher certification to include school nurses.

---

[498] Massachusetts Department of Elementary & Secondary Education, Education Reform, *First Annual*

In the *More than Band-Aids* Fall 1987 issue, President Ann Lowry talked about the strong past role of the school nurse in health education, in the reduction of communicable disease, and decreased absenteeism in the classroom. These elements had been replaced. She related intermittent care, and record-keeping had replaced these elements, whereas, at times, school nurses had ignored preventative care, health education, and community involvement. Further, many school systems had not applied and knew little about the "Standards of Care for School Nursing Practice" they had recently developed.

These omissions, she related, resulted in discrepancies by the many Massachusetts town and cities regarding the ability of nurses to deliver safe and effective care in schools and their current competence in their specialized field. She called on school nurses, despite their disappointments and dissatisfactions, to try to regain the same public trust of nurses that was evident during the early years of public health and to expand the role of the school nurse to make them a vital part of the school team. Lowry reminded them they were one of the key players in the school that could identify early health related problems that can affect a child's school performance. She called on them to bring up these issues before their local school board.

An example of the issues that school nurses faced during contract negotiations appeared in a commentary in *More Than Band-Aids*, Winter 1987, "Negotiations Frustrating for School Nurse." This article related the experiences of school nurse Judith Hodge, BS, RN, a member of the Seekonk Educators Association Negotiation Team. Her position on the team so disheartened her that as a result, unfortunately, she resigned as Seekonk's school nurse. She requested school nurses be put on the same salary scale as teachers with similar education and experience.

The school committee offered a $6,000 salary adjustment, bringing her salary to $17,000. It is interesting to note they offered the same wage to two new school nurses who had no previous experience in school nursing. As Hodge said, "What third-year teacher would accept a first-year teacher's salary?" In comparison, a Boston school nurse with similar experience received about $27,000 in compensation at that time.

Moreover, the intense negotiations resulted in a strike. It boiled down to the school board not giving nurses the same salary as teachers with similar education and experience. Judith Hodge referred to the negotiations as "bittersweet," but had praise for her fellow teachers on the team, who were very supportive, as was MSNO in planning a strategy. Again, though, she urged school nurses to take part in their contract negotiations because no one knows better what a school nurse does than a school nurse.

As Paul Harvey would say, "And now the rest of the story:" The article reported Judy became a visiting nurse and happily worked where her skills were appreciated. Her schedule encompassed working 24 hours every other weekend, getting reimbursed for 40 hours, and not regretting her move.

Salmonsen Awarded Grant

The same newsletter, *More Than Band-Aids*, Winter 1987, continued with an account of MSNO being awarded a grant for $1,250.00 from the MTA to produce a video about the school nurses' role to show to community groups. Future MSNO president, Linda Salmonsen wrote the grant. In addition, she received two more awards, for her research in the field of school nursing. Individual school nurses were performing pioneering achievements.

Evidence Based Practice

More Than Band-Aids, Summer 1988, recorded a "Commentary," by Connie Brown, RN, Public Health Nursing Advisor, Massachusetts Department of Public Health, Western Region. She advised nurses to develop "realistic, attainable, and measurable goals and objectives relative to the needs identified" in their school population. They should write up their plan, involve parents, and demonstrate how this school health program affects the behavior and physical state of the students and the school community. Additionally, she suggested they illustrate the role the school nurse plays in attaining these goals. She followed up urging them to document all they did and evaluate the outcomes. Following these tasks, they should write an annual report, and make suggestions for the following year, based on the findings.

Lastly, she advised school nurses to link and demonstrate what their school health program had accomplished, resulting in positive changes in the behavior and or health status of the school population. Think of the cost effectiveness of their program. For example, how had it affected school attendance, injuries, illness, family stability, visits to the emergency room, and parents' lost days at work? She recommended they provide evidence showing the need for their health program, and to take continuing education courses. "Realize your obligation to control your own practice and upgrade your professional role." Again, Connie Brown, RN, was right on target.

Brown described what is called evidence-based practice. Show what you do enhanced educational outcomes for students. As early as 1970, L.C. Ford observed, "Her (my) frank opinion was that nursing (school nursing) had failed to demonstrate to the public that its services were worth the cost." She is a nationally known nurse educator.[499] Perhaps, in 1970, school nurses did not listen, because nurse educators asked them to do the same thing again in 1988. Granted, that was a tall order for a single nurse in a school system to accomplish. They would require more resources and support. Over the years, the National Association of School Nurses developed toolkits with exact details on topics such as "How to Present to your School Board", "How a Principal Can Evaluate a School Nurse", "Back To School Checklist," and "Ideas on How to Encourage Healthy Lifestyles for Students" to support school nurses and improve student health outcomes.

This *More Than Band-Aids*, Summer 1988 issue, packed with informative information, included an article written by MSNO President, Ann Lowery, "School Nursing- The Curriculum for Caring." She issued a warning that school nursing was on the "critical list" saying there was a role identity crisis due to the wide variation of nursing practice over the state, and role confusion, because of the varied assignments of school nurses in the districts. Lowery discussed the renewed interest in educational reform. However, the Massachusetts Department of Education continued to ignore the social problems that had affected the work of school nurses, counselors, social workers, and other personnel that work outside the classroom.

Lowery continued that school nurses cared for children with AIDS, and children who had benefitted from advances in medical treatments, new technologies, and scientific discoveries. Some students, she said, needed central arterial and venous lines for medication, dialysis or chemotherapy. Other children required respirators, while others needed bladder catheterizations, gastrostomy feedings (a feeding tube that goes directly into the stomach), and tracheostomy care (opens the airway and aids in breathing). She stated many more students had eating disorders, depression, and suicidal ideation than in previous years.

---

499   Wold, S. (1981*). School Nursing, A Framework for Practice*. North Branch, MN: Sunrise River Press. P. 17.

She reported early in 1987, Harold Raynolds Jr., Massachusetts Commissioner of Education, delivered a keynote address to Congress, saying an H symbolizing health should precede the 3 R's. He said this symbol, H-RRR, more appropriately reflected the priority of issues facing schools. Ann Lowry deliberated why school nursing had not experienced reform, upgrading, or improvement in practice over the last 25 years. She called for MSNO members "to support improvement and upgrading of school nurse practice-the curriculum for caring-in Massachusetts."

These reports provided exclusive insight into the obstacles affecting school nursing. Nothing was recorded. Nothing was preordained. School nurses could reverse their slide by making informed choices to promote their specialized branch of nursing. As Pulitzer Prize-winning author, Charles Krauthammer, wrote in his book, *Things That Matter*, "We can follow the advice of Demosthenes when asked what was to be done about the decline of Athens. His reply? 'I will give what I believe is the fairest and truest answer: Don't do what you are doing now.'"[500]

Administration of Psychotropic Medication in School

Again, school nurses faced yet another challenge regarding psychotropic drugs administered in public schools to schoolchildren, as outlined in the Winter 1989 issue of *More Than Band-Aids*. The Massachusetts Law, Chapter 71, Section 54B of the General Laws, stated only a registered nurse or a licensed physician could administer medication, including psychotropic medication in school.

The challenge now came from a surprising source. A pediatrician from Lynn, Dr. Walter Harrison, MD, and a group of concerned parents whose children received Ritalin in school, claimed their children had not received their prescribed medication, because of the scarcity of school nurses. This group wanted the law changed to allow classroom teachers to administer Ritalin (a central nervous system stimulant used to treat attention deficit disorder).[501] Dr. Harrison said he had the backing of the American Academy of Pediatrics and the Massachusetts Medical Society. They wanted the current law amended and filed a new bill with this proposal, Senate Bill 258.

---

500 Krauthammer, C. (2013). *Things That Matter Three Decades of Passions, Pastimes, and Politics*. New York, NY: Crown Forum. P. 365

501 Brener, T., & Doyle, R. (Eds.). (2007). *Nursing 2007 DRUG HANDBOOK*. Ambler, PA. Lippincott Williams & Wilkins. P. 530-531.

The deck was stacked against them as the Massachusetts Department of Public Health and Department of Education supported this proposed new bill to allow other personnel, under the direction of registered nurses and licensed physicians, to give psychotropic drugs in school. This action was practicing nursing without a license. It would be grounds for nurses to lose their RN license. In a letter dated December 30, 1988, to Harold Raynolds, Commissioner, Board of Education, Mary Snodgrass, Executive Director, Board of Registration in Nursing, explained that given the current nursing shortage, she understood how difficult it was to implement the statute (M.GL. Ch. 112, s. 80B). Still, she said, in the letter, "lowering standards of care is inappropriate and possibly dangerous to the health of consumers of health care, even in a nursing shortage."

As a result of this challenge, MSNO hired a law firm, Snyder and Sweeney, to represent them at the State House on this issue. Moreover, the Massachusetts Teachers Association and the Massachusetts Federation of Teachers offered support for the position taken by MSNO. Their newsletter, *More Than Band-Aids*, Winter 1989 issue, contained a timely article about how to write your legislator, the "ABC's of Writing Your Legislator," to motivate nurses to contact their representatives and voice their opposition to this bill. MSNO suggested a solution to this situation: Instead of involving teachers and other school personnel, reduce the school nurse/pupil ratio, and hire more school nurses. Why should teachers be involved in giving meds in a classroom? That takes time away from teaching, their primary concern. The bill did not pass.

The 1990s

The 1990s chronicled the beginning of another decade for MSNO. Now they were going into their 20th year. Michael Stanley Dukakis was in his last year as Governor, and Raymond Flynn was Mayor of Boston. After a booming decade of growth in the 1980s, Massachusetts was going into an economic downturn, with unemployment rising to 6.7 percent. Locally, Boston's Gardner Museum heist occurred, the most significant art burglary in history. The crime remains unsolved, and the museum has never recovered the art works. Boston harbor stopped a centuries old practice of directly dumping sewer sludge in 1991, which made it the dirtiest port in the nation. The Boston harbor cleanup followed restoring Boston's pristine waters.

Construction began in 1991 on the Central Artery/Tunnel Project, unofficially known as the "Big Dig," the most expensive highway project in the United States. School employees working in East Boston who traveled through the tunnel daily desperately sought assignments on the other side to avoid the impending traffic nightmare, as I did. When completed in 2006, Bostonians breathed a sigh of relief after years of rerouted and snarled traffic. Whether or not the Big Dig led to traffic flowing more easily is still debatable, but in the ensuing years, it opened up the city to a boom in real estate development.[502]

A technological and pharmacological revolution hit health care in the 1980s and the 1990s. New cutting-edge technology and new drugs arrived on the scene, aimed at improving patient and student care. School nursing had to meet these new challenges.

MSNO reported a membership of 401 on February 1, 1990. The Board still held their meetings at the MTA Regional Headquarters, Auburn, MA.

School Nurse Activities

On the eve of National School Nurse Day, 1990, as reported in *More Than Band-Aids*, Winter 1990, MSNO celebrated with a dinner attended by 120 school nurses. The highlight of the evening was a presentation by nurse attorney Marie Snyder. She singled out two areas she found to be problematic for school nurses, the administration of medications, and record documentation. In some districts, unlicensed personnel dispensed medications, because, according to Snyder, there were not enough personnel to do the job. She further explained, under the nurse practice act in Massachusetts, nurses could not administer medications in school without a doctor's order, even "over the counter drugs" as Tylenol. Moreover, Snyder said, some school nurses had not done an adequate job of explaining nurse practice to their school administrators.

Regarding documentation, she focused on the need to record negative findings, to use checklists for assessments, and not to draw "conclusions." Let the experts do that, she commented.

In an act of desperation, Linda Salmonsen let it be known in the *More Than Band-Aids*, Winter 1990 issue, that she planned to lead a group of school nurses

---

[502] *10 Years Later, Did the Big Dig deliver?* (2015, December 29). Retrieved from https://www.bostonglobe.com/magazine/2015/12/29/years-later-did-big-digde liver/tSb8PIMS4QJUETsMpA7Spl/story.html

from MSNO who considered filing a class action pay equity suit to bring school nurses up to the teacher's salary scale. Linda would become MSNO president in 1992. A lawyer from the Massachusetts Teachers Association (MTA) promised to investigate the potential possibilities of this case for MSNO. There was no further reference to Salmonsen's request.[503]

For the first time, *More Than Band-Aids* commented on Ann Sheetz, the new Massachusetts Director of School Health. Ann and Christine Robinson, the Director, Division of School Age and Adolescent Health for Massachusetts, met with the MSNO Board of Directors. Christine Robinson emphasized that now the department would make school health a priority. This, of course, was great news to hear. Ann Sheetz checked off a list of what she wanted to accomplish for schools. The medication administration policy headed the list. Other issues included certification and a statewide orientation program for school nurses. Ann became a shining star, a visionary leader for school nurses, and the school health program.

In 1990, Judi McAuliffe, a school nurse at Pembroke Elementary School, became President of MSNO. Besides being MSNO President, McAuliffe also served as President of the South Shore Registered Nurses Association and was active in nursing and several health-related community organizations. McAuliffe admitted her school nurse's office was bustling and wondered how she would find the time to complete the state-mandated screenings. She continued, "the rewards of a smile, a 'thank you it worked,' or someone stopping by to say, 'I'm not sick, I just wanted to say hi, have a good day,' make it all worthwhile."[504] See the image on the next page - President McAuliffe confers with Past President Kinsley.[505]

As the new President, Judi McAuliffe visited the various regional meetings across Massachusetts. Many conversations and exchanges during these visits resulted in a list of issues that were brought up frequently. They were: 1) delegation of nursing functions, 2) administration of medication, 3) policies and procedures, 4) legal responsibilities, 5) wages, and 6) contract negotiations. She pointed out that MSNO wanted to work with the Department of Education and the Department

---

503   Salmonsen, L. (1990, Fall). Strong opposition voiced at hearing. *More Than Band-Aids*, 4 (2), 3.

504   Traylor, J.(1990a). Meet the Board of Directors. *More Than Band-Aids*, 4(1), 2.

505   McAuliffe, J. (1990, Fall). McAuliffe outlines vision for year. *More Than Band-Aids*, 4 (1), 1.

of Public Health in developing appropriate policies and procedures for school nurses and the school health program. At the same time, about the wide gap in salaries that existed across the state, McAuliffe reminded them MSNO was an affiliate of MTA. She hoped as nurses became more active on MTA's boards and committees, as others suggested many times, they would negotiate more fair-minded contracts.[506]

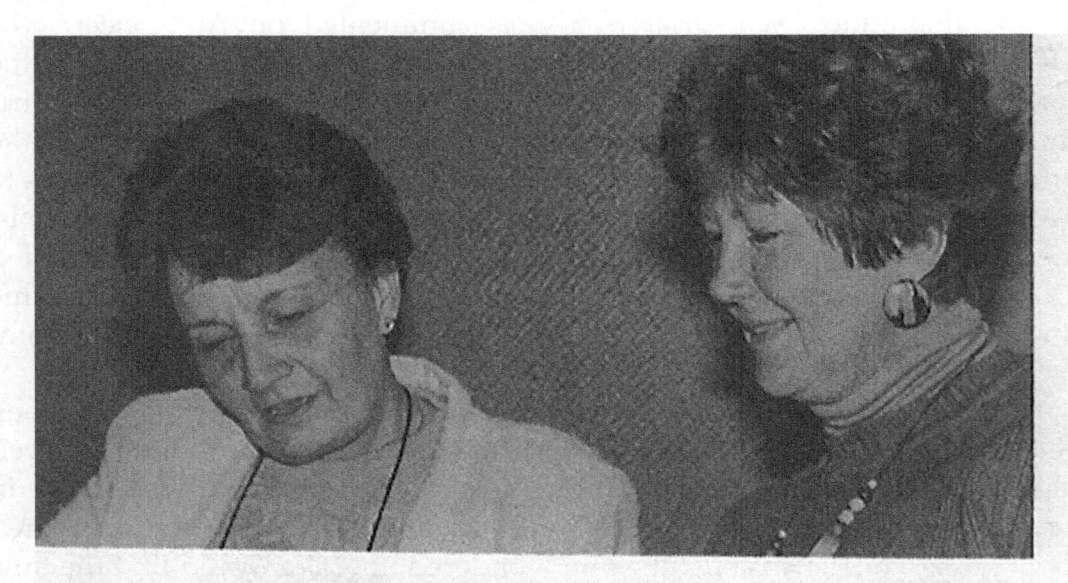

Pres. McAuliffe confers with Past Pres. Kinsley

Photo courtesy of McAuliffe MSNO Album.

Once again, MSNO filed another bill to amend teacher certification to include school nurses through the State Department of Education, HB 4569. It languished in the House Ways and Means Committee. MSNO pleaded school nurses to contact their legislators and voice their support of this bill. State Representative Christopher Hodgkins of Lee, Massachusetts, sponsored this bill. As a result of his work on school nurse certification and for improving the delivery of school health services, he received the Annual Friend of School Nurse Award during their 1990 fall conference. Unfortunately, this bill did not survive the Senate, and they refiled it again in the 1992 session.[507]

---

506   McAuliffe, J. (1990, Fall). McAuliffe outlines vision for year. *More Than Band-Aids*, 4 (1), 1.

507   Traylor, J.(1990b). Christopher Hodgkins receives Friend of School Nurse Award. *More Than Band-Aids*, 4(2), 1.

Advocacy and Legislation 1990

The 1990 Fall issue of *More Than Band-Aids* reported several MSNO members, including Ann Lowry, Judi McAuliffe, and Linda Salmonsen, testified at a Board of Registration in Nursing hearing. These members strongly opposed a proposal to exclude from the legal framework of nursing practice all school nursing procedures and activities performed in schools for special education students. This would allow non-nursing personnel to perform nursing functions. The Board of Registration planned to study this issue to define the range of nurse practice boundaries. MSNO advised school nurses to be aware of the safety and legal liability of their work.[508]

This issue contained another article, "Massachusetts Lags Behind in School Nursing Legislation." It conceded though Massachusetts led in medical care, it fell behind in school nursing. This survey by NASN pointed out some surprising numbers: 16 states medication laws required a doctor's written order, but not Massachusetts; 17 states medication laws required a note from a parent, but not Massachusetts; 8 states mandated or proposed ratios for student/nurse assignments, but not Massachusetts; and finally, 18 states had no qualifications mandated to work as a school nurse, including Massachusetts. These statistics illustrated the need for both more action and advocacy by school nurses, the school community, and legislators on behalf of the school health program.

School Nurse Image

A presenter at their fall conference, 1990, Dr. Christine Bridges, Assistant Professor of Nursing, University of Rhode Island, commented school nurses frequently had an illness orientation approach, rather than a health orientation. Students thought of the school nurse's office, mainly as a place to go when they were sick. The noteworthy part of her presentation, in retrospect, called on nurses to consider their role to include more health promotion and prevention, similar to the goals of the 2010 Affordable Care Act, frequently called ObamaCare.[509]

---

508 Salmonsen, L. (1990, Fall). Strong opposition voiced at hearing. *More Than Band-Aids*, 4 (2), 3.

509 Traylor, J.(1990c). Conflicting health messages hinder children's development. *More Than Band-Aids*, 4(2), 4.

Twentieth Anniversary

Now their first 20 years came to a close. They celebrated their anniversary at a dinner in Shrewsbury on National School Nurse Day 1990. You could feel their joy in the air. Honored guests for the evening were past presidents Martha Rich (1970-1972), Jayne Cash (1978-1980, Jackie Mawhinney (1982-1984), Nancy Miller (1984-1986), Ann Lowry (1986-1988), and Anne Kinsley (1988-1990).

See the image below - Martha Rich says good-bye at Anniversary Party.[510]

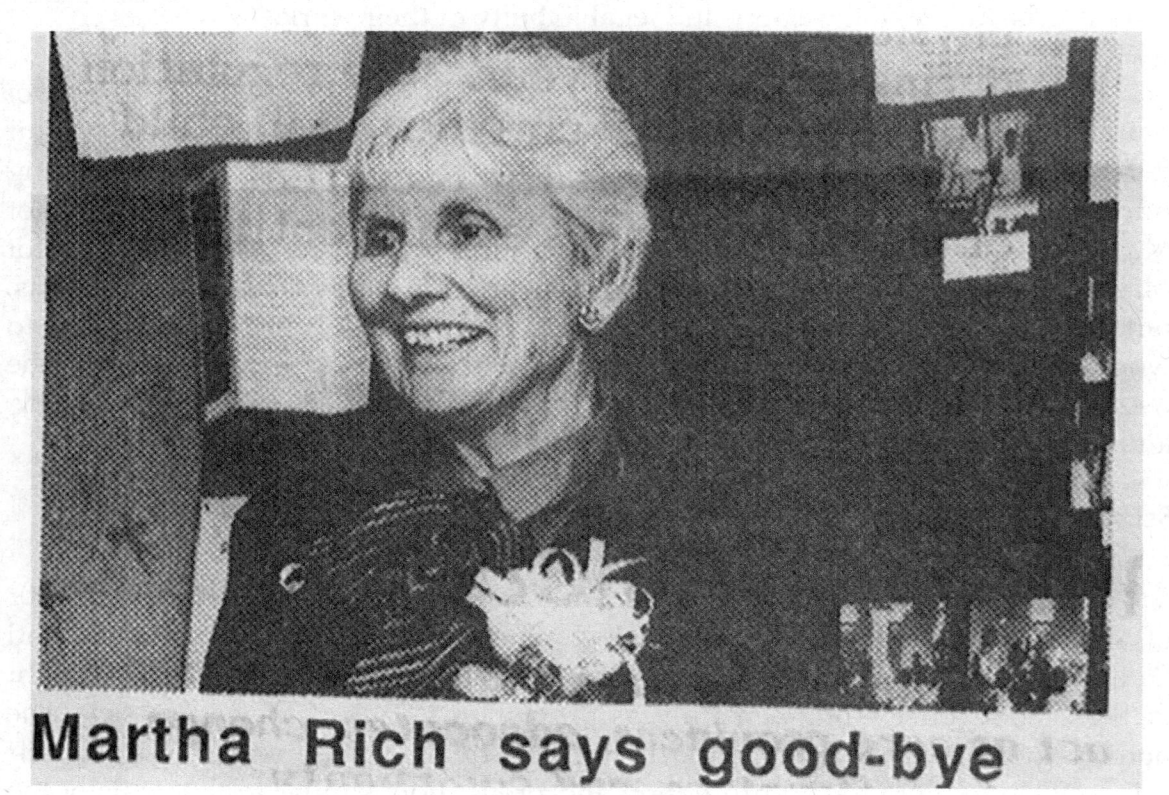

Photo courtesy of McAuliffe MSNO Album.

---

510   Wood, J. (1987) Martha Rich says good-bye. *More Than Band-Aids*, 1(1), 3.

President Judy McAuliffe summarized their many accomplishments along this journey, including the following:[511]

- 1971 First State Certification Bill filed, Martha Rich, president,
- 1972 First New England Regional Conference, Anna Margaret Ray, President,
- 1974 Role of the School Nurse published, RN requirement for school districts, Nancy Wolfe, President,
- 1975 First proclamation of School Nurse Day by Governor Dukakis,
- 1976 Martha Rich elected National President of the Department of School Nursing (DSN)
- MSNO officially incorporated, Gladys Newhall, President,
- 1978 Second State Certification Bill filed; Nurse/Pupil Ratio bill filed,
- Joan Canham edits state Newsletter,
- 1979 Scholarship Committee created,
- 1980 Membership reaches 500,
- Goal to upgrade professional standards. Postural Screening bill passed.
- Susan Kelly, President,
- 1984 Unified with NASN. First National School Nurse Celebration
- Nancy Miller, President,
- 1986 State Certification and Psychotropic Legislation supported, Ann Lowry, President,
- 1988 State Certification and Psychotropic Legislation supported,
- Standards of Practice addressed, Anne Kinsley, President.

The evening concluded with future plans to continue to push for improved standards of practice with supporting legislation, i.e. state teacher certification to include school nurses. During the intervening years, MSNO would address the constantly changing demands of school health, moving beyond their frustrations, and always promoting the health and academic success of the children they served. The further details of these years will be covered in another book, at another time, and by another person.

However, I would be derelict if I didn't include their historic accomplishments in the short years that followed their anniversary dinner; namely, and most

---

511 Traylor, J. (1991). MSNO celebrates 20th anniversary. *More Than Band-Aids*, 4(3), 1.

important, the passage of School Nurse Certification through the Department of Education in 1993 during Linda Salmonsen's term as president; and the passage of An Act Granting School Nurses Eligibility for Professional Teacher Status in 2006, during Marie DeSisto's term as president. These achievements reflected their toil, struggles, togetherness, perseverance, and resourcefulness. Both bills affected all Massachusetts school nurses, but the The Professional Teacher Status Bill raised the salaries of low paid school nurses, regardless if they were MSNO members or union members. MSNO's membership dues paid for all the trips to the State House, and the lobbyists. The phone calls to legislators were legion. If you are a school nurse, and not yet a member, I urge you to do so, as soon as possible, and support the organization.

I cannot paint a future picture for you, but MSNO has dealt with challenges in the past and will continue to do so in the future. So, in closing, here's to an exceptional past, and an exciting, bright, future. I leave you with this thought:

"It is not the strongest of the species that survives, not the most intelligent that survives. It is the one that is the most adaptable to change that survives." Charles Darwin[512]

The train is nearing the station. In our final chapter, you will meet a former acquaintance.

*Many thanks are extended to Judi McAuliffe, who has painstakingly assembled an album of newsletters, important events, and documents of MSNO's early years, from which most of this chapter is drawn.

---

512 Retrieved from http://www.brainyquote.com/quotes/authorship.

Chapter 18

A Midnight Séance

A Midnight Séance

It is a Halloween night, a holiday filled with mystery, magic, and superstition. My husband Jim and I sit on our stoop at our South End, Boston home at nightfall. We greeted and handed out candy to the 100 or more children who annually visit our block to trick or treat amid the ghosts and goblins. Fall leaves swirl in the wind.

Later that night, I wake up suddenly from a hypnagogic state with my mind spinning. Above my head, turbulent air whirls around and around, beckoning me to follow this twirling tunnel up the stairs to the first floor. On my tiptoes, I anxiously ascend the stairs. Immediately afterward, to my astonishment, I find myself entirely dressed and standing in the parlor of my 1860s row house. Food, a large bottle of champagne, and two glasses sit on the dining room table. The sweet aroma of incense is in the air. "What is this? How odd." The knocker on the outside door resounds. "Why don't they use the bell?"

On opening the door, I find a fair-skinned woman of medium height, somehow familiar to me. This woman immediately walks in smiling, saying, "I have wanted to meet you, Mrs. Keeney. You put a nice plaque on my former apartment building over on Washington Street. However, the constant screech, clatter, and soot from the elevated train ran by it. Upon my word, I was glad to get away from it."

My jaw drops, and my eyebrows jump at least an inch. The woman is wearing a white bib apron that covers her long, blue, and white seersucker dress with detachable white collar and cuffs. A broad-brimmed hat covers her brown hair. In her hand, she carries a big, black medical bag. She looks resplendent in her nursing uniform. Yes, this is an IDNA (Instructional District Nursing Association) uniform. Could this possibly be Annie McKay, the school nurse I have been writing about? I can barely utter the words, "Welcome," as I take Miss McKay's hat, and carefully place it in the closet. McKay's pale complexion bears a sharp contrast to the brown hair with wisps of gray piled neatly on her head. Annie McKay strides over to the parlor windows where she can see her former apartment building overlooking Blackstone Park. What kind of mystical power is going on here, I wonder?

As she looks out the window, Annie McKay asks, "There is no more elevated train. What happened to the screeching Orange Line?"

"They removed it in 1985 and replaced the train with Silver Line buses. The old-timers in the neighborhood say the train was faster than these buses. That is progress for you."

An old mahogany grandfather clock sits on the mantel and chimes midnight. I join Annie McKay in the parlor and sit down. Annie McKay looks at me and asks, "Why did you arrange this get-together?"

"Apparently, I have been dreaming about it," and leave it at that. I continue, "very unusual and unexplained circumstances have brought us together. Perhaps the mystery and magic of Halloween played a part; I don't know. However, you apparently have experienced time travel, a trip forward in time to be present here this night in 21st century Boston. I have no idea how long this will last, so let us share our experiences, get to know each other and enjoy ourselves. How do you feel? Let us have something to eat. Do you mind if I call you, Annie?"

"I would be most pleased," she responds.

My guest strolls over to the dining room table and tries some of the appetizers. She calls them interesting. Her gaze travels around the room, noting the high ceilings, intricate crown moldings, and marble fireplaces. She is familiar with the apartment which retains much of its Victorian period authenticity and charm. Shortly, she relaxes, and the dwelling becomes a gathering place, as it has for family and friends for over 150 years.

Annie McKay remarks, "I am curious. How are my former schools doing?"

I beamed. "I am so glad you asked. You served the Quincy, Andrews, and Way Street Schools here in Boston's South End. The old Josiah Quincy School remains on Tyler Street, though now it houses the Chinese Consolidated Benevolent Association of New England. In 2017, it received the distinction of being placed on the United States National Register of Historic Places. The city built a new Quincy School in 1976 and later on added a high school. 'Urban renewal' demolished the Andrews and Way Street Schools."

"If I may inquire, what is 'urban renewal'?"

"'Urban renewal' is what the government called the program of clearing the so-called slums and replacing them with new apartments charging reasonable rents."

"Ah, yes, Way Street was quite an old school."

"Now Annie, when you were a school nurse, what type of activities did you do during the school day?"

"That was a long time ago, but as I recall, I dressed blisters, sores, burns and wounds; I applied fomentations (the application of warm, moist cloths to the body to relieve pain) and poultices, I made up bandages; I kept all utensils clean and disinfected; I supplied fresh air as best as I could, and made accurate observations and reports to the physician. At the end of the school day, I made home visits to talk with parents about various issues, such as immunizations, home care of a sick child, help them understand doctor's instructions, and the need for eyeglasses to improve their child's vision. One of the most important goals of home visits consisted of confirming the sick child dismissed from school was being treated so he/she could return to school. Frequently, when a parent was unable to take a child to the dispensary, with the parent's permission, I would take them instead."

I said, "you certainly kept busy, Annie, but the role of the school nurse has changed. The new Quincy School employs two full-time nurses. They don't visit other schools as your assignment required you to do. Federal legislation, since the 1970s, mandates all children are allowed to attend school, regardless of disability. This law means children who previously attended school in institutions, long-term hospitals, or received home tutoring can attend their neighborhood school."

"Annie, if you were to walk into their school nurses' office now, you might not recognize the names of the conditions that many of these children have. All too often, they have chronic diseases, behavioral, or developmental needs. The nurses from Quincy and other Boston schools would tell you that they deal with students who have asthma, hemophilia, sickle cell disease, cancer, diabetes, pregnancy, autoimmune deficiency, who use orthopedic braces, wheelchairs, walkers, and respirators. They monitor students who are ventilator dependent, have insulin pumps, require daily urinary catheterizations, tube feedings, and administer psychotropic and other medications."

"Other problems that plague our students are: homelessness, drug and alcohol use, HIV, sexually transmitted diseases, lack of exercise, obesity, and poverty. Child abuse, suicide, low self-esteem, family conflict, runaways, gangs, violence, drunken driving, inappropriate Internet use, violent video games, immigration status, and safety issues also afflict them. All of these issues require access to quality student health services. What do you think of this, Annie?"

"Good gracious. Not me so much, but what would Florence Nightingale say about all this?"

"Yes, I wonder if she were here, what would she say?"

Annie continued, "I followed her statements and writings because, as you know, I was a visiting nurse both in Canada and Boston. One of her messages was, 'She shows them in their own home…how they can be clean and orderly, how they can call in official sanitary help to make their poor one room more healthy [healthier].' 'The nurse also teaches the family health and disease-preventing ways.' 'The nurse shows the patient how to be clean.' There must also be, 'School teaching of health rules.'[513] I adopted her theories in my nursing practice. Besides, her theme of cleanliness, prevention, and proper nutrition also included the need for clean air and sunlight."

"Yes Annie, you mentioned nursing theory. Nursing has a distinct body of knowledge that makes it different from other disciplines. Carol Costante, a past

---

[513] Nurse Buff. (2018) *25 Greatest Florence Nightingale Quotes for Nurses*. Retrieved from https://www.nursebuff.com/florence-nightingale-quotes/

president of the National Association of School Nurses, says school nurses "have always delivered components of primary health care and preventive services in a client-friendly community setting, in a cost-effective and accessible manner." Historian Susan Reverby argues that nurses have viewed caring as the basis for their practice. Since we live in a society of instant gratification, I wonder if caring is valued as much as it was in your day, Annie."

Annie continues, "I would take some of the children up to the top floor of the Quincy School, where we could walk out on the roof for some fresh air. Some of the students "have weak, ill-framed bodies and nervous, irritable dispositions, due to living in filthy, ill-ventilated homes, with about half the amount of sleep and nourishment they ought to get. Many of these little children are allowed to sit up until ten or eleven o'clock at night, then dragged out of bed in the morning while still half asleep, given a cup of strong coffee or tea that has been boiling on the stove since their father had his breakfast, some hours before, with perhaps a doughnut to eat, and hurried off to school before they have time to swallow it. ...The school nurse, working with the teachers, has opportunities that are open to few others, for she has a chance to gain the friendship of the children, and it is almost wholly through them that there is any hope of influencing the home life."[514]

I smiled at Annie's remarks about taking the children out on the roof at the old Quincy School. Several years ago, when I visited the old Quincy, I could visualize Annie following a similar plan.

"Another of Nightingale's passions was the observation of the patient, that being part of the assessment, keeping records and data," I add.

"We tabulated every student that we saw and what we did for the student. That took time, and some of us didn't enjoy record keeping."

I continue. "The early period of school nursing sought to reduce student's high absentee rates due to contagious diseases and other physical ailments. Annie, you continued to work with these students and return them to the classroom, using the nursing process of assessment, intervention, and follow-up. These same nursing

---

514 Work in The Public Schools. (1906) *20th Annual Report, Instructive District Nursing Association, Year Ending January 30, 1906.*

services that supported and enhanced school attendance, increased learning potential, and academic success in the 1900s, continues in the 21st century as well, now one of the bedrocks of school nursing practice. That is your legacy. The students are healthy, in school, and ready to learn."[515]

"Annie, do you think you could function now in the Quincy school nurse office?"

"Dorothy, as you well know, nursing is more than performing procedures and tasks. My education, of course, did not include the physiology, pharmacology, and mental health that you know. As for all of the procedures, I would have to do a lot of reading to understand them. But I 'cared' for my students, the same as you do, and the school nurses at the Quincy."

"I hope you don't mind, but your school of nursing sent me a copy of your application. You graduated in 1894. Were you required to sweep and mop the hospital floors as a nursing student?"

"Oh, gracious." Her eyes flickered with merriment. "Not on every shift."

I laugh and reply, "Nurses don't scrub floors anymore. Boston has experienced many challenges and changes since you were here in the early 20th century. Were there nurses of color in the ranks of IDNA (Instructive District Nursing Association) while you were there?"

"I dare say, not that I can recall."

"Were you able to follow your dream? Were all paths open to you as a young girl?"

"Housekeeping, teaching, and nursing were viable occupations open for women. Nursing opened many opportunities for me. I traveled first to New York City, then settled in Boston, and later volunteered as a nurse for the Red Cross in

---

515   Charting Nursing's Future. (2010, August). *Unlocking the Potential of School Nursing: Keeping Children Healthy, In School and Ready to Learn*. Retrieved from A Publication of the Robert Wood Johnson Foundation website: https://schoolhealthteams.aap.org/uploads/ckeditor/files/unlocking-the-potential-of-school-nursingRWJF.pdf

France during The Great War."

"Annie, thank you for your service."

"My home country and my adopted country were in the war. It was the least I could do."

I add, "Again, we can thank Florence Nightingale for making nursing a viable and respectable option for women who wanted to work outside the home. Most importantly, she converted the status of nursing from a household service to a profession.[516] When I had to make a career choice, I could choose from a nurse, secretary, or teacher. That was the extent of it. No doubt, we have come a long way, and now, all careers are open to young women."

"Likewise," I continue, "the United States has made great strides in civil rights and women's rights. It doesn't mean we are perfect. Congress passed legislation that accomplished many reforms:[517]

- 19th Amendment 1920, (Giving women the right to vote),
- Brown v. Board of Education of Topeka, Kansas (De-Segregation in Education),
- Equal Pay Act 1963,
- Civil Rights Act of 1964 (Prohibits discrimination in many settings),
- Voting Rights Act of 1965,
- Americans with Disabilities Act of 1990,
- Family and Medical Leave Act of 1993,
- Obergefell v. Hodges 2015 (Rights of Same-Sex Couples)

However, there are still areas for improvement."

"At this time," I said, "the Boston Public Schools have nurses of color in their ranks. Shirley Erikson Garagna became the first black nursing supervisor. Secondly,

---

516   Gill, G. (2005). *Nightingales the Extraordinary Upbringing and Curious Life of Miss Florence Nightingale.* New York: Random House Trade Paperback Edition.

517   *Civil Rights: Timeline of Events.* Retrieved from https://civilrights-overview/civil-rights-timeline-of-events.html.

they hired male nurses, for example, Leslie Bahadosingh, the first male nurse of color into a predominately white, female profession. Nurses of color and men have shared similar civil rights struggles for equality in the nursing profession. Mary Eliza Mahoney, who in 1879 became the first trained black nurse in the U.S., would have been happy to see this progression. Boston suffered through court-ordered school busing in 1974 to desegregate the schools."

"I think I have been talking too much. We should bring out the champagne. It is time for a toast." As I struggle with the cold bottle of champagne, the cork pops. I pass Annie the flute of champagne with the tiny bubbles rising to the surface. "What shall we toast?"

Annie raises her glass and says, "Let us toast the dramatic challenges school nurses have met, and their significant growth."

"I agree. And may school nurses continue to evolve and keep students healthy and safe, so they are ready to learn."

Annie turns to me, "Thank you, Dorothy, for calling out to me so we could get together."

"I didn't realize I was doing that. But, thank you, Annie, for accomplishing what you did in Boston's pilot project. Your work so impressed the Boston School Committee they decided to adopt the program as their own. You showed results. Without your skilled decision-making, critical nursing skills, and powerful work ethic, the BSC might have delayed establishing the Boston school nurses for several more years. You were strong and overcame difficulties. We thank you."

"Fine kids they were."

"Do you know that two of your Canadian relatives came to Boston from Beaverton to see the building plaque and the area where you served?"

"Yes, I'm aware of that."

"We gave them a tour of the area, showed them the plaque, the old Quincy School, the old section of Tufts Medical Center where you escorted the children for a medical checkup, and finally, brought them back here for lunch. They seemed to enjoy the mini tour. Afterward, they were going to do some sightseeing on their own. Then, last summer, when I was visiting Toronto, I drove past your former school, Jarvis Collegiate Institute."

"Oh, my."

See the image on the following page.

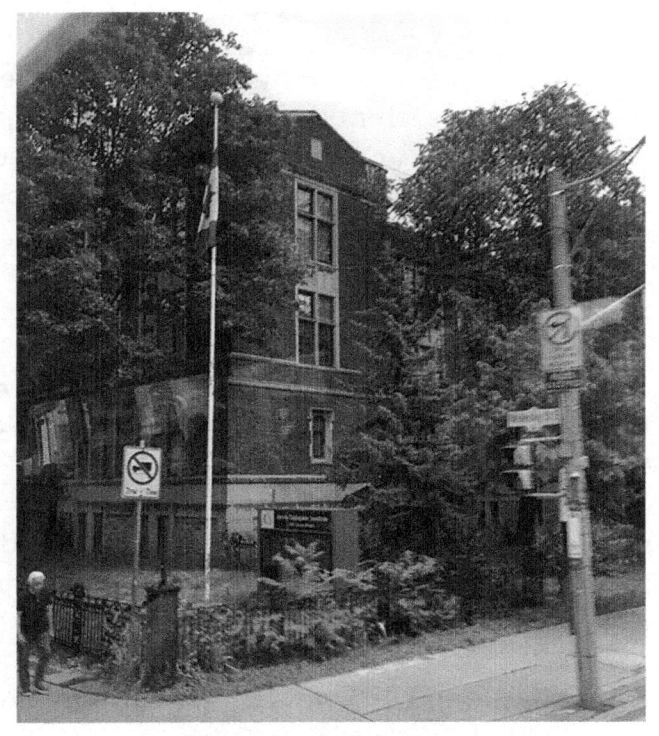

Jarvis Collegiate Institute - Photo by Dorothy Keeney.

The grandfather clock announces 1:30 AM. The night is fleeting. In the far distance, police sirens wail, not unusual for Boston. A dog howls in the night. Annie McKay crosses her legs and then uncrosses them again. I realize time is running out for my guest. Both of us stand up simultaneously. Once again, the smell of incense is in the air. We exchange smiles and acknowledge it is time again to navigate the gateways through time and distance.

As we walk to the door, I say, "How courageous you were. Thank you for your everlasting contributions."

I open the door and immediately see the whirling turbulence in the hallway. I return Annie's hat, and we exchange hugs. "Until we meet again."

Holding back tears, I reply, "Yes. Until we meet again."

As Annie walks into the hallway, she falls under the spell of the electromagnetic field and gingerly steps into the swirling turbulence. With the speed of light, she vanishes.

Now the hallway is quiet again as if nothing transpired here. There is no odor of incense in the air. I stand there, stunned by the events that just unfolded. The police sirens grow louder. A patrol car with flashing lights pulls up to the curb and turns off the sirens. A policeman hops out and walks up the steps to the house.

"Is everything all right here, Miss? We are receiving increased satellite and cell phone activity in this area."

"Everything is fine here, Officer. Nothing to worry about," I reply as I return to my apartment. Suddenly, I feel tired and decide to clean up the dining room table in the morning. I return to bed.

The following morning, I awaken, feeling refreshed, and ready to go. However, I have a lingering sense of a dream involving the school nurse Annie McKay. In this dream, I actually meet her.

"That would be startling," my husband says after I share my story. "How did you recognize her?"

"I recognized her because she wore the uniform of the Instructive District Nursing Association."

I chuckle to myself and continue through my day. Later on, while sitting down in the parlor, I can't stop thinking about the night before. Good grief! Was it a dream? Or did it happen? Was she here? Are there any half-filled flutes on the mantle? "Well, I'll be darned!"

How could I explain or describe the extraordinary situation, but somehow, I answered a call within myself to meet Annie McKay. And, so it was.

EPILOGUE

Endings always prompt thoughts of beginnings. In this chapter, I reacquainted my readers with Annie McKay, a voice that, without the benefit of research, would have been lost to history. Her contributions to school nursing, however, have not gone unnoticed. I have exercised creative license in bringing Annie McKay and Dorothy Keeney together, and have adhered to the historical context of Annie's life and quotes.

This chapter intended to identify the problems and challenges that confronted Boston school nurses and school nursing in the past and to various degrees still persist. Examples are women's rights, voting rights, equal pay, discrimination, desegregation, and removing student's health-related barriers to school achievement. Due to advances in medical science and technology, many of today's students have complex medical and behavioral conditions, chronic illness, and other physical and mental health needs.

Additionally, Florence Nightingale's nursing methods evolved into the nursing process Annie McKay used at her schools and are still practiced by school nurses in the 21st century. New legislation, contracts, and guidance from various public and private agencies also address these problems and challenges in a variety of ways, but this review will not avail itself of that discussion.

I leave you with a thought. What can we take from the history of school nursing as it relates to the future expansion of the profession? The story of school nurses is one of struggle, resilience, and finally, breakthroughs. These skills will sustain school nurses as their roles continue to evolve over time and adapt to new conditions and needs. Without a doubt, school nurses still deal with the effects of poverty on health and educate students and families on the benefits of clean air and nutrition, as they did over 100 years ago. They must continue to work to be an effective bridge between the education system and the health care delivery system, using interprofessional collaboration with the ultimate school nursing objective of positive student outcomes.

Irma B. Fricke, School nurse educator said, "To face tomorrow with the thought of using the methods of yesterday is to envision life at a standstill. To keep ahead, each one of us, no matter what his task, must search for new and better methods — for even that which we now do well, must be done better tomorrow."[518]

---

[518] Fricke, I.B. (1972). School Nursing for the 70s. *Journal of School Health*, 42, 203-206 Retrieved from http://doi.org/10.1111/j.1746-1561.1972.tb08058.x

About the Author

After 20 years working as a nurse in the Boston Public Schools, Dorothy Keeney, MA, BS, RN, has written a book about the history of the Boston public school nurses. Encouraged by the interest expressed when she discovered and wrote about Annie McKay, the first school nurse in Massachusetts, she went on to write this book. Dorothy spent many years researching their history She has published several articles about their complex history that appeared in the *Boston Union Teacher*, and the *South End Historical Society Newsletter*, and in publications of the American Association of the History of Nursing, and the Massachusetts School Nurse Organization.

Dorothy has been the unofficial historian for the Boston School Nurses and the former historian for the Massachusetts School Nurse Organization. Local newspapers also published her articles about good health practices for school children and the documents needed for school, such as immunization records and physical exams.

Born in New York City, Dorothy graduated from Fairleigh Dickinson University, Teaneck, NJ with a BS in Nursing, followed by a Master's in Health Care Administration from Framingham State University in Massachusetts many years later. Massachusetts has been her longtime residence. Dorothy has over four decades of extensive nursing experience including operating room nursing, medical surgical, pediatrics, newborn nursery, public health, and her years as a school nurse with the Boston Public Schools. She lives in Boston with her husband Jim. They have two married daughters and two grandchildren. Dorothy is a former downhill skier and enjoys traveling, reading historical novels, and spending time with her family.

Index

A

Ahearn, Aloysius, 171, 174, 175, 176, 177, 195
Almeida, Carol Fortes 2, 347, 354, 357, 362, 366, 370, 371
Andrews School 62, 197

B

Boston Public School Nurses Club 2, 133, 134, 139, 182, 188, 189, 199, 206, 209, 211, 213, 214, 223, 224, 226, 232, 233, 234, 236, 239, 243, 270, 295, 300, 313, 321, 322, 324, 325, 329, 330, 331, 332, 333, 336, 337, 338, 339, 342, 343, 344, 345, 346, 347, 357, 359, 360, 361, 362
Boston Teachers Union 180, 241, 242, 273, 295, 298, 304, 313, 318, 319, 320, 330, 354, 357

C

child labor laws 19, 20, 150, 152, 153, 177
Clarke, K. Marie 2, 320, 323, 336, 341, 344, 347, 348, 350, 356, 360, 367
coronavirus 39, 40, 139
Curley, James 134, 165, 171, 173, 174, 184, 268

D

desegregation 284, 289, 291, 292, 296, 297, 298, 302, 303, 320, 349, 413

Diphtheria 15, 111, 146, 147
Donovan, Ann 2, 265, 266, 267, 268, 271

F

five-day work week, 1, 134, 181, 183, 190, 191, 199

G

Ganno, Gloria 62
Garagna, Shirley Ericson 2, 285, 288, 289, 409

H

home visits 20, 48, 54, 58, 65, 68, 72, 75, 76, 78, 80, 84, 111, 120, 136, 137, 148, 185, 190, 196, 235, 257, 284, 286, 294, 364, 405

I

Immunization Laws 301, 314
Instructive District Nursing Association 1, 2, 3, 5, 14, 22, 23, 29, 30, 31, 47, 48, 50, 51, 58, 60, 65, 67, 71, 81, 84, 89, 112, 119, 128, 134, 136, 142, 311, 407, 408, 412

J

JK 2, 289, 290, 293, 294, 296, 297

L

legislation 21, 43, 90, 92, 93, 109, 124,

417

125, 128, 270, 296, 330, 355, 380, 381, 401, 405, 409, 413

M

Massachusetts School Nurse Organization i, 1, 3, 13, 25, 334, 356, 372, 375, 377, 389, 415
Medicaid Reimbursement 319

P

Parochial Schools 269, 271
pay equity 1, 14, 113, 181, 397
polio epidemics 2, 134, 246, 247, 259
polio vaccine 259, 287

Q

Quincy 63, 76
Quincy School, 5, 14, 21, 23, 60, 61, 63, 64, 71, 72, 75, 76, 78, 80, 197, 241, 242, 288, 313, 316, 405, 406, 407, 408, 410

R

Racial Imbalance Act 2, 297
Rich, Martha, 375, 376, 377, 378, 380, 400, 401

S

Sabin, Dr. Albert, Vaccine, 216, 259, 294
salaries 2, 105, 109, 120, 140, 142, 144, 157, 163, 168, 211, 219, 220, 224, 225, 228, 229, 233, 234, 235, 237, 239, 241, 243, 262, 276, 282, 304, 307, 356, 378, 388, 398, 402
Salk, Dr. Jonas, Vaccine, 216, 251, 252, 253, 254, 256, 257, 258, 259, 287, 294
School Physicians 89, 90, 107, 163, 337

Spanish flu 135, 136, 139
Strayer Report 213, 218, 219

T

tuberculosis 16, 21, 52, 53, 54, 68, 80, 91, 108, 113, 115, 119, 132, 197, 200, 213, 216, 262, 263, 286, 294, 338, 364

W

Way Street School 21, 61, 62, 70, 71

Made in the USA
Middletown, DE
24 May 2020